Cécile Ernst · Jules Angst

BIRTH ORDER

Its Influence on Personality

Foreword by M. Bleuler

With 86 Tables and 4 Figures

Springer-Verlag
Berlin Heidelberg New York 1983

Dr. Cécile Ernst
Psychiatrische Universitätsklinik
Postfach 68
CH-8029 Zürich 8

Prof. Dr. Jules Angst
Psychiatrische Universitätsklinik
Forschungsdirektion
Postfach 68
CH-8029 Zürich 8

ISBN 3-540-11248-0 Springer-Verlag Berlin Heidelberg New York
ISBN 0-387-11248-0 Springer-Verlag New York Heidelberg Berlin

Library of Congress Cataloging in Publication Data. Ernst, Cécile. Birth order. Bibliography: p. Includes index. 1. Birth order–Psychological aspects. I. Angst, Jules. II. Title. BF723.B5E76 1983 155.9'3 82-19295

Printed in Germany.

Typesetting, printing, and bookbinding: Brühlsche Universitätsdruckerei, Giessen
2125/3130-543210

137
ERN

To our children:
Marianne (1), Andreas (2), Rudolf (3) and
Katharina (4) Ernst
and
Katrin (1) and
Felix (2) Angst,
whose personalities still puzzle their parents

Foreword

This study appears at a time when a decisive turn is due in the research on personality development. After many years of stagnation and misguided research in this field, this book should lead to a thorough revision and a better understanding of current views on the factors which have an influence on personality.

Let us consider the unsatisfactory aspects of the recent developments in personality studies.

At the beginning of this century, the revolutionary insight gained ground that personality is susceptible to various influences, in particular to those resulting from human interaction. This insight swept away many of the old scholastic concepts and gained special importance in the fields of pedagogics and psychotherapy. However, in the wake of every great discovery we find inherent dangers. For years, various claims and creeds on the malleability of personality have been put forward as if they were proven facts. Lay literature, too, was permeated with wrong and distorted information on factors which might endanger child development.

In order to shed light on this unsatisfactory state of affairs, the authors have chosen an impressive example: they investigated the claim that a child's birth rank position should have a decisive and systematic influence on his or her future. They show that the pertinent hypotheses require much more carefully conducted research than that contained in most publications of the past. Many parents will be relieved from worries about a child's future just because he or she is the first- or lastborn, or an only child.

However, the authors do not restrict themselves to opposing mistaken tendencies. They go one step further to uncover what an enormous amount of careful and painstaking work is needed to perceive the relationship between environmental influences and personality development. It is such a large and important task it will require extraordinary dedication, as was the case with the present study.

The future consequences are clearly outlined: research on personality development is certainly rewarding as long as we refrain from premature conclusions based on mere assumptions and statistics. However, valuable results have been achieved in this field, even at the present stage; the authors confirm again that a broken or disrupted home seriously endangers a child's future. Beyond this, however, we can perceive a basic principle: no *single* environmental influence is decisive. The significance of an isolated factor is invariably co-determined by all the other biographical factors and by constitutional predisposition.

The overall result of all this is obvious and simple: however seriously we consider the statistically proved dangers to personal development, the principal task of the investigator still consists in taking into account the individual human being in his or her uniqueness and specific environment. Statistics are not enough to do justice to this aspiration; a feeling heart and critical thought are just as important.

The following significant principle can be derived from this book: science has a justified place in human interaction but it cannot replace our natural humaneness. In this sense the authors' message is truly humanistic.

Zollikon (Switzerland) MANFRED BLEULER

Preface

In part I of this book we have tried to give as complete a survey as possible of studies on the relationship between birth order and socialization, intellectual functioning, and various aspects of personality. The studies considered appeared between 1946 and 1980.

This survey is imperfect for many reasons, some related to the limitations of the author, others to difficulties inherent in the subject. We will start by enumerating the author's failings.

1. Because of the time lag between publication and the appearance of abstracts in scientific periodicals, some recent studies could not be included.

2. The research has not been evaluated for its statistical merits or drawbacks, since a thorough study of statistical methods would have overtaxed our time and capabilities. We have limited ourselves to the much decried "hunt for significance," so nonsignificant trends have not been considered.

3. We have not systematically reported differences in personality or intellectual endowment related to sex of sib, and those that are reported give an incoherent picture.

4. After some attempts, we gave up looking for validity and reliability coefficients of the tests used in the studies. Often they were not reported by the authors, and trying to find data in the pertinent reference works would have protracted our efforts greatly.

5. The studies are grouped first according to areas of behavior, then according to constructs, and then according to the methods used. We do not define these constructs and most birth order researchers also fail to do so: they are nothing more than vague common denominators.

6. The categorization of a given study under a certain construct is to some degree arbitrary. We have followed the authors' intentions whenever they were reported. Other ways of ordering the studies might lead to different results: The differential interest in task and person found in first- and laterborns, for example, has been listed under the heading "Interest and Values," where the majority of data fail to point out birth order differences. It might as

well have been included under "Extra- and Intraversion" to support the opinion of parents that firstborns are more introverted.

7. Studies of a very large qualitative range have been included. Thus it was possible to demonstrate that the frequency of birth order results is negatively correlated to the quality of the studies. On the other hand, the enumeration of unsophisticated research makes tedious reading.

8. Studies in which birth order differences were discovered accidentally have been included. Since they would not have been published if the results had been negative, they bias the survey to some extent. While collecting material for a survey on IQ research we were impressed by the persistent accidental findings of sex differences. Findings that occur repeatedly without being expected are particularly valuable evidence. There are, however, no such trends in accidental birth order results.

9. The evaluation of results is open to criticism as well. We have tried to follow a pattern where studies controlling for social variables or using well-matched controls were given more weight than those using unsophisticated methods, and research on sibs within the same family was considered more extensively than either. Since, however, the latter type of research is missing in many areas of behavior, this procedure has not always been possible.

Other survey writers who evaluate statistical methods, observe trends and interactions, differentiate by sex of sib, and use different evaluation criteria may arrive at different results, particularly in the areas where sib studies are missing. Still. we are convinced that even a survey conducted with better methods will reveal that birth order explains only an extremely small part of variance in the pertinent variables.

So much for the author's limitations. However, there are flaws and grave imperfections in birth order research itself that become apparent when we list the hypotheses examined here:

1. IQ is negatively correlated to birth order in that it is higher in firstborns than in laterborns.
2. School achievement is negatively correlated to birth order in that it is higher in firstborns than in laterborns.
3. Occupational status is negatively correlated to birth order in that it is higher in firstborns than in laterborns.
4. Personality varies with birth order: There is a "firstborn personality."
5. Risk of mental illness varies with birth order.

The vagueness of these hypotheses is not accidental. Everybody agrees that birth order differences must arise from differential socialization by the parents. There is, however, no general theory on how this differential socialization actually works, and how it is related to differentials in IQ, achievement, and personality (Peuckert 1974). Chapter 7 will show the extreme arbitrariness and loose reasoning with which the post hoc theories on socialization and personality are related to differences in variables of birth order that were found with questionable methods. As we will see, Adler is no exception.

Birth order research seems very simple, since position in a sibship and sibship size are easily defined. The computer is fed some ordinal numbers, and it is then easy to find a plausible post hoc explanation for any significant difference in the related variables. If, for example, lastborn children report more anxiety than other birth ranks, it is because for many years they were the weakest in the family. If firstborns are found to be the most timid, it is because of incoherent treatment by an inexperienced mother. If, on the other hand, middle children show the greatest anxiety, it is because they have been neglected by their parents, being neither the first- nor the lastborn. With some imagination it is even possible to find explanations for greatest anxiety in a second girl of four, and so on, ad infinitum.

This kind of research is a sheer waste of time and money. If birth order research is to be continued, coherent theories must be formulated and explicit hypotheses derived. The hypotheses must be tested, taking into account the methodological fallacies that will be described in Chap. 1. We have tried to do this in part II. Most of the hypotheses we examined have been refuted.

Our book aims to put an end to the above-described inadequate kind of research. Perhaps some researchers will take up birth order differences in intellectual development and/or personality afresh; but it may be that having read this survey they will refrain from doing so under the impression that, even with unobjectionable methods, only very modest results can be expected.

Zurich, Psychiatrische Universitätsklinik Burghölzli

CÉCILE ERNST
JULES ANGST

Postscript. The excellent meta-analytic method with which Smith et al. (1981)* conducted their survey only came to our notice when this manuscript was finished. Had we been able to use this method our own survey would have stood on a much firmer footing.

* Smith, ML, Glass CV, Miller TI (1981) The benefits of psychotherapy. Johns Hopkins University Press

Acknowledgments

We wish to thank everyone who helped and counselled us during the long and laborious task of writing this book: First of all we would like to honor the memory of the late Miss Thilde Dinkelkamp, research assistant, who was taken from her work by a sudden and untimely death. Mrs. Anja Dobler-Mikola, sociologist, did the computational work of Part II. Mr. J. Binder, sociologist, and Mr. A. Dittrich, PhD, Mr. M. Sieber, PhD, and Mr. N. v. Luckner, all psychologists, were extremely patient advisers on the problems arising in Part I. Mrs. Hilde Bendel, Mrs. Anja Gubser, Mrs. Francine Lombard, Mrs. Ursula Moser, and Mrs. Martha Sennhauser wrote and rewrote the manuscript with unremitting conscientiousness.

We would further like to thank the editors of the series "Monographien aus dem Gesamtgebiete der Psychiatrie – Psychiatry Series," Professor H. Hippius, Professor W. Janzarik, and Professor C. Müller, for their advice and support.

Last but not least we would like to express our gratitude to our mentor, Professor Manfred Bleuler, Zürich, who taught us to look for the factual basis of even the most popular psychological and psychiatric theories.

Contents

Part I A Survey of World Literature 1946–1980

Chapter 1 Outline of Fallacies in Birth Order Research

Research on birth order and sibship size is carried out with a view to verifying two kinds of hypotheses: psychodynamic theories on the relationship between personality and position in the sibship (Spiegel 1959; Wohlwill 1970) and theories on the role of heredity and environment in psychiatric and somatic diseases (MacMahon et al. 1960). Very often, however, general theories are missing and hypotheses are produced ad hoc, based on vague theoretical reflections (Peuckert 1974). Besides this tendency towards a luxuriant growth of hypotheses, birth order research has another drawback in that, though seemingly simple, it is beset with methodological pitfalls. These must be discussed to some extent in order to justify criticism of many influential investigations.

There are three methods in birth order research:

1. Unrelated individuals to whom a variable pertains are compared with a control group, birth order being the dependent variable
2. Unrelated individuals of different birth order are compared for a variable, with birth order as the independent variable
3. Comparison of sibs within the same sibship by either method.

Fallacies in birth order research will be discussed in relation to these methods.

1.1 Birth Order as Dependent Variable: Problem of Control Groups

Difficulties arise even in relation to a seemingly simple preliminary question: Is a given variable related to sibship size?

1.1.1 The Fallacies in Determining Sibship Size

Sibship Size in Carriers of a Given Variable. In 1914, Greenwood and Yule criticized the research performed between 1907 and 1913 by Pearson, Heron, and Goring, which had apparently shown that individuals who had tuberculosis, who were involved in criminal activity, etc. were, on average, members of very large sibships. In fact, Pearson et al. had neglected to consider that the probability of including in a sample a member of a sibship of a given size is directly proportional to the size of that sibship, e.g., it is seven times more probable that a sib from a family of seven will be included than it is that a single child will be included. The number of „carriers" of a variable in each given sibship size must therefore be divided by the corresponding number of sibs and the sum of these figures divided into the corrected number of sibs in carriers' sibships (which will equal the original total number of carriers) to establish the corrected mean sibship size. This is shown by applying the Greenwood-Yule correction to a hypothetical example:

Sibship size	No. of carriers	Sibs in carriers' Sibships
1	20	20
2	30	60
3	10	30
4	5	20
5	2	10
	67	140

Mean sibship size: 140/67 = 2.1

Sibship size	No. of carriers	Corrected (divided) frequency	Corrected no. of sibs in carriers' sibships
1	20	20.0	20
2	30	15.0	30
3	10	3.33	10
4	5	1.25	5
5	2	0.4	2
	67	39.98	67

Corrected mean sibship size: 67/40 = 1.68

Failure to apply the Greenwood-Yule correction leads to the *overweighting of large sibships and the inflation of mean sibship size*. A consequence will be to *inflate correlations* of variables with sibship size.

Comparison of Sibship Size in a Carrier Population With a Control Group. When census data on the general population are used, comparisons are often made without paying attention to the fact that census data give the number of children per sibship. If sibs per carrier (without the correction mentioned above) are compared with sibs per sibship, a spurious overrepresentation of large sibships and an inflation of mean sibship size in carriers result (Bytheway 1974). Examples of miscalculations of mean sibship size due to comparison of sibs per carrier and sibs per sibship can be found in Kelsall et al. (1972) and Poole et al. (1973, see p. 66).

The comparison of carriers with census data may lead to yet another fallacy since census data include young incomplete families with one or two children. If the carriers are older children or adults, this will again lead to a spurious inflation of their sibship size; the more so the older they are.

Problems Related to Selection of an Adequate Control Group: Age and Social Class. The general trend in Western populations toward diminishing sibship size is illustrated, for example, by Birtchnell's (1970) tabulation of a systematic random sample of the normal population in the northeastern region of Scotland in 1969 (minimum 20 years of age). In this region significantly higher proportions of older than younger subjects are derived from sibships of five and more (68.9% of those born before 1910 in comparison with 28.8% of those born between 1940 and 1949). Differential fertility by social class is also illustrated by the same sample. Sixteen percent of subjects born to parents of social class one but 59.5% of those born to parents of social class five have four or more sibs. If carriers of a variable are not distributed for age and social class in the same way as the general population, comparisons with census data for sibship size will lead to spurious results.

1.1.2 The Fallacy of Comparing Carriers for Birth Order with Their Sibs: Normal distribution of Birth Order

In earlier literature, firstborns were regularly overrepresented among the carriers of a variable. Greenwood et al. (1914) and Lenz (1959) have demonstrated this fact to be a consequence of comparing carriers with their sibs without considering the overrepresentation of sibs in large sibships. The problem has been particularly clearly presented by Lenz (1959).

The following model represents a population containing equal numbers of single children and sibships of two, three, and four (10% of all individuals are carriers of a variable, independent of birth order and sibship size):

x	xo	xoo	xooo	
o	ox	oxo	oxoo	
o	oo	oox	ooxo	
o	oo	ooo	ooox	x = Carriers
o	oo	ooo	oooo	
o	oo	ooo	oooo	o = Noncarriers
o	oo	ooo	oooo	
o	oo	ooo	oooo	
o	oo	ooo	oooo	

Four of the ten carriers are firstborns (40%), three are secondborns (30%), two are thirdborns (20%), and one is a fourthborn (10%). This corresponds to the distribution of first-, second-, third-, and fourthborn children in the population. If, however, only the sibships containing a carrier are counted, the relationship changes. Of 30 sibs, ten are firstborns (33.3%), nine are seconborns (30%), seven are thirdborns (23.3%, and four are fourthborns (13.3%). If we now compare the percentage of firstborns among the carriers and their sibs, firstborns are overrepresented among the carriers.

If, however, the Greenwood-Yule correction for overrepresentation of large sibships is made, we get the following distribution of the carriers and their sibs:

Sibship size	Birth order			
	1	2	3	4
1	1			
2	$2 \times {}^1/_2$	$2 \times {}^1/_2$		
3	$3 \times {}^1/_3$	$3 \times {}^1/_3$	$3 \times {}^1/_3$	
4	$4 \times {}^1/_4$	$4 \times {}^1/_4$	$4 \times {}^1/_4$	$4 \times {}^1/_4$

Birth order in the sibships containing carriers now corresponds to the distribution of birth order in the whole population and to the distribution of the carriers.

The overweighting of firstborns brought about the introduction into birth order research of the *normal distribution for birth order* by Greenwood and Yule (1914). Carriers are supposed to appear at random for each birth order rank within each sibship size. The real distribution is then compared to the expected distribution by means of the χ^2 method.

The Greenwood-Yule distribution of expected birth order has met with some criticism on statistical grounds (Halperin 1953; Sprott 1964; Böök et al. 1950; Keeping et al. 1952) and with some attempts at simplification (Haldane et al. 1948; Bennett 1963; Russel-Davis 1962; Slater 1962; Mantel et al. 1963; Barker et al. 1967 a). The Slater index (Slater 1962) is sometimes used instead; this is an index $n-1/m-1$ where n means the ordinal number of a subject's birth order and m the sibship size. The mean of the Slater indices of a sample of carriers indicates, according to its being smaller or larger than 0.5, whether the earlier or the later half of the sibship is overrepresented.

1.1.3 The Fallacies of the Greenwood-Yule Normal Distribution for Birth Order

The normal distribution starts from the assumption that, within each sibship size, birth order is equidistributed. In this way an artificial control population is created and the carriers are compared with it. Unfortunately, the assumption of equidistribution of birth order within sibships is only true under certain conditions.

The Fallacy of Disregarding Demographic Change

As early as 1914, Cobb warned against expecting normal distribution of birth order in the general population. Barker et al. (1967 b) and, in particular, Price and Hare (1969) (see also Hare and Price 1969, 1970 a, 1974) have extensively discussed the relationship of birth order distribution of *fertility*. The following discussion is very much indebted to their work.

Change in fertility may be due either to a change in the number of families being started or to a change in family size or to both.

Changes in the Number of Families Being Started. This is equivalent to an increase in the frequency of marriage. Let us consider a simplified population in which a first child is born 2 years after every marriage and in which all families are completed within 10 years. During the year $(n-10)$ x marriages are contracted, during the year n $(x+y)$. If in the year $(n+50)$ birth order of all persons born during the year $(n+2)$ is considered, there will be $(x+y)$ firstborns and x lastborns. The firstborn-lastborn ratio is larger than one. Among middle children a similar effect is to be expected: earlierborns will prevail over laterborns. A decrease in marriage frequency, on the other hand, leads to a surplus of lastborns and to an increase in later birth ranks.

Changes in Family Size. In this case the consequences are more complicated. Price and Hare (1969) have given an illustrative sample of a simplified population in which family size is decreasing. It is reproduced here with some slight modifications. Suppose that 100 families are starting reproduction every year. Ninety percent have ten children within 10 years and 10% have 20 children within 20 years. In a given year, the part of the more fertile 10% that is starting reproduction decides to limit fertility to five children within 5 years (see Table 1). During the year

Table 1. Birth order distribution when family size is decreasing

Year				
$n-1$	*Twenty-child families* (10%)		*Ten-child families* (90%)	
	10 firstborns		90 firstborns	
	10 lastborns		90 lastborns	
	Firstborns : lastborns = 100 : 100 = 1			
$n \rightarrow (n+3)$ 4 years	*Five-child families* (starting)	*Twenty-child families* (finishing)	*Ten-child families* (steady state)	
	40 firstborns	0 firstborns	360 firstborns	
	0 lastborns	40 lastborns	360 lastborns	
	Firstborns : lastborns = 400 : 400 = 1			
$(n+4) \rightarrow (n+19)$ 16 years	160 firstborns	0 firstborns	1,440 firstborns	
	160 lastborns	160 lastborns	1,440 lastborns	
	Firstborns : lastborns = 1,600 : 1,760 = 0.9			
	Whole population born during $n \rightarrow (n+19)$			
		Firstborns	Lastborns	Ratio
	Sibships of five	200	160	1.25
	Sibships of 10	1,800	1,800	1.00
	Sibships of 20	0	200	0
	All sibships	2,000	2,160	0.93

$(n-1)$ the population is in a steady state: there are ten firstborn and ten lastborn in large sibships and 90 firstborn and 90 lastborn in the other group.

During the next 4 years the previously more fertile group produces ten firstborns in sibships of five and ten lastborns in sibships of 20 per year. The overall ratio of first- to lastborns is still unchanged, but there is an excess of firstborns in small and of lastborns in large sibships. During the next 16 years the five-child families reach a steady state, producing ten first- and ten lastborns each year, while the 20-child families terminate reproduction with ten lastborns per annum. There is a surplus of lastborns in large sibships, and an overall excess of lastborns. The whole population born during 20 years of diminishing family size has a modest surplus of firstborns in small sibships, a large surplus of lastborns in large sibships, and thus a slight overall surplus of lastborns.

Equidistribution of birth order within sibship size – the fundamental assumption of the Greenwood-Yule normal distribution – can be expected only within a population whose fertility is in a steady state.

The overrepresentation of firstborns in small and lastborns in large sibships has been demonstrated by Hare et al. (1969) in a sample of about 20,000 patients discharged from the Bethlehem and Maudsley hospitals (1958–1966), by the same authors (1974) in a representative sample of the adult population of Great Britain in 1972 ($n = 10{,}053$) and, by Birtchnell (1972), in a sample of the general population registered with practitioners in northeast Scotland during the 1960s. The extent of variation in numbers of marriages and births is illustrated by Fig. 1, taken from Pri-

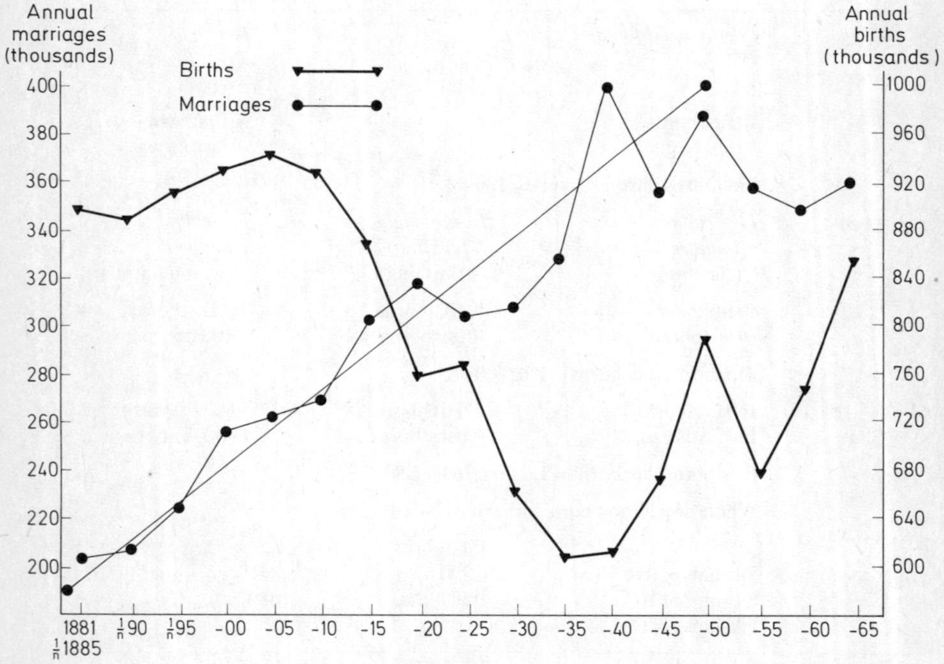

Fig. 1. Marriages and births in England and Wales (1881–1965) (Price et al. 1969)

ce et al. (1969). Rates of firstborns are accordingly unstable: Lenz (1959) found that 40% of all children born in Hamburg in 1939 were firstborns; however, in 1953 the corresponding figure was 53.4%.

The Fallacy of Disregarding Incomplete Sibships

This has been extensively discussed by Price et al. (1969) (Table 2) in relation to the birth order distribution of practically all Scottish 11-year-old school children in 1947, which showed a striking deviation from the normal distribution: Earlyborns in small and laterborns in large sibships are overrepresented and there is an overall surplus of first- over lastborns.

Let us assume for the moment that after some years when all sibships are completed, this population will be in a steady state and normally distributed. The children *most likely* to have other sibs in due course are:

1. Earlier borns in large sibships. If an 11-year-old already has seven younger sibs it is probable that there will be more children and that he will end up oldest of nine or ten.

2. To a lesser degree, firstborns in small sibships. If an 11-year-old is first of one or two sibs, the time which has elapsed since the last birth in his family may still be small enough to make a further birth probable.

The children *least likely* to have other sibs are later- and lastborns in small and large sibships. If 11 years have passed since the birth of the last child, another birth is no longer probable.

Price and Hare (1969) support these reflections with census data from England and Wales: there the probability of a subsequent birth depends on the number and spacing of previous births.

Table 2. Incomplete sibships and birth order in Scottish 11-year-olds in 1947 (Price et al. 1969)

Birth	Sibship size										
rank	1	2	3	4	5	6	7	8	9	10	Total
1	8,239	9,768	5,779	2,766	1,181	454	163	53	17	4	28,424
2		6,998	5,340	3,027	1,672	782	316	102	36	5	18,278
3			4,319	3,055	1,781	1,022	556	204	72	25	11,034
4				2,730	1,822	1,049	624	356	121	48	6,750
5					1,729	1,028	643	407	241	106	4,154
6						1,068	636	423	234	113	2,474
7							660	362	221	119	1,362
8								377	208	138	723
9									226	97	323
10										108	108
Total	8,239	16,766	15,438	11,578	8,185	5,403	3,598	2,284	1,376	763	73,630
									Greater than ten		756
									Not known		825
											75,211

Incompleteness of sibships leads to an overrepresentation of earlierborns in small sibships (whose younger sibs are not yet born) and of laterborns in large sibships (who are not yet outbalanced by earlierborns in large sibships). The effect on a sample is the same as when sibship size is declining (Loxton 1962; Jones 1967; Magaud et al. 1968). On p. 7f. it has been shown that an increasing marriage rate also leads to an overall surplus of firstborns. Price and Hare (1969) explain the present overall excess of firstborns in Scotland by the increasing marriage rate there during the 1930s.

The Fallacy of Disregarding Age and Sex of Subjects

A secular decrease of sibship size having taken place in the West, samples of elderly populations will contain an overrepresentation of laterborns in large sibships, their older sibs being deceased. Young samples, on the other hand, will contain more earlierborns from small sibships. As women live longer than men on average, in female samples laterborns in large sibships will be overrepresented. If, on the other hand, parents tend to stop reproduction after the birth of a son, lastborns may be overrepresented in male samples (Hare et al. 1974).

The Fallacy of Disregarding Social Class

It may be assumed that birth order is differentially distributed over social classes, first- and earlier-borns being overrepresented among middle-class subjects and vice versa. There are several facts which support this assumption.

1. Sibship size is negatively related to social class (see p. 12). Firstborns are biased for small, and laterborns for larger sibships size (see p. 12).

2. In the postwar years, marked by demobilization and high employment in the USA, a spectacular increase in fertility, the „baby boom", took place (Grabill et al. 1958, p. 155). Change in fertility varied with social class (Glass 1970; Rückert 1976; Glick 1975; Bahr et al. 1975; Grabill et al. 1958), in that fertility increased most in wives of professionals and least in wives of unskilled laborers. Occupational differences in fertility were reduced: though remaining the least fertile group, middle-class wives became more similar in fertility to lower-class wives (Grabill et al. 1958, pp. 123, 212; Brown 1971; Kiser 1971; Simon 1974, 1975). The postwar increase in middle-class fertility was not primarily related to larger family size, but to higher marriage frequency (Grabill et al. 1958, p. 368): more women married than formerly, marriage took place at an earlier age, and first births followed marriage more quickly (Grabill et al. 1958, pp. 329, 330, 371). Large family size, on the other hand, remained a lower-class characteristic (United Nations 1973; Kunz 1965; Simon 1974; Hawthorn et al. 1971). A similar class-specific increase in fertility took place in other industrialized nations (Piepmeier et al. 1973; Huback 1957; Gille 1971; Rückert 1976).

3. Social class is related to age, and age is related to birth order. During the 1940s and 1950s, an occupational and educational upgrading took place in that more persons entered skilled occupations and the professions (Grabill et al. 1958,

p. 120). This upgrading mainly concerned younger people. Because of the decrease in sibship size over time, among younger middle-class subjects early-borns will be overrepresented (see p. 7). The fact that small sibship size favors upward mobility has the same effect (see p. 73). In the children of these younger subjects the same overrepresentation of early-borns will be found, because in younger segments of the population incomplete families are more frequent than in older ones.

There is some empirical evidence for the assumption of an early-born bias among middle-class subjects. In a representative sample of 3101 employed American males, Schooler (1972 a) found an overrepresentation of firstborns among subjects from middle-class origins and an overrepresentation of lastborns among men from lower-class origins. In a nationally representative sample of high school males (without control of family size), Jencks (1972, p. 348) found that fathers of firstborns had significantly higher education and occupation than those of secondborns. Higher social class in first- than in laterborn Chicago school children was found by Lessing et al. (1972) and by Wild et al. (1974) in schizophrenics: Being firstborn, being better educated, and having parents living in a city were correlated.

Since there is no control of sibship size in these samples, there is no way of differentiating between the influence of smaller family size in the middle class and of the professional upgrading of the (younger) fathers of first- and earlier-borns. That differences in social class between first- and laterborns may be found even when sibship size is controlled is demonstrated by Jones et al.'s (1974) sample of students at London University and by Douglas's (1964) British national sample of 11-year olds: In the former sample in social classes I and II there was overrepresentation of firstborns of family sizes three and four, while in the latter sample in the lower class lastborns of family sizes two and three were overrepresented.

Differences in background between earlier- and laterborns *within* sibship size may come to light when very large samples of children or adolescents of the same age are compared within gross divisions for social class. There may be appreciable age differences in fathers of subjects of the same age with different birth orders within a certain sibship size (Barker et al. 1967 c).

The Fallacy of Disregarding Population Moves

Most birth order studies are about populations in large cities or in regions with a sufficient number of inhabitants to support colleges and universities (Price et al. 1969). Since World War II there have been two kinds of immigration movements in Western countries: the immigration of workers from underdeveloped countries, and a movement of the native population from economically disadvantaged regions to centers of industrialization and services. Immigrants are mostly young adults with a high marriage frequency. In regions with a rapidly growing population a surplus of firstborns may be expected. In rural regions, on the other hand, there will be a surplus of laterborns in large sibships, because the older part of the population is left there.

The Fallacy of Disregarding Other Social Variables

It has been shown that *religious denomination* is one of the most important factors regulating fertility. In population segments that are predominantly Catholic, larger families can be expected (Westoff et al. 1961). Changes in fertility may be absent or of lesser extent than in non-Catholic populations. Fertility also varies with *urban or rural habitation* and with *ethnicity* (Veevers 1971). Among 14800 gravidae in West Germany small towns, older women with higher parities were found more often than in cities (Deutsche Forschungsgemeinschaft 1977). Fertility also varies with *age of parents*: older parents will have larger families than younger parents (Sweet et al. 1971). In connection with the postwar spread of education and of white-collar occupations, younger parents can be expected to have a higher occupational level (Adams et al. 1968) and to give more education to their children (Hermalin 1967; Lees et al. 1957; Adams 1972; Chen et al. 1960).

Need for Control Groups

These considerations lead to the conclusion that *a normal distribution of birth order cannot be assumed.* A *control group* must be found that is comparable to the sample in parental cohort, locus of habitation, socioeconomic status, ethnicity, race, and religions denomination (Lenz 1959). Equalizing samples and controls for such large categories as "working class" or "middle class" may be insufficient, because subjects of widely varying reproductive behavior are included in these categories. For example, both a Swiss-German foreman with a house of his own and two children and an unskilled Italian immigrant with a large family belong to the working class.

Though research is still being done under the assumption that birth order is normally distributed, claims that carefully selected control groups are necessary have grown in number (Bayer et al. 1967; Bayer 1967a; Folger et al. 1966; Birtchnell 1970, 1971; Breland 1973; Diab et al. 1968; Gregory 1958; Hooke 1966; Jones 1967; Lees et al. 1957; MacMahon et al. 1960; Magaud et al. 1968; Schmidt et al. 1977).

1.2 Birth Order as Independent Variable: Differences Between Firstborns and Laterborns

When individuals of different birth order are compared, the precondition for associating differences with birth order ist that the subjects be comparable for all variables other than birth order. The main body of research, operating with birth order as the independent variable, compares first-, middle-, and lastborns, or simply first- and laterborns. First- and laterborns may be of different social class. Middle- and laterborns are biased for larger sibship size (middle children have at least two sibs, first- and lastborns may have only one). As shown in the preceding paragraphs, large sibship size is related to fertility behavior in certain social classes, in parents of a certain age, and in persons of certain religious denominations, locus of habitation, race, and ethnicity. First- and laterborns within a population are not distributed at random; thus, before comparing them, their comparability ought to be examined.

A large amount of research has been done comparing first- and laterborns among elementary and high school populations and students. Whether results found in children or highly selected groups can be considered valid for other population segments has rarely been discussed, nor has the question of whether first- and laterborns pass through differential selection mechanisms when entering higher education (Jones 1967; Kinsolving et al. 1971; Doren 1972; Sampson 1965; De Avila 1971; Kammeyer 1967).

1.3 Comparison of Sibs Within the Same Sibship

If properly used, this is the most adequate method in birth order research, since between-sibship differences are excluded. Unfortunately, it is rarely applied because of the difficulties in finding large and representative samples. A further problem is that when spacing between sibs is large, the environmental factors (e.g., educational opportunities) bearing on the children may be different. In order to avoid interference of age and sex differences with possible birth order differences in psychological variables, sibs should be examined at the same age and compared within sex. Barker et al. (1967a, c) have extensively discussed the possible fallacies when birth order of carriers of a variable in fraternities is ascertained. As in the literature reviewed on the following pages, studies of sibs within the same sibship usually treat birth order as the independent variable, these methodological difficulties will not be discussed here.

1.4 Conclusions

As will bee seen, most authors relate birth order differences to supposedly differential treatment of first- and laterborns by the parents. It is our opinion, however that subjects of differing birth order and birth rank are characterized by *different social background. We hypothesize that higher IQ and greater socialization in first- than in laterborns are generally not differences between sibs, but between subjects in large and small families, between middle- and lower-class subjects, between subjects of different religous denominations and ethnicity, and between persons living in cities and in the country.*

This hypothesis, rather than the hypothesis of differential parental behavior towards children of differing birth order, will be supported if:

1. Evidence for such behavior is weak
2. Birth order differences between nonrelated subjects tend to disappear with increasing control of social background variables
3. Birth order differences disappear when sibs in the same family are compared

Technical Remarks. As is customary in birth order research, the term "birth order" will be used to indicate the numerical place of a subject in the order of births in his or her sibship. "Birth rank", on the other hand, signifies first child, only child, middle child, youngest child, or later child (Manaster 1977). Unless otherwise stated, the studies discussed were conducted in the USA.

Chapter 2 Birth Order and Biological Differences

2.1 Sex Ratio

Sex ratio by birth order may vary for biological or psychological reasons. Teitelbaum (1970), analyzing all USA births in 1955, found that beginning with birth order 6 there was a small but consistent underrepresentation of male births in comparison with firstborns. There is some evidence that the reduced frequency of male births is correlated with lower social class. Male pregnancies may be more affected by adverse circumstances than female pregnancies and/or there may be antibody formation against the male fetus.

On the other hand, random distribution of sex by birth order was found in large representative samples of Mormon and of Indian families (Greenberg et al. 1967; Pakrasi et al. 1971; Srivastava et al. 1977).

Results for populations practising birth control are different. Anglo-American and Dutch parents tend to have another child – or to consider having one – when the older children are of the same rather than of different sex (Freedman et al. 1960, De Wolff et al. 1957, Lindsay 1971, Wood et al. 1977). In particular, there may be a tendency to look upon a family as incomplete until a son is born, which could lead to an overrepresentation of males among youngest children (see p. 196).

Though the deviations from random distribution of sex by birth order are probably small, their existence justifies the claim that investigators should control for sex when conducting birth order research.

2.2 Prematurity, Gestation Length, Birth Weight, Early Death, and Handicap

The incidence of prematurity, abnormally long or short gestation, and abnormal birth weight may be related to the following variables: maternal age, social class, sibship size, and birth order. These variables are also interrelated, since mothers having their fourth or fifth child will tend to be older and of lower social class than mothers of firstborns. In the following studies, all of which report on large and representative samples, the variables in question are not always separated and weighted.

Birth weight increases with birth order. Holding maternal age and social class constant, this was found by Butler et al. (1966), Crump et al. (1957), Lobl et al.

(1971), and Millis et al. (1954) for English and Welsh, black-American, and Chinese samples. *Abnormally low birth weight* is most frequent in firstborns, particularly if their mothers are under 20 or over 30 years of age (Lobl et al. 1971; black-American sample; Douglas 1950, British sample: Deutsche Forschungsgemeinschaft 1977, German sample). *Abnormally long or short gestation* was most frequently found in very young or older mothers, in those of lower social class, and in fifth and later births (Day 1967, Scottish sample; Butler et al. 1966, English and Welsh sample). Thus two groups seem to be particularly exposed to dangers connected with abnormally low birth weight and abnormal gestation length: firstborns and children of high birth order.

Early fetal loss (before week 20 of gestation) seems to be independent of birth order (Day 1967). *Later fetal loss* is U-shaped: risk is greatest in first- and in fourth- and laterborns, and at maternal age below 20 and over 35 years (Yerushalmy 1945, Selvin et al. 1976; the samples were the entire populations at risk in Hawaii and New York State respectively). *Stillbirths* have the same U-shaped incidence: holding maternal age and social class constant, first- and fifth- and laterborns were at greatest risk (Butler et al. 1966, English and Welsh sample; Yerushalmy, cited in Day 1967, USA sample). *Neonatal death* (death during the 1st month of life) follows the same pattern as stillbirth (Selvin et al. 1976; Butler et al. 1966; Yerushalmy cited in Day 1967; Shapiro et al. 1965; Harlap et al. 1977; all studies based on entire populations).

Postneonatal death and death in early childhood, on the other hand, have a different risk distribution Risk is highest in laterborns of young mothers (Newcombe 1962, population of British Columbia; Morris et al., cited in Wray 1971, population of England and Wales; Yerushalmy cited in Day 1967, population of Hawaii). *Death due to severe malformation* decreases with birth order, which may be due to the parental decision to stop reproduction after such a birth (James 1969, Morris cited in Wray 1971).

In Douglas's (1950) British and Yerushalmy's Hawaian sample (Day 1967), risk factors were related to *spacing* between births. British children born less than 2 years after their older sib had significantly more often a low birth weight than those born after longer intervals. Early fetal death was most frequent at pregnancy intervals of less than 1 or more than 2 years; later fetal death, stillbirths, and death in early childhood increased with decreasing pregnancy intervals in the Hawaian population.

Newcombe (1964; 1965; Newcombe et al. 1964) related to birth records data from all children of British Columbia up to the age of 5 years of age who were registered as *handicapped*. Holding maternal age constant the following birth order effects were found:

1. Firstborns are at greatest risk of intracranial and spinal birth injuries.
2. Third- and laterborns are at greatest risk of asphyxia, tuberculosis, and infantile paralysis (this birth order effect is strongest among children of very young mothers).
3. Handicaps due to maternal-fetal incompatibility increase with birth order.
4. Mental deficiency and cerebral spastic paralysis are independent of birth order (but increase with maternal age). Among children of very young mothers, however, laterborns are at greatest risk.

Comparing all institutionalized children in Baltimore with an IQ below 80 with a well-matched control group, Lilienfeld et al. (1956) found that risk increased with birth order and was greatest in children of very young and older mothers.

2.3 Birth Order and Risk at Birth and in Early Childhood

While early fetal death is independent of birth order, risk during later pregnancy, at birth and shortly after birth is greatest in firstborns (particularly if their mothers are very young or middle-aged) and in children of high birth order (particularly if born to young mothers). The disadvantage of firstborns is certainly an authentic birth order effect, being due to *biological* factors. Laterborns in large sibships – particularly those of young mothers – may have developed under suboptimal intrauterine conditions because of short spacing. The number of previous children and their spacing may be related to the mother's health, e.g., to her nourishment and to the medical help she obtains during pregnancy and at birth. Young mothers with large families are likely to be underprivileged (Day 1967); *so biological and social* reasons for greater risk in laterborns interact.

Death after the 1st month and during early childhood, on the other hand, is more frequent in laterborns in large sibships. These children may be insufficiently nourished or looked after or may be more exposed to infection via older sibs (see Newcombe's data on p. 16). Morris et al. (cited in Wry 1971) found, in all social classes and for each maternal age, an increase in postneonatal death by infection in higher birth orders, but particularly so in families of semiskilled and unskilled workers, whose resources are particularly strained by a large family. Here *social* reasons for a differential risk by birth order prevail. The findings summarized here *confirm the social background differences between first- and laterborns* discussed on p. 10.

2.4 Does Birth Weight Mediate an IQ-Birth Order Correlation?

Since birth weight increases with birth order and since in large samples birth weight is correlated to IQ at school, lower IQ in firstborns might be expected.

In the British National Child Development Study (Davie et al. 1972) birth weight and length of gestation were correlated to results on a reading and an arithmetic test and with ratings on social adjustment at 7 years of age. Birth weight gave an independent but exceedingly small contribution to the variance of test results and ratings when a number of other independent variables such as social class, sex, and number of older sibs were controlled. The same result was obtained in the follow-up of a population of pregnant women in the USA. At 4 years of age, the IQ of their children was mainly influenced by socioeconomic status and education of the mother. Neonatal variables such as weight at birth made negligible contributions to the variance (Broman et al. 1975). Similarly, in a retrospective study of South Carolina firstgraders birth weight did not contribute to the variance in verbal and nonverbal IQ and in visual-motor coordination. These were strongly influenced by maternal race and education. When, on the other hand, the children scoring one standard deviation or more below the mean were compared with those scoring at the mean or higher, birth weight contributed significantly but still not strongly to the variance (3% or less) (Ramey et al. 1978).

Among four complete age groups of Birmingham school children, verbal IQ was positively correlated with birth weight when gestation length was controlled. When, however, pairs of sibs were compared, weight differences of less than 1,500 g did not influence IQ. In addition, a positive correlation of gestation length with verbal IQ (birth weight being controlled), which was found in the whole sample, was not present in the subsample of sibs (McKeown 1970).

We may conclude that positive correlations between IQ and birthweight – and between IQ and gestation length as well – are the result of *between-family differences*. When evident abnormalities are excluded, the influence of birth weight upon IQ in the normal range is negligible. Thus in normal populations a lower IQ in first-borns because of their lower birth weight is not to be expected. It will be seen that the case may be different for monozygotic twins at least during their childhood (see p. 23, 24).

2.5 Birth Order and Minimal Brain Damage

First children and those of high birth order have been shown to be at greater risk of pregnancy and birth complications than middle children. If, among the former group, an increased prevalence of minimal brain damage were found, differences in personality and social adaptation might be expected. Left-handedness is taken by some authors as an indicator of minimal brain damage (Coren et al. 1980).

In large samples of university students Bakan (1971, 1977, Bakan et al. 1973) found a higher proportion of first- and fourth- or laterborns among left-handed subjects than among right-handers. Left-handers also reported adverse perinatal conditions more frequently than did right-handers. Satz (1973) suggested a model on the basis of minimal early brain damage to explain these results. Hubbard (1971) analyzed a similar sample and found, on the contrary, more second- and third-borns among left-handers than among right-handers. Birth order differences between right- and left-handers disappeared entirely, however, when the Bakan and the Hubbard samples were pooled. As university and college students may be selected for absence of minimal brain dysfunction, Teng et al. (1976) investigated a large sample of Taiwan school children and also a large university sample. In both groups left-handedness was independent of birth order. Schwartz (1977) found handedness and reported perinatal risk without correlation with birth order in a large sample of undergraduates. Hicks et al. (1978) pooled five studies and obtained the same result; their work was, however, critized by Bakan (1978), because the populations from which the samples were drawn were not equal in socioeconomic level and hence in perinatal risk in general. Hicks et al. (1979) divided a large sample of college students by birth order (1, 4+) and age of mother at birth (less than 20, 30+) into a high- and a low-risk group. Handedness was not differentially distributed between the groups, and controlling for sex did not change the result. A study by Leviton et al. (1976) which replicated Bakan's findings among elementary school students has been criticized by Annett et al. (1980) for methodological reasons. These authors personally interviewed volunteer families with two, one, or no left-handed parent (471 subjects). The rate of children for whom birth stress was reported by the mother – a more reliable source than self-reporting – was equal in right- and left-handers. In parents of either sex and in sons birth order did not vary with handedness; in daughters, birth orders 1 and 4+ were slightly overrepresented among left-handers. The authors conclude that, besides a pathological left-handedness, a natural (genetic?) left-handedness also exists and that in samples that have no known abnormalities left-handedness appears independent of birth stress and birth order. In large samples of Canadian adolescents and adults interrogated by means of a questionnaire, Coren et al. (1980) found left-handedness to be independent of birth order; this was also the case in the Searleman et al. (1980) sample, which consisted of over 1,000 USA high school college and university students.

The evidence is similar for other indicators of minimal brain damage. In a representative sample of British 11-year-olds, stammering and stuttering was unrelated to birth order (Calman et al. 1976). While Bassett et al. (1977) found that among all 578 first graders of one school system firstborns (particularly males) were lower on motor coordination, figure-ground perception, and visual constancy, according to Ramey et al. (1978) scores on a test of visual motor integration given to 1,000 randomly selected first graders were dependent on race and education of the mother but independent of the number of older sibs at birth.

In conclusion, there is at present no evidence that among normal subjects minimal brain damage is differentially distributed by birth order.

2.6 Birth Order and Height

Height is considered here because it is strongly influenced by environment. If a birth order–height correlation were found, this would indicate that some aspects of environment are more favorable for certain birth ranks than for others.

There is a well-established correlation of *social class and family size* with height: Height decreases with social class and, within social class, with sibship size (Tanner 1966). Wray (1971) analyzed the data of the British National Child Development Study on children born in 1946 and followed up to 15 years of age: There was a consistent social class gradient in height, but no class differences were found between only children. The negative correlation of height with sibship size was not found in the upper middle class but increased with each step down the social scale. In the sample of the Scottish Council for Research in Education (1953) – representative of 11-year-olds born in 1936 – the negative height-sibship size correlation did not appear in the professional and managerial class or in farmers children (Tanner 1966). Further evidence of the height-social class-sibship size correlation in large representative samples is given by Scott (1962) for London children; by Davie et al. (1972) for British children; by Neligan et al. (1976) for an age group of Newcastle children; and by Trémolières et al. (1950), Udjus (1964), and Belmont et al. (1975) for French, Norwegian, and Dutch inductees (see also Keddie 1958, Benech et al. 1960).

A survey of older literature on *birth order* and height is given by Meredith (1950). Firstborns were, as a rule, found to be taller than laterborns; as the former are biased for smaller sibship sizes this result is based on height differences between smaller and larger sibships. The opposite result, a small positive correlation of height with birth order, laterborns being taller, was found in the Welsh subsample among six age classes of female university entrants (1959–1964) at Swansea, social class and sibship size being accounted for (Dann et al. 1969). In the whole sample, including both Welsh and English girls, this laterborn advantage did not appear.

Grant (1964) analyzed in 1960 growth records over 9 years of 1310 London working-class children, a particularly underprivileged group that had to be rehoused through the London County Council. The usual decline of height and weight with increasing subship size was found. The investigation is exceptionally valuable because the author was able to *study sibs*. In family sizes of two to five the author compared 621 consecutive sib pairs, 7–10 years of age, at exactly the same age with all London school children of the same age in terms of average height. There was a trend for the younger sib to be taller, the mean difference being 0.8 cm. Only children were, on average, taller and heavier than children with sibs. On the other hand, in a much smaller sample of 90 pairs of brothers drawn from an American university student population and *not* measured at the same age, Howells (1948) found no significant difference between older and younger brothers.

That the negative correlation of height with sibship size within social class is due to differences in nourishment and health care can be seen from the fact that the correlation is not found in upper-middle class subjects. Two studies, one of them concerning sibs, might lead to the general conclusion that the presence of younger sibs impairs care and nourishment of the older ones. However, the subjects of both samples were born during the austere war and early postwar years in London and Wales. In the U.S.A. sample no difference in height was found between older and younger brothers. Earlierborns', disadvantage may be restricted to times and social classes where insufficient nourishment is a problem.

2.7 Birth Order and Age at Menarche

Tanner (1962) gives evidence from earlier investigations that, during 1800–1950, age at menarche was positively correlated with social class, in that girls from higher social classes menstruated earlier. However, Dann et al. (1969), Douglas (1966), and Nisbet et al. (1963) found that in their samples (born in the 1940s and 1950s) age at menarche was independent of social class. The British National Survey sample, born in 1946 (Douglas 1966), was studied for age at reaching puberty. (Since the children were followed up for many years, the data for girls seem reliable.) Though independent of social class, age at menarche varied with *family size*. The rate of early maturers (i.e., menarche at less than 13 years of age) was negatively correlated with number of sibs. Only children hat the highest percentage of early maturers. Social class and family size being held constant, there was no birth order difference (measured summarily by comparing the percentage of early and late maturers in first- and laterborns). Health of the girl, age of parents, and maternal care in infancy were not related to age at menarche. Spacing, on the other hand, may be of influence, since in families of two the percentage of second girls who were early maturers was higher if the age difference from the older sib was 6 years or more.

Early maturers have, throughout the school ages, a consistent superiority in IQ and school achievement over late maturers (Douglas 1966; Nisbet et al. 1963), even when family size and social class are controlled. Douglas (1966) did not find this correlation in only children. The fact that social class differences in menarche have disappeared over time, while differences related to sibship size have not, again points to *the importance of controlling sibship size* if between-family differences are to be minimized.

2.8 Conclusions

Firstborns and laterborns in large sibships are at highest risk of unfavorable biological influences during pregnancy, at birth, and during early childhood. There is, however, no evidence that this risk expresses itself in hampered intellectual development within the normal range. Consequently a biological basis for possible IQ differences by birth order can be excluded. Nor is there any evidence that within normal populations minimal brain damage is differentially distributed by birth order.

If, on the other hand, height and age at menarche are taken as an indicator of an environmental advantage (particularly regarding nourishment), there is evidence in one large underprivileged sample of sibs that – at least under conditions of insufficient resources – younger children are better fed than older ones. However, the conclusion that this result indicates a generally differential attitude of parents to their children by birth order would not seem justified.

One conclusion, on the other hand, becomes apparent throughout the study of biological differences, be it risk at birth, height, or age at menarche: Children from small and children from large sibships do not have the same background and do not live under the same conditions. Since firstborns are biased for small sibships, this signifies that comparisons between subjects of different birth order that disregard sibship size will show *interfamilial differences*.

Chapter 3 Research on Twins and Only Children

Research on twins and only children is of particular interest. Possible differences between children of different birth order have usually been ascribed to their differing relations with parents. Firstborn children have, until a second child is born, a monopoly on relationships and resources. Only children can be considered as extreme cases of firstborns in that they have the parents to themselves during their entire childhood. Laterborns, on the other hand, enjoy only divided parental attention and live in the company of their sibs. Twins can be considered as extreme cases of laterborns; since the spacing between them is zero, relations between twins are usually close and they are often treated as a unity. Differences between twins and singletons that are not reducible to biological differences may throw some light on the psychological importance of spacing.

3.1 Studies on Twins

3.1.1 Biological Differences Between Twins and Singletons

In any child samples tested for IQ, twins score somewhat lower. The difference usually amounts to about 5 IQ points (Scottish Council 1953; Tabah et al. 1954; Zazzo 1960; Husen 1960; McDonald 1964; Koch 1966; Record et al. 1970; McKeown et al. 1971; McCall et al. 1972). Twins have a considerably higher risk at birth than singletons. Incidence of twinning rises with maternal age (Butler et al. 1966; Scottish Council 1953; Koch 1966) and twins have lower average gestation length and lower birth weight for each gestation week. Mortality at birth and during the first years of childhood is higher for twins than for singletons. Secondborn twins are more disadvantaged than firstborn twins, and monozygotic twins (MZ) more so than dizygotic twins (DZ) (Butler et al. 1966; Scottish Council 1953; Record et al. 1970). Left-handedness and stuttering are found more frequently in twins than in matched singletons (Koch 1966, for further references).

3.1.2 Is Lower IQ in Twins Related to Lower Birthweight?

Record et al. (1970) studied over 2,000 twins, born between 1950 and 1957 in Birmingham, at 11 years of age. In comparison to singletons, their mean verbal reasoning score (obtained at the 11+ examination) was 4.4 points lower. A significant difference in favor of singletons still remained when the samples were equalized for length of gestation and birth weight. For 857 twin pairs it was possible to relate IQ scores to birth weight. Only with a difference in birth weight of 650 g or more was a substantial difference in scores found. Exactly the same result is given by Schmidt et al. (1978) for a representative sample of twins born at Nuremberg and followed up at 10 years of age: IQ was lower only when there was a difference in birth weight of 650 g and more. In smaller samples this independence of IQ of small differences in birth weight is confirmed (Babson et al. 1964; Churchill 1965; Matheni et al. 1971; McDonald 1964). In a representative sample of Swedish male adult MZ, Tienari (1966) did not find a correlation of the adult IQ with birthweight, though there were reported childhood differences in dominance, strength, and school achievement favoring the heavier twin. The author concludes that birth weight influences are of a transient nature and not found in adults.

Weight differences seem to affect MZ more than DZ. Kaelber et al. (1969) studied all twin births in four major Boston hospitals during 1952–1960. The children were followed up to the ages of 6–16 years. When large birth weight differences between the twins were considered (300 g or more), there was a mean IQ difference of 5 points in MZ pairs, but no significant difference in same-sex DZ pairs.

3.1.3 Is Lower IQ in Twins Related to Social Background Variables?

Husen (1960) compared to a random selection of singletons, 634 twin pairs found among a full age class of 12-year-old Swedish pupils given an achievement test. The twins' scores were consistently lower in four subtests, the difference corresponding to 3–5 IQ points. Twins' results were, however, normally distributed, which speaks against twin inferiority being caused by an external influence, such as premature birth or brain lesion.

The probability of twinning increases with the age of the mother and the number of previous births (Record et al. 1970; Tabah et al. 1954). As large sibships are biased for lower social class and as social class is correlated with IQ, differences in test scores between twins and singletons may disappear when social background is controlled.

Among all 11-year-old Scottish school children given a group intelligence test in 1947, there were 525 twin pairs (MZ and DZ not differentiated). Their mean IQ was 5 points lower than singletons' mean IQ, but there was no evidence that twins originated from larger sibships. Holding maternal age and social class (nine categories) constant, there still remained a small significant IQ difference, which was considered by the authors to be due to some factor inherent in twinning itself (Scottish Council 1953). In 1944 a representative sample of 95,000 6- to 12-year-old French children took a nonverbal intelligence test (Tabah et al. 1954). Among them, 325 twin pairs were found (MZ and DZ not differentiated). The twins' mean IQ was 10 points lower than that of singletons. When, however, sibship size and social class were controlled, the difference remained significant only for twins in sibships of three. In sibships of two the IQ difference was reduced to a nonsignificant 2 points when twins' IQs were compared with the IQs of narrowly spaced children.

Control of background variables such as social class, sibship size, and maternal age appreciably reduces the twin-singleton difference in IQ, but the latter does not quite disappear.

3.1.4 Is Lower IQ in Twins Related to Interaction with a Partner of the Same Age?

According to Zazzo (1960) and Luria et al. (1959) intellectual retardation in twins is mainly verbal and due to their interaction, which shields them from acquiring higher levels of language through contact with parents or older sibs. "Spacing zero," according to this theory, is thus the cause of an intellectual retardation. In the sample described on p. 22, Record et al. (1970) controlled for sibship size and age of the mother. The twin-singleton difference in IQ was reduced from 4.4 to – still significant – 3.9 points. When, however, twins who had grown up alone because of the death of their cotwin were compared with singletons, the IQ difference decreased to 0.7 points. The authors consider this result to be a confirmation of the hypothesis that twins' intellectual development is impaired by their close relationship with their cotwin. As there was no control for social class and birthweight it is, however, possible that the pairs in which one twin died were different in one or both of these variables from the other twin pairs. McDonald (1964), in a representative sample of low weight multiple births, controlled for birth weight, social class, and sex, after which the higher IQ in twins with a dead cotwin was reduced to nonsignificance. The same result was obtained by Myrianthropoulos et al. (1976) in white and black twins analyzed separately.

Only one investigation has been found by us in which twins were individually matched to singletons. Koch (1966) compared 35 MZ and 55 DZ pairs of white suburban middle-class families in Chicago with 360 singletons, individually matched to the twins for age, sex, sex of sib (all children had only one sib), and social class. The children were 5–7 years old and represented a highly selected research group of 540 subjects. Zygositity was carefully diagnosed. All children were given the Primary Mental Abilities Test (PMA) and, in order to analyze language, the Childrens Apperception Test (CAT).

The only significant difference was between male MZ and their controls, where twins were five points lower on the PMA. They scored lower on the verbal, quantitative, and spatial subtests. Female MZ and all-male DZ were nonsignificantly lower merely on the verbal subtest; mixed-sex DZ did not differ at all from singletons and all female DZ were even higher than singletons on the verbal subtest.

Interviews with the children, their mother, and their teacher did not elicit any differences between twins and singletons in terms of frequency or kind of contact with adults. Female MZ appeared even more eager to form contacts with other children than singletons. Neither kind and frequency of contact with nonsibs nor closeness to cotwin were related to IQ in the twins. When the groups were equalized for "severe prematurity," i.e. for a birth weight of 2,000 g or less, all test differences disappeared (mean birth weight in Western countries is 3,200–3,400 g). These differences were mainly caused by male MZ with low birth weight, who were much more linguistically retarded than subjects with normal birth weight, but, at the same time, were reported to have especially narrow contacts with adults. This latter fact was probably the consequence of their helplessness but did not seem to influence their linguistic capacities.

3.1.5 Conclusions

That only large birth weight differences in twins are related to differences in IQ fits well the data on singletons presented on p. 17. A part of the twin-singleton difference in IQ is explained by a twin bias for lower social class and larger sibship size. That having a partner of the same age hampers intellectual and particularly linguistic development is not supported by Koch's careful study, in which verbal capacities and IQ were found to depend mainly on sex and zygosity and to be independent of contacts with adults and other children and of closeness between twins. Significant IQ differences were seen in male MZ, a group which by zygosity and sex is at a particular risk. In this group lower IQ and lower verbal capacity is related to a birthweight of 2,000 g or less. The study, however, cannot claim representativity. It leads to the preliminary conclusion that, when social class, sibship size, and sex are controlled for, IQ differences of twins are due to biological rather than psychological differences between twins and singletons, which mainly appear in groups at special risk.

3.2 Studies on Only Children

3.2.1 Character Development

The Burke (1956), Bossard et al. (1960), and Howe et al. (1975) surveys of the literature on single children reported that studies conducted before 1945 generally stressed the abnormality of only children's familial situation and the probability of their being egocentric and unhappy personalities and of having a higher risk of psychiatric disorders. More recent literature on the only child, though generally less negative, has often failed to meet scientific standards (Cutts et al. 1954; Bossard et al. 1960; Van Krevelen 1946; Taylor 1945). Thompson (1974) surveyed popular ideas on desirable family size and on only children. The latter are stereotypically described as "generally maladjusted, self-centered and self-willed, attention seeking and dependent on others, temperamental and anxious, generally unhappy and unlikeable." Almodowar (1973) demonstrated the relationship between negative "scientific" opinions on only children and public propagation of fertility.

Studies comparing only children with matched children with sibs, had, however, already been written at a time when purely ideational literature was still predominant (Fenton 1930; Guildford et al. 1930; Hooker 1931). Dyer (1945) paired 100 college females without sibs by age, education and occupation of parents, home locality, and high school activities with girls having sibs. Results on the Bell adjustment inventory and on college achievement tests did not differ. Similar scores on the Minnesota Multiphasic Personality Inventory (MMPI) were found by Burke (1956) in well-matched pairs of college women with and without sibs. More recent studies using personality tests found that female undergraduates without sibs were more confident and less dependent than firstborns (Feldman 1977) and that among undergraduates of either sex only children were less influenced by group decisions than subjects with sibs but were equally popular (Falbo 1977). Welch (1977) compared only children, firstborns, and laterborns using an undergraduate sample. Only children were not more anxious or guilt-ridden, nor did they feel more "unique" than the other birth ranks. All these studies may be objected to because they were done with small numbers of subjects. But Payne (1971), using the Edward's personal preference schedule (EPPS), found no difference in need for affiliation and achievement between only children and children with sibs among over 1,000 Air Force Academy freshmen; and only children were rated highest for leadersib by their peers.

The following studies refer to psychiatric disorder in only children in comparison with children with sibs. A systematic household sample in Buffalo was interviewed for behavior deviations in children (Lapouse et al. 1964). Mothers' reports of only children and children with sibs did not differ when age, sex, and race were controlled. Howe et al. (1975) compared 115 records of only children attending a London mental health clinic with those of a random sample of children with sibs matched for age. Only children were treated at a younger age and returned more frequently, and the staff more often described their parents as overprotective. Only children were less often juvenile delinquents than children with sibs. Apart from these points, differences in psychiatric disturbance were small.

In 1946 Wattenberg studied previous investigations that had found inconsistent results concerning the rate of only children among delinquents and concluded that social background was a far more important influence in delinquency than the number of sibs. This opinion is confirmed by Matejcek et al. (1978). The authors compared representative samples of well-matched children with mothers who had applied for an abortion and of children where this had not been the case. In the unwanted group (containing a high rate of broken homes), only children scored higher than children with sibs on a maladaptation score, while in the other group the result was reversed.

Among Dutch inductees only children were overrepresented among subjects whose father's occupation was unknown because of illegitimity or death (Belmont et al. 1976). According to USA census data of 1970, 17% of mothers of one child are widowed or divorced vs 10% of mothers of at least two children. The probability of growing up in a broken home is higher in only children than in children with sibs (Falbo 1978). In studies not matched for home background, only children may therefore appear disadvantaged. In well-matched samples, on the other hand, differences between only children and children with sibs are small or nonexistent.

3.2.2 Intellectual Development

The question of whether being an only child leads to better intellectual development due to stimulating contact with adults is difficult to answer. If an intellectual

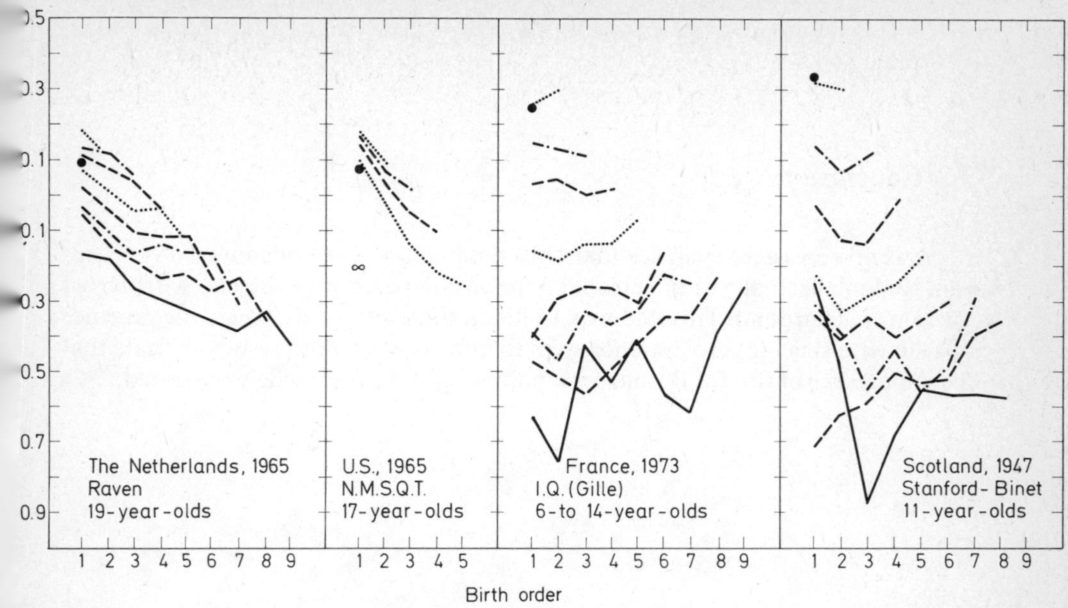

Fig. 2. Birth order and IQ in four national samples. Intellectual performance of four large populations, plotted as function of birth order and family size. Separate curves in each graph represent different family sizes, which can be read from the last birth order on each curve. *Solid circles* represent only children. The *double open circle* in the USA data represents twins. The years show when data were collected. The means of the Dutch, American, French, and Scottish data sets are 2.82, 102.5, 99.2, and 36.74 respectively. The corresponding standard deviations are 1.43, 21.25, 14.53, and 16.10 (Zajonc 1976)

advantage is expected in firstborns because, at least at the beginning of life, they have the full attention of their parents, it would be logical for only children to have a higher IQ than children with sibs, because they enjoy this undivided attention during their entire childhood. Zajonc (1976) has grouped studies in IQ of large populations in France, USA, Scotland, and the Netherlands (Scottish Council 1949; Enquête Nationale 1973; Belmont et al. 1973; Breland 1974). Figure 2 demonstrates that only children's rank is by no means uniform. Further analysis of the samples shows that even *within* these populations their rank is different at each social level. The same variation of only children's IQ with social background was demonstrated by Page et al. (1979) in a large representative sample of USA high school graduates and by Steelman et al. (1980) in elementary students of the Health Examination Survey.

This inconsistency may be related to the various reasons leading parents to have one child (notwithstanding social pressure for larger families), such as broken homes, illness, financial difficulties, working mothers, ideological motives, and immigration. Every such reason could be differentially related in different social strata to the biological and cultural endowment of the parents. As long as only children are compared with children with sibs without better control for social variables than a very gross subdivision into social classes, the question of whether their more narrow contact with parents is related to a particularly advantageous intellectual development must remain open. At present there is no evidence for an affirmative answer.

3.3 Conclusions

There is no consistent evidence that only children are either advantaged or disadvantaged intellectually or in personality when compared with subjects with sibs of the same background. This finding parallels results with twins, where the presence of a sib with spacing zero does not seem to influence IQ. Both results indicate that the importance of sibs for IQ and personality may have been widely overrated.

Chapter 4 Birth Order and IQ

4.1 Introductory Remarks

Since Sir Francis Galton's study on English men of science (1874), it has frequently been upheld that firstborns are more often eminent or more often take part in higher education than laterborns generally and middle children particularly (for a survey see Altus 1965 a, b, 1966 a, b). As the use of intelligence tests increased, the hypothesis was examined that oldest children have higher IQs than their sibs because of their closer contact with parents. Zajonc's famous "confluence hypothesis" (see p. 39 f.) then extended this theory of a firstborn advantage to a model of a largely environmental determination of a child's IQ by his position in the sibship.

IQ as a variable in birth order research needs some comment. IQ will be understood as the result of an individual or group test of intelligence, ability, or aptitude. The reliability of the accepted and widely used intelligence tests is high. Their significance for such important biographical items as years of schooling and income has been thoroughly discussed by Jencks (1972). Though IQ explains only a part of the existing variance in education and income, the validity of intelligence tests and similar measurements is still higher than the validity of any other known psychological test.

It will be seen that as IQ is correlated with variables like social class and sibship size, overlooking these correlations leads to fallacious birth order effects. If members of large sibships have a different social origin and a mean lower IQ than those of small ones, any arrangement of mean IQs by birth order will lead to a stepwise decrease in IQ favoring firstborns. A difference between sibships will, in this way, appear as a difference within sibships.

4.2 The IQ-Social Class Correlation

It is one of the best-established facts in IQ research that in children and adults, mean IQ declines with social class (Eells et al. 1951; Anastasi 1958; Cropley 1964; Illsley 1967). Jencks (1972, pp. 78, 185) gives a zero-order correlation of children's IQ with their father's occupational status of 0.35 and of nonfarmer white men's IQ with their own status of 0.5.

4.3 Differential Fertility by Social Class

The literature showing differential fertility by social class is extensive (Cook 1951; Westoff et al. 1961, 1963; Benjamin 1966; Nisbet et al. 1967; Davies et al. 1972). Large sibships are reported to be raised more frequently by parents with small incomes and little formal education. Since World War II, the linear relationship between social class and fertility has become attenuated. The postwar increase in fertility has affected the middle and upper-middle classes more strongly than the other classes (see p. 10 f.). There is also a general trend towards decreasing fertility in the Western nations due to an increasing opportunity for birth control, which may finally lead to the disappearance of differential fertility by social class.

4.4 Sibship Size and IQ

When among unselected child or adolescent populations the subjects' IQs are correlated to the number of their siblings, a negative correlation is found, ranging usually between −0.2 and −0.4. One of the rare studies of adults shows that it persists in grown-up women (Scott et al. 1955). But IQ is not merely negatively correlated with the size of the family of origin. In a representative sample of completed Minnesota families the correlation between the average parents' IQ and the number of their offspring was −0.3 (Reed et al. 1965). The negative correlation of IQ with family size has been discussed since the beginning of IQ research as "differential fertility for IQ." A large amount of evidence for differential fertility was collected by Nisbet (1953, 1958) and Nisbet et al. (1967).

Anastasi (1954) has reported on the methodological problems connected with differential fertility. Individual large families living under special conditions may be overweighted, particularly when the age range of the sample is small (McCall et al. 1972). On the other hand, the inclusion of incomplete families (children from incomplete, potentially large sibships appearing together with those from small ones) could obscure a correlation between IQ and sibships size. There may be cohort problems, in that a layer of younger, better-educated, incomplete families may superpose older, less-educated, complete ones (e.g., when a suburb absorbs a former village). In this case, a spurious correlation between IQ and sibship size could appear but subsequently disappear after completion of the newcomers' families. Maxwell (1969 b), in his national Scottish sample, observed a transitory correlation between IQ and number of offspring due to subjects with higher IQ starting their families later.

A factor contributing to the negative correlation between IQ and sibship size is parental age at birth. There is evidence that children's IQ correlates positively with the mother's age at birth (Illsley 1967; Lobl 1971). In the Maxwell (1969) sample of Scottish children followed up to adulthood, higher IQ, longer education, delayed marriage, and higher occupational class clustered together. Also, among all Amsterdam inductees with one sib there was a modest correlation between the mother's age and the son's IQ when social class and birth interval between first and second child were controlled (Zybert et al. 1978). Older mothers have a restricted fertility span and, on average, fewer children. According to Bumpass et al. (1977), age at first birth is one of the most important determinants of fertility.

4.4.1 Is the IQ-Sibship Size Correlation Spurious?

If IQ declines with social class and fertility increases with declining social class, then it is possible to hypothesize that the negative correlation between IQ and sibship size is an artifact which should disappear when social class is held constant (Kennett et al. 1970; McCall et al. 1972). Should this prove true, some light would be cast on the possible causes of the negative correlation between IQ and sibship size. Different hypotheses have been advanced:

1. Less intelligent parents make less use of birth control and genetically transmit a lower IQ to their children.
2. Less intelligent parents make less use of birth control and give their children a less stimulating environment.
3. Children growing up in large sibships have less opportunity for adult contact, with the consequence that their intellectual development is retarded.
4. The distribution of human beings into social groups is dependent on many biological, psychological, and social influences, IQ and education explaining only about half of the variance (Jencks 1972). Within social groups, habits, norms, and pressures concerning fertility (Westoff et al. 1961; Griffith 1973; Thompson 1974) influence group members, to a large extent independently of IQ.

Hypotheses 1 , 2, and 3 imply that within social class the negative correlation between IQ and sibship size persists. Hypothesis 4 implies that within well-defined and homogeneous social strata the IQ-sibship correlation should become insignificant. The evidence will be discussed in the next paragraphs.

4.4.2 Differential IQ by Sibship Size Within Social Class

Samples Consisting in or Representative of Entire Populations

Illsley (1967) gave a group test for nonverbal intelligence to 11,280 7-year-old children born in Aberdeen between 1950 and 1955. Using five social categories, he found, in each class, lower scores with increasing sibship size. The decrease was slightest in class I and most marked in classes III, IV, and V. Nisbet et al. (1967) confirmed this finding in successive age groups of the same population, as did Oldman et al. (1971).

The Scottish Council for Research on Education (1949) gave a group intelligence test to 75,000 11-year-old children in 1947. The correlation of IQ with sibship size was −0.28. An individual test given to a representative sample of 1,110 children resulted in a correlation of −0.32. Nine occupational classes were distinguished and each showed a clear downward trend in scores with increasing sibship size.

In an investigation of all children born during 1 week of 1946 in England and Wales (Douglas et al. 1968) and tested when 8 and 11 years old, the ususal decrease in a composite ability-achievement score with increasing sibship size was found. A subsample of 3,626 children tested when 8, 11, and 15 years old did not indicate a change over time in this association. It was stronger in working- than in middle-class children, stronger for verbal than nonverbal skills, and stronger in children of older rather than younger parents.

The same result was found in the investigation of the French Institut National (1959) when a sample of 66,000 French elementary school children were given a group intelligence test in 1944. The inquiry was repeated in 1965 (Enquête Nationale 1973). On six social levels, a decrease of IQ with family size was least pronounced in the professional and managerial class and in farmers' children.

In the following studies regression analysis is used and the sibship size influence on IQ weighted. A nationally representative sample of over 7,000 elementary school children investigated in the course of the USA. Health Examination Survey was studied by Svanum et al. (1980). When social class was controlled, sibship size was negatively correlated with IQ but explained only slightly less than 3% of the variance. Steelman et al. (1980) selected from the Health Examination Survey material over 3,000 elementary school children living with all their sibs and both parents at home, no other adults being present. The subjects were divided into those from families above and below poverty status. In the former group the zero-order correlation coefficient of birth order with IQ was −0.13, in the latter −0.23. After a regression analysis, with income, birth order, and mother working held constant, the partial correlations were −0.12 and −0.18. Sibship size and birth order together accounted for 6.1% of the variance in the below poverty group and for 2% in the above poverty group, sibship size explaining the majority of the variance. Income contributed most to the variance.

Another sample representative of all USA high school graduates, and consisting of over 20,000 subjects, was investigated in the context of the National Study of Educational Effects by Page et al. (1979). Sibship size explained 4% of the variance in IQ. When, however, race and social class were controlled, birth order and sibship size together explained less than 0.5% of the variance. Decreasing IQ with increasing sibship size was found neither in white graduates of the upper and middle classes nor, when data on white and black subjects were put together, in the 25% of subjects with the highest socioeconomic status. The authors were able to prove that the IQ-sibship size correlation is due to between-family differences: The rate of upper- and middle-class subjects at each sibship size had a linear correlation of 0.95 with the IQ of each sibship size group.

A study from a developing country gives a similar picture. Velandia et al. (1978) studied the IQ of 36,000 Columbian college applicants. Among those representing the top 25% on a socioeconomic scale, IQ was highest in sibships of three; among the middle 50% in sibships of three and four; and among the lowest 25% in sibships of four to seven. At each social level IQ was lower both in smaller and larger sibships than those mentioned above. With control of socioeconomic status, sibship size just failed to explain 1% of the variance in overall ability. It explained even less variance in mathematical and reasoning ability and slightly more than 1% in verbal ability.

The study with the largest sample did not use sophisticated statistical methods. The IQs of almost 400,000 Dutch inductees (Belmont et al. 1973) born between

1940 and 1944 were analyzed by siships size and three social classes. IQ fell with sibship size strongly in the manual, less strongly in the nonmanual class, and not at all in the farmer group. When Marjoribanks et al. (1975b) reanalyzed the material they found a raw regression weight of −0.035 for sibship size.

Smaller, Socially Homogeneous Samples

No significant correlation of IQ with sibship size was found in participants in a longitudinal child development study (Rees et al. 1970), in a sample of high school girls born during the 1930s (Damrin 1949), in sixth graders from a middle-class area (Cicirelli 1967), in Canadian middle-class high school students (Kennett et al. 1970), in Jewish high school students (Romanoff 1976), in Cambridge middle-class adolescents (Mascie-Taylor 1980), or in Manchester University students born during the 1930s (Warburton 1951). A smaller than usual correlation (−0.13) was found in London students born during the 1920s (Himmelweit 1948).

Three studies have used samples from developing countries. Sibship size was not correlated to IQ in a sample of Indian high school students (Chopra 1966). In a random sample of 10- to 11-year-old Samoan children, sibship size was curvilinearly related to IQ: Members of sibships that significantly deviated in size from the mean of the whole sample (6.5 children) had lower scores on a test standardized on the Samoan population (Ranking et al. 1979). A similar curvilinear association was found by Ho (1979) in over 1,600 Hong-Kong Chinese high school students: Subjects with two to four sibs scored higher than those with more or fewer sibs. Sibship size explained less than 2% of the variance in IQ.

McCall et al. (1972) sampled 750 males and 680 females from the second to sixth grades and different school systems in an American state. The authors argue that samples matched for age introduce a bias for large families of lower social class since their children have shorter mean birth intervals than those of smaller families with higher-class background and are consequently more likely to enter a sample. For each subject there was an "early" and a "late" IQ. Using multiple regression and analysis of variance and holding paternal occupation constant, there was no influence of sibship size on IQ either at the same or at variable age levels. Social class proved the strongest contributor to variance in IQ.

Evidence from an Adoptive Study

In a volunteer sample of 120 natural and 104 adoptive families in Minnesota, Scarr et al. (1979) found the usual correlation of IQ with sibship size in natural children (−0.21), but IQ in the adopted children was not correlated to the number of children in the family.

4.4.3 Conclusions (Table 3)

In studies where social class is used as a gross division forming groups that are not culturally homogeneous, within social classes a negative correlation between IQ and sibship size appears. Usually it is smallest or zero in the highest social class

Table 3. Sibship size and IQ in samples consisting of or representative of entire populations. Control of social class

Author	Country	*N*	Age	Negative Correlation
Illsley (1967)	Scotland	11,280	7 years	+
Scottish Council (1949)	Scotland	75,000	11 years	+
Douglas et al. (1968)	England and Wales	3,676	8, 11, 15 years	+
Institut National (1959)	France	66,000	Elementary school	+
Enquête Nationale (1973)	France	103,781	Elementary school	+
Svanum et al. (1980)	USA	7,000	Elementary school	+ Explained variance 3%
Steelman et al. (1980)	USA	3,428	Elementary school	Explained variances 2%/6%
Page et al. (1979)	USA	20,000	High school graduates	Explained variance 0.5%
Velandia et al. (1978)	Columbia	36,000	College applicants	Explained variance 1%
Belmont et al. (1973)	Netherlands	367,398	Inductees	Raw regression weight −0.035

and sometimes in the class of farmers as well. In studies where statistical methods allow the influence of sibship size to be weighted, the explained variance reaches at most 6% and is usually smaller. Race and social class are the main contributors to IQ variance.

Investigations from the developing countries are particularly instructive. There IQ is highest in children of medium-sized families, and the linear decrease with increasing number of sibs, typical for many Western samples, is not found.

The IQ of adoptive children appears uninfluenced by the number of sibs they grow up with. And, similarly, if care is taken to have socially homogeneous samples, IQ is independent of sibship size.

Thus the evidence points to a *spurious IQ-sibship size correlation*. Large sibships do not necessarily impede intellectual development. In populations in which birth control is not in general use, sibship size may be an indicator of the genetic and environmental conditions parents transmit to their children. But where, as among Western middle-class parents, a large family may be planned or, as in developing countries, a small family may indicate some disadvantage, the negative IQ-sibship size correlation disappears. It is a consequence of between-family differences.

4.4.4 Research on Direct Influences of Sibship Size on IQ

Hunt (1966) was of the opinion that in large sibships, individual children do not receive the same amount of stimulation as in small sibships. Nisbet (1953), Nisbet et al. (1967), and Scott et al. (1955) tried with different methods to prove that the negative correlation of verbal IQ with family size increases with age because of a cumulative deficit. The results were not consistent, but there was a general tendency for IQ to correlate more strongly with sibship size when it was measured verbally rather than nonverbally.

Higher correlations of verbal than nonverbal tests with sibship size were also found by Douglas et al. (1968) in the British National Child Development Study, and by Marjoribanks (1972) in a random sample of 11-year-old Canadian boys.

Language may be more amenable to environmental influence than other skills. Scarr et al. (1979) found a very modest correlation of adoptive children's verbal IQ with the mean IQ of their adoptive parents, while nonverbal scores were not correlated. Before accepting that large sibship size hampers linguistic development because of insufficient contact with adults, it must be remembered that social class differences are also largest for verbal tests (Jencks 1972, p. 78), and that social class differences in behavior toward children are most evident in language (Lukesch 1976, p. 151; Tulkin et al. 1970). A much more careful ascertainment of differences *between* sibships seems necessary before accepting the hypothesis that sibship size per se influences verbal IQ (Henry in Institut National 1954, p. 95).

4.4.5 Birth Intervals and IQ

Spacing may be more important for intellectual development than sibship size. Children born at small intervals share a low language level, while much older sibs may be more adequate models. Large sibships have, on average, smaller birth intervals than small sibships. Only when social class and sibship size are controlled can the influence of birth interval be differentiated from the IQ-sibship size correlation (Dandes et al. 1969). Oldman et al. (1971) controlled both variables and calculated a family growth rate. The nonverbal IQ of a subsample of all children born in Aberdeen and tested when 7 years old was negatively related to family growth rate within sibship size. The difference between the „quickest" and the „slowest" quartile was 4.3 IQ points. On the other hand, the authors found the IQ of firstborns within social class to be somewhat lower if conception had taken place *before* marriage (the difference was 2.8 IQ points), so that some doubt remains as to whether spacing itself influences IQ within social class and sibship size, or whether spacing is merely an indicator of other sociocultural and biological variables. A nationally representative elementary sample was studied by Svanum et al. (1980) (see p. 32). A density index was created by dividing the number of years the subjects' parents were married by the number of the subjects' younger sibs. IQ was independent of this index.

Douglas et al. (1968), in the sample mentioned above, compared test scores with spacing in children from middle-class sibships of three (see p. 37). There was no correlation between birth intervals and nonverbal IQ, but scores in reading and vocabulary were lower in narrowly spaced sibships. In middle- and working-class boys from same-sex sibships of two, test scores were highest when birth interval was 2–4 years. Longer and shorter intervals were related to lower results. Verbal tests were more sensitive to spacing than nonverbal tests.

Belmont et al. (1978) studied the influence of spacing in a subsample of their inductee population: men with one sib living in Amsterdam. The sample contained large numbers of brothers. The IQ of first- and secondborns was independent of spacing. In a large sample of Kalamazoo brother pairs tested at grade 6, the IQ of adjacent brothers did not vary with spacing (Olneck et al. 1979).

Four less representative samples give conflicting results: Marjoribanks (1978), using regression surfaces, found that IQ was positively related to spacing to younger sib in 500 11-year-old Australians. Among over 1,000 undergraduates with one sib, females with a sister scored higher on an intelligence test at narrow than at large spacings, while males with an older brother did better at large spacings (Rosenberg et al. 1969). Nuttall et al. (1979) studied suburban adolescents with one or four and more sibs. Only among the larger sibships was there a significant *negative* correlation of IQ with spacing. In his large Jewish middle-class sample, Romanoff (1976) found that narrow spacing was associated with higher IQ.

It seems decisive that in a sample of adoptive children spacing was unrelated to IQ (Grotevant et al. 1977).

There is no evidence that spacing is associated with IQ at small sibship sizes, though IQ may be lower in narrowly spaced subjects with many sibs. The U-shaped curve found by Douglas et al. (1968) and the slightly lower IQ found in premaritally conceived children on the one hand, the negative correlation between spacing and IQ in the Jewish sample and the missing spacing effect in adoptive children's IQ on the other, seem to indicate that *spacing is an indicator of background factors* influencing intelligence rather than an autonomous influence. The data on twins (see p. 22ff.) confirm this view.

4.5 Birth Order and IQ

4.5.1 Birth Order as the Independent Variable

For the reasons set forth above, it is evident that subjects of different birth order compared for IQ should be as similar as possible in terms of social variables, sibship size, parental cohort (see p. 10ff.), and birth intervals. Completeness of sibship must be considered as well. In incomplete sibships, differences between earlier- and laterborns may be obscured by between-sibship differences. In 7-year-old children in sibships of two, secondborns represent complete sibships, as the probability of another child being born after 7 years is small. Firstborns, instead, can represent complete as well as incomplete sibships (Lees et al. 1957; Scottish Council 1949).

4.5.1.1 Nationwide Samples

The Scottish Council for Research on Education (1949) analyzed scores on an individually given Binet-Terman intelligence test in a subsample of 1,100 11-year-olds representative of all Scottish school children of that age. When sibship size was controlled, there was some evidence that lastborns were superior. In a later publication (Scottish Council 1953) this was not upheld: The authors stated that there was no clear association between IQ and birth order.

The National Child Development Study (Douglas 1964) describes a representative sample of all children born in England, and Wales who were given a combined intelligence-achievement test at 8 and 11 years of age (4,195 subjects). In sibships of two and three from the middle and the lower classes, there was no consistent difference in scores between first- and laterborns. Firstborns tended, however, to improve their scores between 8 and 11, while the scores of laterborns tended to drop. The differences are in the range of 0,5–1 IQ points. Same-sex sibships of two and three were again studied at 15 years in the same sample, which had decreased to 3,626 (Douglas et al. 1968), without control of social class. In sibships of two the first boy scored slightly higher on verbal IQ (amount not given) than the second boy, while results on a nonverbal test did not vary with birth order. In female sibships of two, the younger sib scored better on IQ as well as on achievement tests. In sibships of three, firstborn boys had the same advantage over laterborns as in sibships of two. For females there was no consistent difference. The advantage of the firstborn seems to be restricted to boys and to verbal IQ. Possible cohort and cultural differences between parents of firstborns and those of laterborns were not considered.

In 1965, a sample of 103,781 French children representative of all 6- to 14-year-old school children were given a nonverbal intelligence test (Gilles' Mosaique). Corrections for differences in age were carefully made. In the highest social class IQ declined with birth order in sibships of four or more; in smaller sibships there was no difference. In the other five social classes IQ in sibships of six or more rose with birth order (Enquête Nationale 1973) (Fig. 2). The authors consider these IQ differences to be spurious as the highest social class contained very heterogeneous occupations and large sibships were rare. Also in the other classes, among earlierborns of small families there were children in incomplete sibships who, given the negative correlation of IQ with sibship size, depressed the scores of earlier-borns in complete sibships.

There are two further arguments for the higher IQ in laterborns of large sibships being due to interfamilial differences: (1) Earlierborns who, when young, have many sibs must live in narrowly spaced sibships, while for laterborns this is not necessarily the case (see p. 35f. for a possible association of low IQ with narrow spacing); and (2) in large sibships, parents of laterborn children are on average appreciably older than parents of earlierborns. The former may be a cohort to whom contraception was unfamiliar, while the latter may have undergone a differentiation for use of contraception according to cultural und perhaps biological variables. The higher IQ of laterborns would then reflect differences between parental cohorts.

Gill (1976) discusses the results of the Irish standardization of Raven's Progressive Matrices and of the Mill Hill vocabulary test with stratified samples of 3,695 6- to 11-year-old school children, representative of 380,000 Irish children in non-private schools. A multiple regression analysis was carried out, and a former study of Kellaghan et al. (1972) was replicated inasmuch as sibship size, number of older sibs, and „modified ordinal position," i.e., birth order expressed as a fraction of sibship size, were introduced as predictor variables. The age factor explained most variance, and social class, urban and rural habitation, and sibship size followed. Sex, social class, sibship size, and modified ordinal position *together* explained 1%

of the variance in the nonverbal test and 4% in the verbal test; for the 9- to 11-year-old children (a group where variance was homogeneous, which was not the case for the whole sample), they explained 4% and 6%, respectively.

There are some studies on birth order effects which have been carried out with the large „Project Talent" sample of USA high school students. Burton (1968) analyzed a national sample of 43,352 high school seniors tested in 1960 by Project Talent. Social class was very carefully ascertained by a mailed questionnaire which, due to self-selection, gives the sample some degree of bias. The sample was weighet for type, localization, and size of school to represent a national sample. The IQ had verbal and nonverbal components. The authors concluded that a decrease of IQ with birth order predominates, in that firstborns score higher than middle children, who in turn score higher than lastborns. This was, however, only true in 15 of 32 possible comparisons. Among 16 comparisons involving first, middle, and last children in sibships of four and five, the latter had higher scores than at least one of the other groups in seven. The tendency for an IQ upswing in laterborns of large, lower-class families (Enquête Nationale 1973) appeared in this investigation as well (see p. 37). The mean difference in IQ between first- and lastborns was found to be 3 points.

McCall (1973) investigated a 1% subsample of the Project Talent national high school sample ($N = 3{,}308$), and a correlation of -0.26 was found between a composite IQ and birth order. The correlation was reduced to -0.17 (explaining 3% of the variance) when sibship size and social class were controlled.

Jencks (1972, p. 348) gives data on a nationally representative sample of 6,379 men who were tested by Project Talent in 1960 in the 11th grade of high school and followed up in 1966. A comparison was made of first- and secondborns in sibships of two and more (the subjects were not brothers). There was evidence of differences between fathers of the subjects, in that, on average, fathers of firstborns were better educated and had higher occupations than those of secondborns ($P \leqq 0.001$). The difference was primarily due to the fact that no control was made for sibship size; this caused secondborns to be biased for larger sibships, since the larger the family the more narrow the spacing and the higher the probability that the second son would be included in the sample. It is also possible that the educational and professional upgrading of younger fathers contributed to the difference. Firstborns' mean verbal IQ was 3.57 IQ points higher, which is a small but highly significant difference ($P \leqq 0.0001$). The difference in nonverbal IQ was nonsignificant, that of firstborns being 0.36 points lower than that of secondborns. This study, incidentally, demonstrates the differences in familial antecedents between firstborn and secondborn sons of the same age and attending the same type of school.

Glass et al. (1974) studied a nationally representative population of 10th and 17th graders corresponding to the Project Talent sample, and selected subjects with one or two sibs. With control of the fathers' education, birth order explained less than 1% of the variance in verbal IQ.

Three studies involving samples representative of USA children and adolescents have used regression analysis. In an investigation of elementary school children. Svanum et al. (1980) found that 0.1% of the variance in mental ability was explained by birth order. Steelman et al. (1980) found a partial correlation of

0.03 of birth order with IQ in above poverty status subjects and no significant correlation for below poverty status subjects. In the Page et al. (1979) study of over 20,000 high school graduates, the variance explained by birth order was 0.5%.

Among over 36,000 Columbian college applicants the birth order contribution to the variance in mental ability studied by the same method was zero (Velandia et al. 1978). In each of these four studies social class and/or ethnicity were the best predictors of IQ (see p. 32).

4.5.1.2 The Dutch Inductee Study and Zajonc's Confluence Model

Belmont et al. (1973) divided the entire population of 19-year-old Dutch preinductees born between 1940 and 1944 into three social classes on the basis of paternal occupation: sons of nonmanual workers, sons of manual workers, and sons of farmers. Scores on Raven's Progressive Matrices, transformed into a 6-point scale, were used as dependent variable. For the 367,398 subjects on whom complete information was available, scores decreased in each class within sibships with increasing birth order. The effect was regular and systematic in sibships of two, three, and four; in larger families it was inconsistent. In farmers' sons, IQ had a tendency to increase in the later birth orders of large sibships (see Fig. 2).

In a study of this size any difference between variables attains significance. Notwithstanding this, there are two objections:

1. The method used in transforming Raven's scores into a 6-point scale is not given. It is questionable whether, after transformation, scores are still normally distributed, and it is not possible to translate differences in scores into IQ points. The authors themselves are of the opinion that differences for birth order within sibship size are „small." An analysis of the contributions of social class, sibship size, and birth order to the total variance would have been helpful.

2. The social class subdivision is very sweeping. Different sibship sizes within social class may signify different parental age, different parental cohort, different habitation, different denomination, and different interest and opportunity for schooling; in short, different backgrounds hidden behind the broad classification.

Marjoribanks et al. (1975 b) reanalyzed the Dutch data using hyperbolic regression equations and constructing regression surfaces. The resulting raw regression weight of test scores on birth order was −0.078.

Zajonc et al. (1975) based their famous „confluence model" on the Belmont et al. (1973) data. The model postulates that intellectual development is to be understood entirely as a consequence of the mutual influence among children and of the average of the family members' „absolute intellectual levels." If two parents, both gifted with an absolute intellectual level of 100, are joined by a newborn, whose absolute intellectual level is zero, the resulting average for the child's environment is 67: $(100+100+0)/3$. At the birth of another child – the first one has reached a level of 40 – the environment becomes even less inspiring: $(100+100+40+0)/4 = 60$. In this way the decrease of IQ with sibship size and with birth order is explained. If, however, spacing between the sibs is so large that the firstborn is at a level of, for example, 80 at the birth of the second child, the latter's environment will be 70. Large gaps between children improve the environment so that younger sibs may surpass the older. The effect of spacing is independent of social class.

Spacing is thus pivotal for the confluence theory. Sibship size and birth order acquire a negative impact for IQ only if spacing is small. Zajonc constructed a regression equation on the basis of average intellectual level and age of a child that explained 97% of the variance in the Dutch data, and where IQ decline by birth order in later children of large sibships is zero and then changes into an increase.

In a later study (1976) Zajonc used investigations from Scotland, France, and the USA in addition to the Dutch data to prove that changes in test scores were associated with changes in the spacing of sibs. Hypothetical spacing differences were inferred from national birth rates. Regional IQ differences in France, racial differences in IQ in the USA, and even sex differences in the American national data on the Scholastic Aptitude Test (SAT), which is given to high school absolvents, were thus explained.

In the Dutch study, the data on only children and lastborns did not fit the confluence theory, according to which only children should obtain the highest scores as they have the best intellectual environment, and last children in large sibships should surpass penultimates. To explain these findings, Zajonc introduced another theoretical postulate, the „teaching hypothesis," which suggested that only children and lastborns are disadvantaged because they do not have the opportunity to teach younger sibs. The relationship between the opposing influences of teaching and/or the dilution of the intellectual environment by a younger sib was not clearly defined.

In 1979 Zajonc et al. explained incoherent data on IQ differences between first- and secondborns by an age factor: At elementary age the confluence effect of the younger child predominates and the firstborn's IQ is depressed. In adolescence the teaching effect predominates and firstborns score higher than laterborns. In 1980 Zajonc et al. demonstrated that aggregate data of six national surveys were consistent with the confluence model.

Refutation of the Confluence Model

The Zajonc et al. (1980) Investigation of Scholastic Aptitude Test (SAT) Results. In 1976 the decline in national SAT results had been connected by Zajonc with increasing birth rates and thus presumably lower spacing. In 1980 the author of the confluence model studied two cohorts (1973/4 and 1976/77) by means of a regression analysis. The total variance explained by birth order, sibship size, cohort, and family income was 8% in verbal and 6% in nonverbal scores. The partial correlations of sibship size with verbal and quantitative scores were −0.04 and −0.03, thus explaining negligible parts of the variance. The author concluded that family factors may be quite minimal and the SAT sample of more than 5,000 students too small to display the trend.

Data Presented in Sects. 4.4.3 and 4.4.5. On pp. 32, 35 f. research on the IQ-sibship size and the IQ-spacing correlations was presented, demonstrating that the amount of variance in IQ explained by sibship size is extremely small, that a decrease of IQ with sibship size is due to between-family differences, and that there is no consistent evidence that small spacing depresses IQ.

Refutation of the Zajonc Model by Individual Authors. Page et al. (1979) showed in their high school graduate sample that the position of the single child in relation to children with sibs varies with social class and ethnicity and that his/her low position in aggregate data is due to the fact that among single children the proportion of lower class subjects is particularly high. The same variation of the single child's position by income was found by Steelman et al. (1980). Svanum et al. (1980) tested the Zajonc (1979) hypothesis that the position of the first – in relation to the secondborn child varies with age (see p. 40) and were unable to support it. These authors, as well as Velandia et al. (1978), demonstrated in their material that the use of aggregate data leads to a very much higher rate of explained variance than when individual data are used. Melican (1978) demonstrated with data of the Iowa High School Testing Program that there was no regular association of spacing with achievement scores within sibship size. In a sample of adolescent adopted and natural children representing 101 adoptive middle-class families, the adoptive parents' IQ was entered in the Zajonc et al. (1975) equation for the calculation of the intellectual environment. Birth order, sibship size, and spacing together then explained 2% of the variance in IQ of the natural and 1% of the variance in IQ of the adopted children (Grotevant et al. 1977).

Defects of the Confluence and Teaching Theory.
1. Nonenvironmental (e.g., genetic) factors are not considered.
2. The calculation of the mean intellectual level of the environment shows that the intellectual level of the newborn child is taken as a part of his/her environment (Olneck et al. 1979).
3. Environmental influence is seen in a completely mechanistic way as a kind of „contagion“: All members of the household have the same impact on the child. A mother with an IQ of 50 and a father with one of 150 would thus produce the same environment as parents with an IQ of 100 each (Page et al. 1979; Ho 1979).
4. The teaching effect seems to be introduced ad hoc. It is improbable that being taught by parents, as is the case for the only child, could be completely counteracted by the absence of the opportunity to teach.
5. Lastly it seems improbable that effects of processes within the family should appear only in the statistical treatment of very large populations and then to a very low extent (Svanum et al. 1980).

Disregarding all biological and social variables in favor of a psychological theory of confluence does not seem helpful. This was made particularly evident when Zajonc (1976) found an almost perfect negative correlation between measures of reading comprehension in school children of different countries and the birth rate in these countries (Sweden ranking highest for scores and lowest for birth rate and Iran the opposite). General poverty and scarcity of good schools in underdeveloped, densely populated countries are more probable reasons for low reading scores than the decrease in intellectual level of families with many children. It may be a sign of the general lack of adequate theorizing in birth order research that Zajonc's confluence model has won wide recognition in spite of such evident weakness.

The McCall Model

McCall (1980) constructed a simulated population model of 100 completed families with one to six children. The distribution of sibship size and occupational level was taken from USA census data. IQ values followed the normal distribution and were made to correlate negatively with social class (−0.4) and with sibship size (−0.25). For the whole sample a partial IQ/birth order correlation of +0.06 resulted when sibship size and occupation were controlled. When single age samples were used the partial IQ/birth order correlation was in most cases significantly higher and uniformly negative. Thus the IQ decrease with increasing birth order appears as an artifact of the single age sample.

4.5.1.3 Samples Consisting of or Representative of Smaller Populations

In two studies of IQ at 4 (Broman et al. 1975, 26,000 subjects) and 6 years of age (Ramey et al. 1978, 1,000 subjects) was correlated to the number of sibs at the time of the subject's birth. The variance explained by this variable amounted to 2% and 1% respectively, the main contributors being race, social class and education of the mother. The former sample was part of a large perinatal project, the latter, representative of North Carolina.

Studying 9,523 7-year-old Aberdeen school children who were given a nonverbal intelligence test, Illsley (1967) (see p. 31) found no difference by birth order when sibship size and social class were controlled.

In the Newcastle survey of child development (Neligan et al. 1976), of all children born over a period of 2 years ($N = 3{,}442$–$4{,}651$), a composite IQ was taken at 5 and 10 years of age. When sex, social class, and care of child were controlled, scores were not related to the number of older sibs. Farley (1976) studied all eight and ninth graders from two small towns in Ohio ($N = 1{,}186$). Previous significant birth order differences in composite IQ disappeared when sibship size was controlled.

In the Ho (1979) study of Chinese Hong Kong pupils (see p. 33), birth order was not significantly correlated to IQ. McCall et al. (1972) sampled 1,430 male and female students from all elementary and high school grades and a wide range of social classes and habitations in Illinois. Two IQ tests were given, one at the beginning of elementary and one at the beginning of high school. Controlling for seven social classes, sibship size, and testing age removed associated variance between IQ and birth order.

4.5.1.4 **Conclusions** (Table 4)

Table 4. Birth order and IQ in nationally representative samples (A) and smaller populations (B)

	Author	Country	*N*	Age	Superiority
A	*No Control of Sibship Size and Social Class*				
	Jencks (1972)	USA	6,379	11th grade	Firstborns (3.57 IQ points, verbal)
	Control of Sibship Size				
	Scottish Council (1953)	Scotland	1,100	11 years	–
	Douglas et al. (1968)	England Wales	3,626	15 years	Firstborn boy (verbal), secondborn girl
	Control of Social Class and Sibship Size				
	Enquête Nationale (1973)	France	103,781	6–14 years	–
	Gill (1976)	Ireland	3,695	9–11 years	Extremely small part of variance explained
	Svanum et al. (1980)	USA	7,000	Elementary school	Explained variance 0.1%
	Steelman et al. (1980)	USA	3,428	Elementary school	Partial correl 0.03
	Burton (1968)	USA	43,352	High school seniors	Earlierborn (3 IQ points)
	McCall (1973)	Subsample of the above			Explained variance 3%
	Glass et al. (1974)	USA	2,532	High school seniors	Explained variance 1%
	Page et al. (1979)	USA	20,000	High school graduates	Explained variance 0.5%
	Belmont et al. (1973) (Statistical treatment by Marjoribanks et al. 1975b)	Netherlands	367,398	19 years	Regression weight birth order −0.078
	Velandia et al. (1978)	Columbia	36,000	College applicants	Explained variance 0%
B	Broman et al. (1975)	USA	26,000	4 years	Explained variance 1%
	Ramey et al. (1978)	USA	1,000	6 years	Explained variance 1%
	Illsley (1967)	Scotland	9,523	7 years	–
	Neligan et al. (1976)	England	3,424–4,651	5 and 10 years	–
	Ho (1979)	Hong Kong	1,965	High school	–
	McCall et al. (1972)	USA	1,430	Elementary and high school	–

On the evidence of these large studies and particularly of those using regression analysis it has to be concluded that *the influence of birth order on IQ is negligible*.

4.5.1.5 Smaller and Less Representative Studies

In view of the overwhelming negative evidence presented in the foregoing sections, the following studies will be summarily treated. They can be divided into those that control sibship size and social class and those that omit controlling either or both of these intervening variables (Table 5).

Table 5. Birth order and IQ in smaller samples. No control of social class and/or sibship size (A) and social class and sibship size controlled (B)

	Author	*N*	Age	Highest IQ
A	Lobl et al. (1971)	3,263	4 years	–
	Baughman et al. (1968)	200	Elementary school	Firstborns, lastborns
	Dandes et. al. (1969)	184	Elementary school	–
	Start et. al. (1974)	157	Elementary school	–
	Cropley et. al. (1975)	124	Elementary school	Only children
	Zielinsky (1966)	800	Fourth grade	Oldest, middle, last, according to sibship size
	Adams et al. (1972)	370	Fourth and fifth grades	Firstborns
	Blustein et al. (1968)	350	Fourth and sixth grades	–
	Eysenck et al. (1969)	4,000	11 years	Earlierborns (Sibship sizes four and six)
	Marjoribanks et al. (1975a)	185	11 years	Firstborns
	Chopra et al. (1966)	1,359	High school	–
	Oberlander et al. (1967)	313	High school	Firstborns
		357	High school	Firstborns
	Lunneborg (1968)	5,000	High school	Firstborns
	Lunneborg (1971)	896	High school	Firstborns (males)
	Stroup et al. (1965)	1,560	College	–
	Payne (1971)	574	College	Only children
		499	College	Firstborns
	McCutcheon (1977)	291	College	–
	Biegelsen (1976)	1,813	Freshmen	–
	Macbeth (1975)	716	Undergraduates	Firstborns (3.9 point)
	Altus (1959a, b)	1,300	Adults	Firstborns, lastborns
B	Koch (1954)	360	6 years	Secondborns
	Miller et al. (1976)	1,760	First grade	–
	Cicirelli (1976)	614	Sixth grade	Firstborns, secondborns (interaction sibship size and sex)
	Cicirelli (1976)	603	11–12 years	–
	Oberlander et al. (1970)	318	High school	Firstborns (3 IQ points)

Table 5. (continued)

Author	N	Age	Highest IQ
Murray (1971)	709	Secundary modern school	–
Romanoff (1976)	770	11th and 12th grades	Firstborns, laterborns (interaction sibship size and sex)

Among 20 samples where background was not controlled, there was an unequivocal superiority of firstborns in six; however, among seven samples with some control of background such superiority was found in only one. This is evidence that *birth order differences in IQ are artifacts*, due to inadequate methodology.

4.5.2 Birth Order as the Dependent Variable

Terman et al. (1925) found, in a classic study of highly gifted Californian children, 56.6% firstborns from sibships of two, 36.9% from sibships of three, and 33% from sibships of four. This overrepresentation of firstborns among the gifted was confirmed by Sheldon (1954) and Kincaid (1969). There was no control group, making it impossible to isolate the effects of demographic change, incomplete families, and differences in IQ by social class and sibship size.

The control of all these variables, though in a small sample, is the merit of the following study: Schlichting (1968) selected from 187 West German high school students (all sons of professionals) 20 pairs matched for age and family size, but different in IQ (127 or more versus 107 or less). There was no difference in birth order between the groups. Kellaghan et al. (1971, 1972) selected from Irish 11-year-olds who had been given an intelligence test 100 subjects with a verbal IQ of 119 or more and compared them with 461 children of average ability. The former subjects significantly more often came from somewhat smaller families of good social standing and living in town. There was no significant difference in birth order between the two groups; the bright group contained 32% firstborns, the less bright group 27%.

Conclusions

The studies in which birth order is the dependent variable again demonstrate the necessity of a control group. The Irish study found no significant differences in the birth order distribution between a mainly urban and a mainly rural population because, as the authors remark, in catholic Ireland well-situated families have almost as many children as the poor.

4.5.3 Comparison of IQ Between Sibs in the Same Family

4.5.3.1 Need of Correction of IQ for age Differences

The first studies of large numbers of sibs in the same sibship usually demonstrated an increase of IQ with birth order (Arthur 1926; Thurstone et al. 1931). This was recognized to be a consequence of a negative correlation of IQ with age (Hsiao 1931; Richardson 1936). Later comparisons of large samples of older and younger sibs in the same sibship did not result in any IQ differences by birth order (Hsiao 1931; Finch 1933) when IQ was corrected for age. The IQ-age problem has been extensively discussed by Roberts (1947) and Kamin (1974).

4.5.3.2 Large Representative Studies

Roberts (1947) tested five yearly groups of children born in Bath, England, at the ages of 11–13 years. Among them he found 504 pairs of sibs. There was a non-significant IQ difference of 1 point between the older and the younger sib.

Tabah et al. (1954) found, in the French national sample (see p. 32), 6,222 sibships of two. Birth order explained no variance in IQ when sex, social class, and urban or rural residence were controlled.

Jensen (1974) identified all sibships from kindergarten to sixth grade in a Californian school district. There were 3,174 families where at least one comparison between sibs was possible. For white children in sibships of two to six, there was only one significant birth order effect: In sibships of four, firstborns had higher scores. In black sibships there was no birth order effect at all. The independence of birth order was the same for verbal and nonverbal IQ with the exception of black only children, who had a higher verbal IQ than children with sibs. Sex of sib explained no variance.

In 50,000 children born in Birmingham (1950–1954) and tested there at age 11 for verbal reasoning (Barker et al. 1967; Record et al. 1969; McKeown 1970), 5,094 consecutive sibs were compared with social class controlled. The mean difference between the older and the younger sib was 0.7–0.8 IQ points in favor of the older sib. Since there was no control for sibship size, the laterborn members of adjacent pairs were biased for larger family size. In Aberdeen the whole elementary school population was tested when 7 and again when 11 years old with a nonverbal intelligence test (Oldman et al. 1971). Sibship size was controlled. In 1,326 comparisons between consecutive sibs there was evidence for a slight advantage at 7 years for the younger and at 11 years for the older sib. This was mostly due to younger girls in sibships of two having lower scores than their older sib. The largest difference observed was 2.2 IQ points.

In the Scottish national representative sample, the 1,215 children, born in Scotland in 1936 and tested individually at 11 years of age (see p. 36), had 17,554 younger sibs who were tested at the same age (Maxwell et al. 1960; Maxwell 1969). The mean IQ of all younger sibs was 5 IQ points lower than that of all firstborns. Younger sibs are biased for large families, whose sibs have more chance of being sampled than children from small sibships. If for each sibship the average IQ of the younger sibs is used for comparison, the difference disappears (De Avila 1971). When analysis of variance between and within each position in birth order for each family size was performed, there was no association between IQ and birth order. In a sample of 90 families with four or more sibs and where the sample member was a firstborn, there was a median maximum difference between sibs of the same sibship of 26 IQ points and no evidence for an association of IQ with birth order (Maxwell 1969). Olneck et al. (1979) studied 346 pairs of brothers – a part of the sample of the Kalamazoo follow-up study of former male public school students – using their sixth grade aptitude tests given in the years 1928–1950. Without control of sibship size and testing age, each succeeding birth order was associated with a two point decrease in IQ. With control of these variables this difference was reduced to 1.4 points. For brothers within the same family there was an insignificant decrease by birth order of less than one point.

Belmont et al. (1978) studied an inductee subsample of brothers in all-male sibships of two living in Amsterdam (535 pairs). IQ was slightly higher ($P \leqq 0.05$) in the older sib. Unfortunately no details whatsoever are given.

4.5.3.3 Smaller Studies of Sibs at the Same Age

In the Fels longitudinal study of child development (Sontag et al. 1958), comprising 140 children from 89 sibships, 62 sample children were compared with a sib, mostly first- or secondborn in a two-child family. Change in IQ was not related to birth order. Schoonover (1959) compared all sib pairs in an elementary school. In 59 pairs, each child had at least four scores. Earlier- and laterborn sibs were not different in their deviation from age norms. Scores were not influenced by spacing. Children with a male sib, however, scored higher.

Bartelt (1973) studied 129 sib pairs (first- and secondborns in sibship sizes two to eight) selected from southern New Jersey town high schools. All combinations of sex and sex of sib were equally represented, as well as two social classes. There was no difference for IQ taken in school. Laniel et al. (1975) selected younger children in sibships of two from the seventh year school population in a Canadian town. The sample comprised 84 children, whose older sib had taken the same intelligence test at the same age as the younger sib. There was no significant difference in IQ between the sibs. The sample was subdivided by spacing. At a spacing interval of up to 36 months there was a slight significant difference in favor of firstborns ($P \leqq 0.05$), which was due to firstborn girls followed by a brother. Dolph (1966) compared first- and secondborn ninth graders from 36 sibships of three for IQ tests taken in school at the same age and found no difference by birth order. Wolf (1967) compared sibs in 83 sibships of three who were attending public schools in one USA town. When sex was controlled, IQ did not vary with birth order. In the course of the Scarr et al. (1979) adoption study, Grotevant et al. (1977) found birth order effects on IQ in 143 adolescent natural children of 72 adoptive families to be nonsignificant.

4.5.3.4 Conclusions (Table 6)

Table 6. Birth Order and IQ in sibs in the same family: large, representative studies (A) and smaller studies (B)

	Author	Country	Age	N	Superiority
A	Roberts (1947)	England	11–13 years	504 pairs	Firstborns 1 point (NS)
	Tabah (1954)	France	6–14 years	6,222 pairs	–
	Jensen (1974)	USA	Elementary school	3,174 families	Firstborns with 3 sibs
	Barker et al. (1967)	England	11 years	5,094 sibs	Earlierborn (0.7–0.8 points; sibship size not controlled)
	Oldman et al. (1971)	Scotland	7 years 11 years	1,326 comparisons	Older sib of two with sister
	Maxwell et al. (1960) (analyzed by De Avila 1971)	Scotland	11 years	2,769 sibs	–
	Maxwell et al. (1969)	Scotland	11 years	90 sibships of four	–
	Olneck et al. (1979)	USA	Sixth grade	346 pairs	Earlierborn 1 point (NS)
	Belmont et al. (1978)	Netherlands	19 years	535 pairs	Firstborn ($P \leq 0.05$)
B	Sontag et al. (1958)	USA	Whole childhood	62 pairs	–
	Schoonover (1959)	USA	Elementary school	59 pairs	–
	Dolph (1966)	USA	Ninth grade	36 families	–
	Bartelt (1973)	USA	High school	129 pairs	–
	Laniel et al. (1975)	Canada	Seventh grade	84 pairs	–
	Wolf (1967)	USA	Public school	83 families	–
	Grotevant et al. (1977)	USA	Adolescents	72 families	–

Considering the total evidence presented by the nine large-scale studies of sibs, the earlierborn child appears to have an extremely slight advantage. It is of one point or less and does not appear in smaller samples. The smallness of the birth order difference agrees well with the extremely small amount of variable explained by birth order when regression analysis is used on large samples of nonsibs. *Birth order differences in IQ are negligible.*

4.5.4 Birth Order and Linguistic Skills

The usual explanation for higher IQ in first- or earlierborns is that they become more proficient in linguistic skills because of their narrower contact with adults in early childhood. Associations of family variables with IQ or achievement are more often found in verbal than nonverbal tests (see p. 35). Later, evidence will be presented – by the comparison of sibs as well as of nonsibs – that firstborn infants are more often spoken to and more encouraged to make sounds or speak than laterborns (see pp. 89, 90). As the rate of early development depends on stimulation, the developmental quotient (DQ) is slightly higher in first- than in laterborns. In a nationwide 1- to 15-month-old USA sample, Bayley (1965) found a noncumulative firstborn advantage in mental tests in four of 15 age levels. The finding was supported in a random sample of Cardiff infants (Bryant et al. 1974). There is some evidence that at a later age older children tend to monopolize the conversation with their parents and that younger children are excluded (Bosshard 1945).

Only a few authors have studied the question of whether stronger verbal stimulations of and higher verbal skills in firstborns persist after infancy. In 32 mother-child pairs the complexity of the mother's speech to her preschool child was rated during a play session. It was found to be dependent on the child's age but independent of his/her birth order (Fraser et al. 1975). Similarly, linguistic skills in 96 elementary school children who had to explain pictures to another child were correlated with age and verbal IQ but not with birth order (Dickson 1974). Winett et al. (1978) gave two linguistic tests to 123 3- to 5-year-olds. Unexpectedly, the youngest children scored highest.

There is at present no evidence that after infancy a linguistic advantage of firstborns persists. It is surprising that this widely accepted hypothesis has not been more thoroughly examined.

4.6 Conclusions

There is no evidence that the well-known negative correlation of IQ with *sibship size* is due more to a less stimulating environment and diluted adult contacts in children with many sibs than to biological and cultural differences between parents of large and small families. When social background is controlled, IQ differences by sibship size become negligible.

There is no evidence that the relationship of *narrow birth intervals* with lower IQ is caused by understimulation rather than parental characteristics.

In extremely *large and representative samples* IQ differences by birth order approach zero when background variables are appropriately controlled.

The study of *smaller samples* leads to the conclusion that an advantage of firstborns in IQ tends to disappear with increasing control of background variables and more sophisticated statistical methods.

The comparison of *sibs within the same sibship* excludes interfamilial differences and is of paramount importance for assessing whether birth order differences in IQ between unrelated sibs are within- or between-family differences. Among sibs within the same sibships birth order differences near zero. Where they appear, they amount to 1 or 2 IQ points and are either sample-specific or due to disregarding the fact that when sampling younger sibs, those of large, narrowly spaced sibships are more likely to be included.

There is as yet no evidence that a linguistic advantage or firstborns due to increased stimulation persists after infancy.

Chapter 5 Birth Order and School Achievement

5.1 Introductory Remarks

In most studies, school achievement is measured by one or another of the following variables:

1. School grades
2. Standardized achievement tests
3. Educational attainment

These measures have been extensively discussed by Jencks (1972).

1. School grades are of low reliability and validity and are influenced by many factors other than mastery of the subject they relate to. As achievement tests and educational attainments both correlate with social class, school grades, by correlating with both and influencing attainments, may also be expected to vary with social class. Sex influences school grades in that female students are reported to achieve higher grades than male students.

2. Standardized achievement tests are highly reliable and valid (Jencks 1972, p. 55; Süllwold 1971, p. 356; Kline 1976; Buros 1972). If items specific to certain curricula rather than to others are not included, these scores correlate stronly with IQ. Achievement tests vary with social class in the same way as IQ (Jencks 1972, p. 78).

3. Educational attainment means level of school attended or examination passed. It implies a higher degree of adaptation to an existing school system than achievement tests, and correlates strongly with social class and extraintellectual personality variables. Jencks (1972, p. 138) gives a correlation of 0.55 of children's educational attainment with father's income and occupation. Educational attainment varies by sex. The expectations for men and women may vary by different classes and different cohorts. For example, up to 1950 American women had an educational advantage over men, but since then sex differences in education have been reversed (Lloyd et al. 1976, p. 101). Since World War II an educational upgrading has taken place in many countries, putting educational attainment within the reach of social classes formerly excluded. Children of younger parents will have profited most from this change. Educational attainment predicts occupational status in adult life better than school grades or achievement tests do (Jencks 1972, p. 202). For this reason we consider it the most important measure of school-related achievement. Evidence for birth order differences in educational attainment will lead to the expectation of birth order differences in social status as well.

5.2 Sibship Size and School Achievement

5.2.1 School Grades

Kunz et al. (1973) studied a very large random sample of high school students from 27 USA schools, correlating self-reported school grades to sibship size. A significant association was not found. The same was true for grade point average (taken from university records) in over 1,000 Mormon students. In 1977 Kunz et al. published data on self-reported grade point averages of a large sample of high school adolescents from 46 high school representing all major regions of the USA. Sibship size contributed 0.002% to the explained variance in grades, while social class contributed 6%.

Nuttal et al. (1976) controlled IQ in high school students of middle class families in a Boston suburb. Sibship size accounted for 2% of the explained variance in school grades of males.

In a random sample of Indian high school students of one district, school grades decreased with sibship size only in sibships of six and more (Chopra 1966). Similarly, in a sample of Hong Kong high school students mean academic performance was highest in sibship sizes three to six, and sibship contributed slightly less than 2% to the explained variance (Ho 1979) (see pp. 33, 42).

5.2.2 Standardized Achievement Tests

There are four studies on nationally representative samples and one on the whole 11-year-old population of the Isle of Wight. In the latter Rutter et al. (1970, p. 71) traced reading retardation with a group test and confirmed the diagnosis with an individual test. Within social class and by comparison with a control group, reading retardation was found more frequently in children from large sibships.

In their national British sample tested at 15 years of age, Douglas et al. (1968) found that in middle-class girls scores on an arithmetic test decreased with increasing number of sibs.

The following studies allow the influence of sibship size to be weighted. Davie et al. (1972) followed up the sample of the British National Child Development Study at 7 years (see Butler et al. 1966, p. 15f.). When sex, five social classes, mother's age at birth, and birth weight were controlled, the number of older sibs contributed 6.5% and the number of younger sibs 1.5% to the explained variance in a reading test (having more sibs being correlated to lower scores), while the scores on an arithmetic test were independent of sibship size. In the nationally representative USA sample of elementary school children investigated by Svanum et al. (1980) (see p. 32, 38). 2% of the explained variance was attributed to sibship size. In the Zajonc et al. (1980) study of the Scholastic Aptitude Test (SAT) scores of a nationally representative sample of USA high school absolvents, the contribution of sibship size to the explained variance was negligible (see p. 40).

5.2.3 Educational Attainment

Here a very large West German sample is instructive. Jürgens (1967) investigated some 500,000 senior high school and first-year university students; the entire population of this description in a West German province. In the highest and lowest classes, educational attainment was independent of sibship size. In the upper-middle, middle, and lower classes, however, it correlated negatively with sibship size. In large towns the influence of sibship size was almost insignificant, while in small towns and in the country it was consistent but small.

Two British studies are particularly valuable in that they study the association of sibship size with educational attainment while controlling for IQ. Floud et al. (1956) investigated entrance into grammar school in two English countries. Within four social classes the rate of 11-year-olds entering grammar school tended to drop with increasing sibship size when IQ was controlled.

Douglas (1964) obtained the same result with the 11-year-olds of his national British study (see p. 31) when controlling social class at two levels. Following up these children when they were 15 years of age, he found that, at the same level of intelligence, staying on at school and obtaining a final certificate was less frequent in sibships of four than in smaller ones (Douglas et al. 1968).

Adams et al. (1968) studied educational attainment in a random sample of the white adult population living in one town of North Carolina and consisting of sibs. Sex and two levels of social class wer controlled, but there was still a sizeable negative effect of sibship size on college attendance.

Belmont et al. (1976), in their Dutch inductees sample (see p. 39), studied school failure rather than educational attainment in 200,000 subjects (omitting farmers' sons). Within the manual and the nonmanual social class both the frequency of having attended a special school and of having failed elementary school increased with family size. The risk of failing was four times higher for manual than for nonmanual subjects. The Blau et al. (1967) nationally representative sample of USA male civilians is extensively described on p. 59f. in connection with birth order. With control of the father's occupation, sibship size and birth order together explained 2.77% of the subjects' educational attainment.

5.2.4 Conclusions (Table 7)

It is evident that sibship size is negatively correlated to school achievement. But when large and representative samples are studied, the influence of sibship size on school grades and test scores is found to be exremely restricted – just as in the case of IQ. That educational attainment, on the other hand, ist curtailed by the presence of many sibs is demonstrated even in those studies which involve a large sample of sibs or control for a measure of ability as well as for social class. Unfortunately the size of the impact of sibship size on educational attainment has been estimated in only one study, and it could be little larger than in the case of school grades and test scores.

Table 7. Sibship size, and school achievment: School grades (A), standardized achievement tests (B), and educational attainment (C)

	Author	Country	*N*	Age	Negative correlation
A	Kunz et al. (1973)	USA	1,153	High school	–
		USA	1,226	University	–
	Kunz et al. (1977)	USA	6,642	High school	Explained variance 0.002%
	Nuttall et al. (1976)	USA	210	High school	Explained variance 2% (males only)
	Chopra (1966)	India	1,359	High school	–
	Ho (1979)	Hong Kong	1,695	High school	Explained variance 2%
B	Rutter et al. (1970)	England	227	11 years	+
	Douglas et al. (1968)	England and Wales	3,626	15 years	+ (Females)
	Davie et al. (1972)	England	6,057	7 years	Explained variance variance 6,5%, 1,5% (reading test)
	Svanum et al. (1980)	USA	7,060	Elementary school	Explained variance 2%
	Zajonk et al. (1980)	USA	7,192	High school	Regression coefficients −0.03; −0.04
C	Jürgens (1967)	West German province	500,000	Senior high school, 1st year university	Limited to small towns and country
	Floud et al. (1956)	England	2,494	Grammar school entrants	+
	Douglas (1964)	England and Wales	4,195	11 years	+
	Douglas et al. (1968)	England and Wales	3,626	15 years	+
	Adams et al. (1968)	USA	1,442	Adults	+
	Belmont et al. (1976)	Netherlands	201,801	19 years	Positive correlation with school failure
	Blau et al. (1967)	USA	20,700	Adults	+ Explained variance 2,7% (together with birth order)

5.3 Birth Order and School Achievement

5.3.1 Birth Order as Independent Variable

5.3.1.1 School Grades

Large and Representative Samples (see Table 10 A, p. 60). In the Kunz et al. (1977) nationally representative sample of USA high school students (see p. 51), grade point average tended to decrease with increasing birth order at each sibship size, as was the case with IQ in the previously discussed large Dutch sample (Belmont et al. 1973; see p. 39). Using multiple regression analysis, Kunz et al. found birth order to add 0.003% to the explained variance. Similarly, in a large population of Hong Kong Chinese high school students (Ho 1979) birth order was not significantly associated with mean academic performance or with grades in several academic subjects, though the author reports that the traditional importance of primogeniture is still alive among Hong Kong Chinese (see p. 51).

Among a large populaton of firstgraders, school grades were not correlated to birth order when sex, race, social class, and sibship size were controlled (Miller et al. 1976). In all junior high school students from two American towns previous birth order differences in grade point average disappeared when sibship size was held constant (Farley 1978 b). The same negative result was found by Johnson (1973 b) in all students of three Midwestern high schools, and by Macbeth (1975) in two populations of undergraduates. Datta (1967, 1968) studied male high school seniors representing th top 20% of those participating in a science talent search. Within this group qualifications for scientific work were independent of birth order.

The results of *smaller samples* are presented in Table 8.

Table 8. Birth order and school grades in smaller samples

Author	*N*	Age	Social class controlles	Sibship controlled	Highest grades
Cicirelli (1977)	90	Sixth grade	+	+	–
Adams et al. (1972)	370	Elementary school	+	–	Firstborns
Oberlander et al. (1967)	313	High school	+	–	Firstborns
	357	High school	+	–	Firstborns
Eisenman et al. (1968)	131	College	–	–	–
McClure (1969)	173	College	–	–	–
McClure (1971)	372	College	+	–	–
Krumboltz et al. (1958)	426	College	–	–	–
McGlynn (1969)	306	University	–	–	–
Blustein (1967)	350	Fourth to sixth grade (one sib)	–	+	Firstborns
Edwards et al. (1979)	326	Freshmen (one sib)	–	+	–

Though most of these smaller investigations are methodologically unsophisticated, the majority find no birth order differences in school grades, which could be due to the low reliability and validity of this measure.

5.3.1.2 Standardized Achievement Tests

Nationwide Samples (s. Table 10 B). From the British National Child Development Study (Douglas et al. 1968) males and females in same-sex sibships of two and three were selected (see p. 31). At 8, 11, and 15 years the older boy was consistently superior on a reading test in both sibship sizes (the mean difference from the second boy corresponding to 4.9 IQ points). The girl's tests did not vary significantly with birth order. Social class was not controlled. In their Health Examination Survey Sample of 7,000 children at elementary school age (see p. 32), Svanum et al. (1980) found that in an achievement test birth order did not contribute to the explained variance. Social class was the main predictor.

In 1962 and 1965 participants in the National Merit Scholarship Examination were studied by Breland (1972, 1974). These are 17-year-old high school students who take a nationwide test that may entitle them to a college scholarship and that covers five school subjects. In 1962 a random selection of participants (670 subjects) and all participants scoring 2 SD or more above the mean (1,147 subjects) were sent a questionnaire. In 1965 all participants answered a questionnaire before the examination (almost 800,000). In all three samples, the unweighted mean examination score was listed by birth order and sibship size. The same stepwise decrease in scores was found as in the Belmont et al. (1973) Dutch sample (see p. 39); scores decreased with sibship size and, within sibship size, with birth order (Fig. 2). Higher achievement in earlierborns remained significant when social class (based on education of parents) and age of mother were controlled.

A step-down analysis, demonstrated that all birth order differences were reducible to differences in *one test score:* word usage. Zajonc et al. (1980) calculated the regression coefficient for birth order, which corresponds to 1.5 IQ points.

In relation to the Breland (1972, 1974) study, the McCall (1973) investigation is of interest since the subjects were high school students of about the same age as those in Breland's investigation. The author analyzed a 1% subsample of the national Project Talent sample of 400,000 9th to 12th graders. In the subsample, elimination due to missing information left over 3,308 male and female subjects. Seven achievement tests were given, including tests on vocabulary, English, and arithmetic, which are similar to the topics of the National Merit Scholarship examination. Social class was determined by a socioeconomic index. Partial correlations and multiple regression were used. Test scores were negatively correlated with birth order, with highest correlations for verbal and lowest for nonverbal tests. When sibship size and socioeconomic index were controlled, birth order accounted for 2% of the variance in English and vocabulary and for less than 1% in arithmetic and the other four nonverbal tests. When IQ was controlled as well, birth order accounted for less than 1% in any of the tests.

The Zajonc et al. (1980) study on nationally representative SAT results has been reported on p. 40. There the regression coefficient of birth order corresponds to 0.5–1 IQ point. The study by Davis et al. (1977) on four annual sets of Israeli eighth graders (1966–1970, almost 700,000 subjects) deserves special attention. This population was subdivided according to sibship size and the father's origin from a Western or an Oriental country. There was no control of social class, but Israeli immigrants from Oriental countries are known to have a lower mean social level than European immigrants. Achievement scores in the European group were found to drop quite regularly with sibship size and at each size with increasing birth order.

The picture in children of Oriental origin was somewhat different. In sibships of two and three, scores fell with increasing birth order. Second-, third-, and last-borns in sibships of four were almost level, but in larger sibships scores increased with birth order. The authors discussed the ability of Zajonc's „confluence model" to explain this reversal (see p. 39f.). As large Oriental families are not likely to have large birth intervals, which is the condition mentioned by Zajonc for scores to increase with birth order, the authors offered another explanation: In large Oriental families older sibs help younger sibs with their schoolwork and in this way compensate for the latter's educational disadvantages. This is a „being taught hypothesis" in opposition to Zajonc's „teaching hypothesis." (The latter is refuted by the fact that in sibships of four or more children the youngest child has a higher score than the next-to-last child.) It is, however, not evident why older children, even though teaching, should remain less efficient than those they teach. An explanation by cohort differences between parents seems more appropriate in an Oriental immigrant population. Parents of laterborns in large sibships are considerably older than parents of earlierborns. They belong to a cohort that has lived in an environment where birth control was unknown, that perhaps needed a large number of children to subsist, and in which the number of children may even have been positively correlated to IQ.

In this study, the largest difference in scores between subjects of different birth order corresponds to 3 IQ points. However, apart from ethnicity, no other sociological variables were taken account of. Thus the negligible birth order differences in investigations that control background more stringently are indirected confirmed.

Entire Populations of Smaller Units. In the entire junior high school population of one American state, Wark et al. (1974) found firstborns to achieve better results on a scholastic aptitude test, not controlling for sibship size or social class. In the high school population of two small American towns previous firstborn advantages in achievement disappeared with control of sibship size (Farley 1978b). Investigating the entire population of third to sixth graders of a Southern town by means of regression analysis. Touliator et al. (1978) found that ordinal position explained 1.5% of the variance in each of three achievement tests of language, reading, and mathematics.

Smaller Studies. In view of the negative evidence in the previously described large and representative samples, less representative or less sophisticatedly treated samples are merely presented in Table 9.

Table 9. The birth order-achievement test relationship in less representative samples with no control of sibship, size and/or social class (A) or with sibship size and social class controlled (B)

	Author	Country	*N*	Age	Highest achievement scores
A	Adams et al. (1972)	USA	370	Elementary school	Firstborns
	Start et al. (1974)	Canada	157	Elementary school	–
	Zielinsky (1966)	West Germany	800	Fourth grade	–
	Blustein (1967)	USA	350	Fourth–sixth grades	Firstborns
	Eysenck et al. (1969)	England	4,000	11 years	Earlierborns
	Marjoribanks (1978)	Australia	500	11 years	Earlierborns
	Lunneberg (1968)	USA	5,401	High school	Firstborns (males only)
	Lunneberg (1971)	USA	896	High school	Firstborns (males only)
	Oberlander et al. (1967)	USA	302	High school	Firstborns
			357	High school	Firstborns
	Oberlander et al. (1970)	USA	962	High school	Firstborns (interaction with tests)
	Krumboltz et al. (1958)	USA	426	College	–
	Altus (1963)	USA	1,120	College entrants	Firstborns
	Altus (1965 c)	USA	1,432	College entrants	Firstborns (females only)
	Walker et al. (1967)	USA	142	College entrants	Firstborns (females only)
	Lemay (1970)	USA	Annual set	Female freshmen	Firstborns
	Biegelsen (1976)	USA	1,883	Freshmen	–
B	Doren (1972)	USA	1,442	First grade	First- and lastborns (interaction sibship size)
	Gustin (1972)	USA	344	Second grade	–
	Levinson (1963)	USA	816	Third grade	First- and laterborns (interaction level of IQ, sibship size)
	Solomon et al. (1972)	USA	149	Fifth grade	Firstborns (interaction sibship size)
	Cicirelli (1967)	USA	614	Sixth grade	First- and secondborns (interaction sibship size, sex)
	De Avila (1969)	USA	165	Sixth grade	–
	Hall (1963)	USA	104	College	Firstborns
	Rosenberg et al. (1964)	USA	377	College entrants	Firstborns (males only)
	Rosenberg et al. (1969 a)	USA	1,013	College entrants	–

An unequivocal superiority of firstborns was found in eight of 17 samples where there was insufficient control of background variables, but in only one of nine samples with control of social class and sibship size. Results are similar to those found in smaller studies of IQ (see p. 44).

5.3.1.3 Educational Attainment

Nationwide Samples (s. Table 10c). In the Douglas (1964) national British sample, entrance into grammar school was compared by birth order – two social classes, sibship size, and a mixed ability-achievement score being held constant. In both classes male firstborns with one or two brothers entered grammar school more frequently than male laterborns. The birth order difference was strongest in the middle range of scores. A cohort hypothesis can be upheld, since firstborns on average may have been children of younger parents in urban or suburban surroundings who make more use of new schooling opportunities. In comparison with firstborns, only children with comparable scores were disadvantaged in obtaining grammar school places. The author concluded that younger sibs have a stimulating influence. As homes broken for reasons other than illegitimacy were not excluded, the question of whether some of the only children were hindered in their school careers by emotional drawbacks remained open.

At 15 years of age, the oldest of two boys had obtained more and better certificates and stayed longer in school than either the younger boy or the only boy (Douglas et al. 1968). This time there was no control for social class (see p. 37 for IQ).

Bayer (1966) analyzed college attendance in 80,000 former high school students who had participated in Project Talent. The sample was the same as Burton's (1968) (see p. 38). One year after leaving high school, 45,855 subjects returned a questionnaire. Four social classes were carefully defined on the basis of nine variables, and male and female subjects were investigated separately. Unfortunately the author did not differentiate for sibship size within social class, so the result was the expected one: First- and lastborns had equal chances of going to college within each social class. The chances of middle children (being biased for large sibships) were considerably lower. In all social classes only children were most advantaged for going to college. Hermalin (1967) objected to inappropriate weighting in this study, and Bayer (1967b) in his answer admitted that the study of *sibs* was decisive. Schooler (1972a) quotes the USA National Occupation Study in which 3,101 men were interviewed. According to the author, college-goers were equally represented in all birth orders when sibship size and father's education were controlled.

Jencks (1972, p. 348) compared 6,379 firstborn and secondborn men for educational attainment. They had been part of the nationally representative Project Talent sample in the 11th grade, and were followed up after 6 years (see p. 43). Education at 22 years, expressed in number of years of schooling, was slightly higher in firstborns. The reasons for a secondborn bias to larger sibships have been discussed (see p. 46), and so at least a part of this difference would probably have disappeared if sibship size had been controlled.

Belmont et al. (1976) studied a subsample of their Dutch inductee population for attendance at a special school and having failed elementary school. When both forms of school failure were tabulated together for firstborns, middleborns, and lastborns within each sibship size, the manual class showed a linear rise of failure rates with birth rank, i.e., from firstborns to middle children to youngest children. In the nonmanual class, however, firstborns and middleborns had the same failure rates, but the lastborns' failure rate was significantly higher. The authors concluded that the relationship between school performance and birth order within sibship size reflected the distribution of measured intelligence which they had formerly established (see p. 39).

Blau et al. (1967) studied educational attainment in a sample of 20,000 men representing all civilian, noninstitutionalized males in the USA in 1962 (Fig. 3). Education was measured on an 8-point scale (mean 4.43). For sibship size the sample was divided into two categories: smaller sibships with one to four sibs and large sibships with five and more sibs. Father's occupation was held constant. The followed deviations from the sample mean were found:

Smaller sibships:	Only son	+0.55
	Oldest son	+0.47
	Youngest son	+0.39
	Middle son, no older brother	+0.22
	Middle son with older brother	+0.16
Larger sibships:	Youngest son	−0.01
	Oldest son	−0.33
	Middle son, no older brother	−0.46
	Middle son with older brother	−0.41

It is evident from Blau et al.'s findings that sibship size contributes far more than birth order to differences in educational attainment. Middle sons were at a disadvantage in both sibship size groups because of their well-known bias toward larger sibships. In large sibships, last sons had an advantage over oldest sons: In this context the authors mentioned demographic changes leading to a reduction of

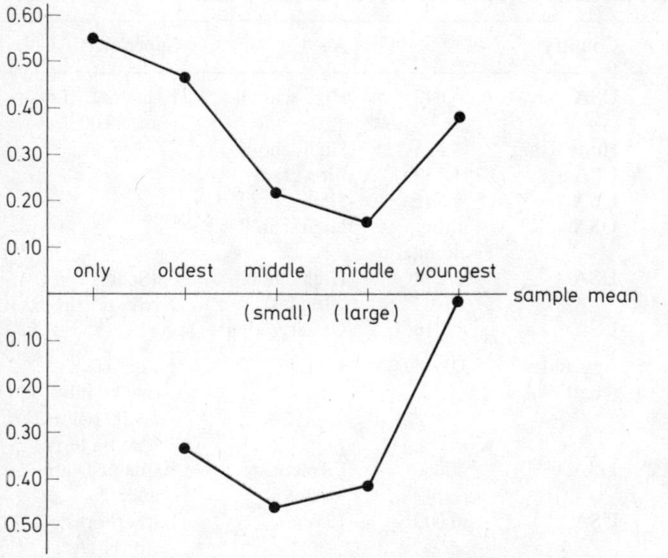

Fig. 3. Educational attainment in an American sample (Blau et al. 1967)

sibship size over time. The youngest in large sibships will probably be older, on average, than the oldest in large sibships and descend from less atypical families (see p. 56). In smaller sibships oldest sons have an educational edvantage over last sons; the former may be younger, (because smaller families get more frequent over time) and have fewer sibs on average. Unfortunately no indices for age differences in the different birth order categories were given and including sibships of up to four in the „small sibships" may have obscured differences.

Within smaller sibships, middleborns were advantaged when there was no older brother, i.e., when there were fewer sibs (the probability of having an older brother increases with sibship size). Within sibships of five and more, middle sons belonging to larger sibships were advantaged. One is reminded of the studies where, in large sibships, a reversal of the usual stepwise decrease of IQ or achievement scores becomes apparent (see pp. 56, 37, 38).

Education and occupation of the father explained 27.94% of the variance in the son's education; sibship size and birth order together explained 2.77%. It is evident that most of this variance was due to sibship size, so that birth order influences per se must be minimal (see p. 52).

Smaller Studies. Among 306 university students (McGlynn 1969), firstborns did not pass examinations in greater numbers than laterborns, and among 347 18- to 60-year-old participants in a course for ameliorating occupational skills who were all of lower class and large families, dropping out of the course was not correlated to birth order (Forbes 1974).

5.3.1.4 **Conclusions** (Table 10)

Table 10. Birth order and school achievement in samples consisting of or representative of entire populations: School grades (A), achievement test scores (B), educational attainement (C)

	Author	Country	*N*	Age	Superiority
A	Kunz et al. (1977)	USA	6,642	High school	Explained variance 0.003%
	Ho (1979)	Hong Kong	1,695	High school	–
	Miller et al. (1976)	USA	1,750	First grade	–
	Farley (1978 b)	USA	1,186	High school	–
	Johnson (1973 b)	USA	Eintire population	High school	–
	Datta (1967)	USA	578	High school (males)	– (Scores research project)
	Macbeth (1975)	USA	716	Undergraduates	–
B	Douglas (1964), Douglas et al. (1968)	England and Wales	3,000–4,000	8, 11, 15	Firstborns (males only, 4.9 IQ points, reading test)
	Svanum et al. (1980)	USA	7,060	Elementary school	Explained variance 0%
	Breland (1972, 1974)	USA	800,000	15 years	Earlierborns, word usage, 1.5 IQ points

Table 10. (continued)

	Author	Country	N	Age	Superiority
	McCall (1973)	USA	3,308	9th–12th grades	Explained variance 1% (control IQ)
	Zajonc et al. (1980)	USA	5,000	18 years	Regression coefficient amounting to 0.5–1 IQ point
	Davis et al. (1977)	Israel	191,933	Eight grade	Mathematics: largest difference equivalent to 3 IQ points
	Population of one state or town				
	No control of sibship size or social class				
	Wark et al. (1974)	USA	25,000	Junior high school	Firstborns
	Control of sibship size				
	Farley (1978 b)	USA	1,126	Junior high school	–
	Control of sibship size and social class				
	Touliator et al. (1978)	USA	637	Third to sixth grades	Explained variances 1.5%
C	Douglas (1964), Douglas et al. (1968)	England and Wales	3,000–4,000	11, 15	Firstborns
	Bayer (1966)	USA	45,855	18–19 years	Firstborns and lastborns
	Jencks (1972)	USA	6,379	22 years	–
	Belmont et al. (1976)	Netherlands	201,801	19 years	Earlierborns; first- and middleborns (interaction social class)
	Blau et al. (1967)	USA	20,700	Adults	Firstborns and lastborns. Explained variance minimal
	Schooler (1972 a)	USA	3,101	Adults	–

Birth order does not have a larger impact on school achievement than on IQ. This is true for school grades and achievement tests and for educational attainment as well. Whenever the statistical treatment of data reports the amount of explained variance contributed by birth order, it is extremely small.

5.3.1.5 The Comparison of School Achievement Between Sibs in the Same Family

School Grades

In his high school sample of 129 pairs of first- and secondborns in two social classes and of sibship sizes two to eight (see p. 47 for IQ), Bartelt (1973) found no difference in school grades. Chittenden et al. (1968) compared school grades of first- and secondborn sibs in the fourth and fifth grades (62 pairs) and in the seventh and eighth grades (67 pairs) in two school systems. Sibs were always compared for grades in the same year and there was a correction for age. Firstborns had better grades in 63% of the pairs in the younger group and in 69% of the pairs in the older group (50% chance). Firstborn superiority was particularly frequent when the first sib was female and in sibs close in age. Unfortunately, data on the *size* of birth order differences were not given.

Standardized Achievement Tests

Schoonover (1959, see p. 47) compared all sib pairs found over 22 years in one elementary school who had at least four achievement scores. Numbers of sib pairs per subject varied from 38 to 64. In none of seven tests was there a difference between older and younger sibs in terms of deviation from age norms. Sibs with a brother scored significantly higher than those with a sister. In the Chittenden (1968) sample mentioned for school grades in the last paragraph, however, firstborns scored higher on an achievement test in 58% of the younger and in 64% of the older group. Again, data on the *size* of differences are missing.

Dolph (1966) compared first and second sibs in 36 sibships of three. The sample was taken from all ninth graders in a school system and sibs were compared at the same school year. There was no significant difference in achievement scores between first- and secondborns, though there was a trend toward lower scores in secondborns, which was due to younger girls with an older sister.

Wolf (1967) compared sibs in 83 sibships of three, who were attending public schools in one American town, on an achievement test. Within sex, first- and secondborn children were not different, while third girls scored higher than second sibs of either sex.

Kinard (1975) analyzed 170 pairs of first- and secondborn sibs from lower-class backgrounds. There was no difference between sibs on a verbal and nonverbal achievement test.

Educational Attainment

Smelser et al. (1968) followed up the sample of the Berkeley Guidance Study on Child Development when the subjects were in their early thirties. The 155 subjects and 122 spouses were interviewed about their own and all their sibs' educational attainments. The 277 sibships comprised 616 subjects, all white and predominantly middle class. Sibships of five and more were rare and not included in the study. The dependent variable was years of schooling. In sibships of two and three, male and female firstborns graduated more often from college and went more often to graduate schools than lastborns. However, differences between sibs were not significant, though all tending toward the same direction.

A further analysis of sibships of two showed that the difference between older and younger sibs was due to sibs of different sex. While same-sex sibling had equal educational attainment, the older sib, independent of sex, had more schooling than the younger sib in mixed sibships. The data are based on 45 pairs of the same sex and 61 of different sex. The difference is again not significant.

Adams (1969) and Adams et al. (1968) investigated a random sample of white once-married subjects who had finished their education and lived in one American town. The 779 respondents answered a questionnaire for themselves and for the sib next to them in age. Data were thus analyzed for 1,442 persons and the dependent variable was any college attendance. When the sample was analyzed without control for social class, firstborns were found to have attended college more frequently than laterborns. When, however, social class on two levels, sex, and sibship size were controlled, there was no difference for college attendance by birth order.

The particular merit of this study is the stress on sociological variables. Large sibship size was found to be prohibitive for college attendance, but more so in blue-collar than in white-collar sibships. When the sample was analyzed for parental age, children of older parents were more often in blue-collar occupations than children of younger parents – a consequence of educational upgrading since 1920, and a hint at the importance of cohort differences. There is also some evidence for the importance of considering sex in assessing educational attainment: In blue-collar sibships college attendance of females decreased with rising numbers of brothers. In 178 sibships of two, same-sex sibs were not different in educational attainment, but first- and secondborn males had higher attainment when their sib was female. This finding is, incidentally, opposed to that of Smelser et al. (1968).

Inbar et al. (1976) analyzed a sample of Israeli immigrants. The subjects reported on 238 of their children at college age. First- and laterborns did not differ for college attendance. Olneck et al. (1979) studied years of schooling in 346 pairs of brothers who had frequented the Kalamazoo public schools. Educational attainment was independent of birth order when sibship size and age at follow-up were controlled.

Conclusions (Table 11)

Table 11. Birth order and school achievement in sibs in the same family: School grades (A), achievement tests (B), Educational Attainment (C)

	Author	Country	Number	Age	Superiority
A	Bartelt (1973)	USA	129 pairs	High school	–
	Chittenden et al. (1968)	USA	129 pairs	Elementary and high school	Firstborns
B	Schoonover (1959)	USA	38–64 pairs	Elementary school	–
	Chittenden et al. (1968)	USA	129 pairs	Elementary and high school	Firstborns
	Dolph (1966)	USA	36 sibships	Ninth grade	–
	Wolf (1967)	USA	83 sibships	Public school	Third girl
C	Inbar (1976)	Israel	238 subjects	College	–
	Smelser et al. (1968)	USA	616 subjects	Adults	Firstborns(NS)
	Adams (1969)	USA	1,442 subjects	Adults	–
	Adams et al. (1968)	USA			
	Olneck et al. (1979)	USA	346 pairs	Adults	–

One study in ten found a significant firstborn advantage in grades and achievement tests and another a nonsignificant advantage in attainment. Sib studies confirm the results of the large methodologically sound studies of nonsibs: *Birth order effects on school achievement are negligible*.

5.3.2 Birth Order as Dependent Variable

5.3.2.1 Standardized Achievement Tests

In a very influential study Nichols (1964, 1968) selected from male college seniors, representing the whole graduating population of 1961 in USA, 3,397 average students. This group was compared with 1,184 National Merit Scholarship semifinalists, representing the upper 4.5% of all high school students. In the semifinalist group there was a significantly higher proportion of firstborns. From this group a subsample of 334 students was matched to the average group for sex, father's occupation and income, parents' education, and size of hometown, so that for these variables the mean was within 2% of the mean of the average group. The overrepresentation of firstborns among the semifinalists was found again. Schooler (1972 a) has very pertinently criticized the missing subdivision for family size. According to him the semifinalists were born around 1947, while graduating college students are 8–10 years older. Semifinalists will have, on average, younger parents with smaller families. The overrepresentation of firstborns among the semifinalists could be a consequence of the control group not being adequately chosen.

5.3.2.2 Educational Attainment

Most of the following studies stressed the overrepresentation of firstborns for a given level of attainment. They did not compare subjects with a control group, but with the normal distribution of birth order within sibship. The necessity of a control group matched for social class, sibship size, and parental cohort was demonstrated by Sutton-Smith et al. (1970). In an elementary school situated in a new neighborhood with many young families, he found 50% firstborns in sibships of three. This is, incidentally, the same proportion as in Nichol's semifinalists mentioned in the last paragraph.

Breland (1974) also listed seven samples not distinguished by particular achievement. In five of them there were more firstborns in sibships of two and in four of them in sibships of three than could have been expected in chance distributions.

Studies Without Control Groups

As is to be expected, among populations born in the years after World War II and taking part in higher education, firstborn rates amounting to 50%–60% were found. This was the case in the famous Altus (1965 b; 1966 a, b) studies of university entrants, in the Alexander (1966, 1968) study of male college attenders, and in the Sharan et al. (1969) study of entrants into an Israeli officers' training school. Diab et al. (1968) obtained opposing data from the University of Beirut (Lebanon), where the firstborn rate among freshmen was slightly more than 25%, and explained the difference by the demographic data of a developing country. Jones et al. (1974) demonstrated that rates of firstborns varied with social class among London college entrants.

Three studies investigated birth order in populations with learning difficulties, i.e., in children from outpatient clinics and special schools. An overrepresentation of lower-class children and, therefore, of laterborns in large sibships is to be expected where there is a reduction of fertility, and equidistribution where this is not the case. Overrepresentation of laterborns was accordingly found by Greer et al. (1971) and Harris (1961) and equidistribution of birth order by Vockell et al. (1972) and Hodges et al. (1961).

In Kenya 331 eighth and ninth graders (a highly selected group for educational attainment) were investigated by Munroe et al. (1971). In sibships of three to ten, firstborns were overrepresented, but this was not so in sibships of 11 and more. No subject had less than two sibs. Possible social and demographic reasons were not considered, though equidistribution by birth order was mentioned in a very small sample of students attending a school of lower standing.

Studies Using a Control Group

Control Group Not Fitted to the Sample (see p. 12). Schachter (1963) collected studies on college populations with a proportion of firstborns of 50%–60%. His control group was the population of Minnesota born in the same year as the students, and the entire population of the USA. In both control samples, proportion of firstborns was 32%–37%. Both control samples deviate from the subjects at least in social class and probably in other variables also. Coker et al. (1959) compared students in eight randomly selected medical schools with the USA population born in the same year and found that of the students, 50% were firstborns, but of the general population only 33%. Bayer (1966), in the sample already mentioned (see p. 58) for college attendance, found that 48% of 88,000 12th graders in high school were firstborns. In the subsample attending college 1 year later this percentage increased to 55%. The same author (1967) elicited information from all USA students who had attained a doctorate in 1962, and 8,124 subjects gave sufficient information on birth order, sibship size, and paternal education as indicator of social class. Of this sample, 50% were firstborns, while in the USA population born in the same years as the graduates there were 23% firstborns. The author rightly rejected this control group as not corresponding to the sample in social class and sibship size. When the sample was analyzed for sibship size, firstborns were overrepresented in sibship sizes two to four. In larger sibships firstborns as well as lastborns were overrepresented in comparison with a chance distribution. When the sample was divided into those subjects whose father had more and whose father had less than 8 years of education, there was an overrepresentation of firstborns in the former and an overrepresentation of youngest children in the latter group.

This is exactly what would be expected on the basis of differential demographic change by social class and differential occupational upgrading by age of parents. The result confirms the Blau et al. (1967) study, (see p. 59) which found highest educational attainment in firstborns in smaller, and lastborns in larger sibships.

Bradley et al. (1969) compared the birth order of 1,505 high school students (corresponding to the most successful 1% over 10 years) with the USA population born in the same years. In the high school sample firstborns were overrepresented in 9 years out of 10.

Shaver et al. (1970) compared the birth order of 50% of Gothenburg's medical students (those returning a questionnaire) with the birth order of the entire Swedish population born in the same years. In the student sample firstborns were highly overrepresented.

Greene et al. (1968) compared birth order data of Mexican university freshmen with census data. In 168 Anglo-American students firstborns were overrepresented in comparison with the general population, while in 180 Spanish-American students they were underrepresented owing to larger sibship sizes in this group.

In 1966 Poole et al. (1973) sent a questionnaire to 10,000 men and women who had graduated in 1960 from a British university and 8,284 subjects answered (born around 1938–1939). A control group was found in the census data of 1951: Completed fertility ascertained for social class in a national sample of married women born between 1903 and 1906. This group is probably 5–10 years older than the graduates' mothers. In the two lowest social classes the graduates were very significantly more often members of sibships of two. In the two highest classes graduates were less often only children and more often members of sibships of two, three, and four than the national sample. The Greenwood-Yule correction for sibship size was not applied when comparing sibship size found by sampling mothers with sibships size found by sampling sibs (see p. 4). Among the graduates there was a strong overrepresentation of firstborns in comparison with the general population born during the same years. In each sibship size and for two social classes (manual and nonmanual), firstborns were overrepresented and youngest underrepresented in comparison with chance expectation. Both comparisons (the one with mothers for sibship size and the one with a chance distribution for birth order) are fallacious.

Control Group Adequately Selected. Lees et al. (1957) compared birth order in different types of secondary schools in an English „small city“ and a „midland borough“. In the whole school population there was an overrepresentation of firstborns, confirming the Hare et al. (1974) findings in an English population sample (see p. 8). As to be expected on the basis of the assumption that different social classes with different sibship sizes are differentially distributed over the school types, the proportion of firstborns in both sexes declined and the proportion of intermediate children increased as one steps down from grammar school (the most exacting school type) to technical school and then to secondary modern school (the least exacting type). In „A-forms“ (classes with highly achieving students), firstborns and only children were overrepresented among boys both in grammar and secondary modern schools, while for girls this was true only in secondary modern schools. The authors concluded that the study provided evidence for the superiority of firstborns, with youngest ranked second and middle children last. As social class and sibship size were not controlled, this conclusion seems unwarranted.

Carlson (1970) compared female psychology graduates with a sample of graduates in various subjects of both sexes. Among female graduates, firstborns were overrepresented. Possible differences in sibship size were not considered (on average, female graduates may be from smaller sibships because of differential selection by sex). On the other hand, female doctoral and master's degree students in psychology had the same proportion of firstborns, though the former is a more highly achieving group.

Epstein et al. (1972) compared a stratified sample of 1,500 students, representing 13,000 American university freshmen of autumn 1965, with two successive samples of freshmen entering a New York university in 1969 and 1970 (2,010 and 892 subjects respectively). As not all students returned the questionnaire, there is some degree of sample selection. In 1965 52% of USA freshmen were first and only children, but in New York 44% (1969) and 42% (1970). The 1970 sample did not deviate from chance proportions when it was subdivided for sibship size and oldest, youngest, and middleborns. The authors consider this to be a consequence of the entrance requirements being less exacting in 1970, thus giving access to entrants from lower social strata and larger sibships than before. In universities avoiding this policy firstborn ratios remained high, as demonstrated by Layman et al. (1978). The authors compared 270 successful New Jersey Medical School applicants with 2,100 unsuccessful candidates. In both groups oldest sibs were strongly overrepresented in comparison with youngest children, and the ratio increased with sibship size. In the accepted group the oldest-youngest ratio was slightly higher than in the rejected group. The difference was due to a particularly strong overrepresentation of oldest sibs among successful female and minority applicants. An inspection of the tables demonstrates that, among successful minority applicants, two-thirds had one or two sibs; among the unsuccessful this figure was only 45%, while one-fourth had five or more sibs.

5.3.2.3 Conclusions

Failure to control for social class, sipship size, denomination, and ethnicity explains the uniform advantage of firstborns when populations with higher education are compared with general populations.

The overrepresentation of firstborns is not found in Hispanic and Oriental high achievers, where large families are common. In an African population, where both family size and marriage frequency are increasing, firstborns of all sibship sizes are overrepresented. Studies of a New York university and a New Jersey medical school demonstrate how the birth order distribution of a high-achieving population is dependent on admittance policies. Entrance into higher education may be easier for lower class and minority students if their background has the qualities where of small sibship size is an indicator.

5.4 Birth Order and Over- and Underachievement

In the following paragraphs IQ, school grades, and achievement tests will be considered in relation to each other and to birth order. Overachievers are students who perform better in school than would be expected by their IQ, and the reverse is true of underachievers.

Myers (1952) constructed an „achievement index," relating the scores of 355 female freshmen on a scholastic aptitude test to their grade point averages during the first year of college. Sibship size did not influence this index, but youngest girls were higher achievers than middleborns, firstborns, or only children. Krumboltz et al. (1958) compared an intelligence score with high school rank in 426 college entrants, and analyzed over- and underachievers (the upper and lower 25%) separately. The groups did not differ by birth order or sibship size. Pierce (1959) chose from 215 high school students those above the 70th percentile on several intelligence tests. Achievement was measured by school grades. High and low achievers were defined as being below or above the median discrepancy between intelligence and achievement. High achievers were found more often to be first- than laterborns, from smaller sibships, and from higher social class. Possible correlations between these variables were not considered.

Kanter (1970) selected from 2,250 sixthgraders within a school system 56 overachievers and 55 underachievers. The IQ of both groups was 90–110. Achievement was measured by a mean achievement test score. The groups were similar for birth order. First graders (97 black and 127 white) in a rural Southern elementary school were compared by the correlation of IQ given in school and a school achievement test (Asbury 1973). Over- and underachievers were defined as deviating more than 1 SD from the correlation between IQ and achievement predicted on the basis of the scores of 50 subjects stratified for race and sex. Over- and underachievement in three verbal tests were not correlated with birth order, but with race and sex. Overachievers in arithmetic, however, were more frequently earlierborns than underachievers. The correlation of overachievement with birth order on this subtest was weak. Sibship size and social class were without influence, which was probably due to the social homogeneity of the sample.

An Indian random male high school sample (Chopra 1966) yielded the result that IQ and scores on the high school examination were independent of sibship size up to six. When IQ was held constant, examination scores decreased with increasing sibship size. An influence of birth order was not found.

Conclusions (Table 12)

Table 12. Birth order and overachievement

Author	*N*	Age	High achievers
Kanter (1970)	111	Sixth grade	–
Asbury (1973)	224	First grade	Earlierborns (arithmetic)
Pierce (1959)	215	10th to 12th grades	Firstborns
Myers (1952)	355	18 years (females)	Youngest
Krumboltz et al. (1958)	426	18 years	–
Chopra (1966)	1,359	High school males	–

There is no consistent evidence of overachievement in firstborns.

5.5 Conclusions

School-related achievement is measured by grades, scores on achievement tests, and educational attainment (level of school attained or examinations passed).

School achievement is negatively correlated with sibship size. When background variables are controlled, *the impact of sibship size is minimal.*

School grades do not seem to be connected with birth order, which may be due to their low reliability and validity. Differences in *achievement tests* by birth order may be largest in verbal tests. Birth order explains a very small part of the variance. The same is true *for educational attainment*. The identical results appear when sibs within the same family are compared.

The many studies demonstrating an overrepresentation of firstborns among persons with high achievement scores or of high educational attainment have not used adequate control groups and are methodologically inadequate.

There is no evidence that firstborn subjects are more often overachievers than subjects in other positions.

Chapter 6 Birth Order and Occupational Status

A large amount of literature published before 1946 claimed that firstborns reach higher social status than laterborns (Galton 1874, 1887; Clarke 1916; Ellis 1926; Cattell 1917; Cattell et al. 1921; Apperly 1939). Most of these studies were based on the birth order of scientists and other eminent men whose names were found in biographic dictionaries or encyclopedias. The result was invariably that firstborns were overrepresented among the outstanding (for surveys, see Chen et al. 1960; Stroup et al. 1965; Sutton-Smith et al. 1970). Fallacies, e.g., different family sizes in different social classes, different occupational expectations for sibs of different sex, and (until some time ago) different rights of succession for first- and laterborn sons (and therefore different financial opportunities) were disregarded. As will be shown, this type of study was still being pursued in the 1970s, though it has always drawn criticism.

If evidence were produced for differences in occupational status for persons of different birth order who have spent their childhood under similar or possibly equal social conditions, this would prove birth order to be an extremely important influence on human lives. Such evidence is not, however, easy to find. In the previous chapter we mentioned the upgrading of schooling after World War II. An upgrading in occupation has also taken place through expansion of the tertiary sector and, in many industrialized countries, through immigration, the immigrants filling positions at the bottom of the occupational scale. Older persons, then, can be expected to have a lower mean social status than the younger generation. This is a cohort difference which has frequently been disregarded in birth order research.

On the other hand, within cohorts occupational status tends to rise with age, some well-paid and highly considered positions being reached only after many years of occupational activity. This is particularly true of middle-class occupations. Consequently subjects of different birth order should be compared for occupational status at the same point in life.

Since birth order research started with studies using birth order as the dependent variable, investigations of this type will be reviewed first. The importance of a control group of the same social class and same cohort has already been discussed.

6.1 Birth Order as Dependent Variable

6.1.1 Studies Without Control Group

In all studies in which middle-class occupations have been investigated, there is an overrepresentation of firstborns in comparison with chance distribution, which may be supposed to be due to class differences in birthrate trends and sibship size (Schooler 1972a). Dubno et al. (1969, 1971) found no significant difference in the proportion of firstborns between two large groups of top- and middle-level managers in 500 USA industrial corporations, but among college-educated top managers firstborns were overrepresented. An overrepresentation of firstborns among samples of jet pilots, lawyers, psychologists, and psychiatrists was found in the studies by Reinhardt (1970), Kardener et al. (1972), and Bruce et al. (1974); this was also the case among students taking up teaching (Angers 1974) and taking examinations in medicine (Cobb et al. 1966). In a sample of Israeli women in high positions, firstborns were overrepresented in small sibships and youngest children in large ones, exactly as would be expected on the basis of demographic change (Padan 1972). Firstborns were also overrepresented in 485 USA women in academic positions (Monson et al. 1976). Stewart (1970) and Wagner et al. (1977) analyzed the birth order of USA presidents, vice presidents, and nominees for both positions. First and third sons were overrepresented (statistical significance not given). A sample of candidates for a USA state senate was equidistributed for birth order, but in the subjects elected to office, first- and lastborns were overrepresented (Forbes 1972). Perry (1965) found 80% firstborns among highly achieving military pilots and Farley et al. (1974) found a greater proportion of firstborns among officers than among enlisted soldiers. Visher (1947, 1948), Roe (1953), and Helson et al. (1970) demonstrated an overabundance of firstborns among eminent scientists and mathematicians; West (1960) found the same for research personnel, whether eminent or not, and Bullough et al. (1971) for famous Scotchmen of the eighteenth century.

Among nurses, second borns in sibships of two and firstborns in sibships of four were overrepresented (Fischer 1962), as were, in another sample, firstborns from sibships of two and four, and, in nursing students, firstborns in families of three and four (Baker 1963). Social class was not given, though nursing might be taken up by girls from lower middle-class families with younger parents in the course of an occupational and educational upgrading. A short study by Skipper et al. (1970) has become quite famous: Investigating 35 stripteasers from all over America, he found 74% firstborns and 14% only children. Evidently, firstborns can also overrepresented in occupations not distinguished by scientific or literary eminence. In this context, it may be mentioned that firstborns were also overrepresented among 205 unwed mothers (Horn et al. 1975).

6.1.2 Studies With Inadequate Control Groups

Very et al. (1969, 1970, 1973) compared the birth order distribution of small samples of lawyers, beauticians, and Carmelite nuns with census data for the birth years of subjects. As expected assuming different social class, different cohorts, and different denomination, among lawyers firstborns were overrepresented, but among beauticians and nuns second- and thirdborns. Stone (1963) compared freshmen in five departments of Kansas University for birth order (1,631 subjects). In each department, first- and early-borns were overrepresented. This was particularly so in students of enigneering architecture. The difference is explained by a particular affinity of firstborns to conformity, possible class and sibship size differences being disregarded. Cleland et al. (1967) compared personnel in an institution

(363 subjects) for tenure and participation in night shifts. Laterborns from large families had longer tenure and participated more in night shifts. This leads to psychological explanations: Differences in age and schooling, which may lead to different occupational mobility and to differential assignment to night shifts, were not controlled – a typical example of the quality of some birth order research. Studies with adequate control groups have not come to our notice.

6.2 Birth Order as Independent Variable

One of the most important studies was conducted by Blau et al. (1967) in 1962; it involved 20,700 USA men representative of all male civilians between 20 and 65 years of age (see pp. 39, 59).

Occupational status was measured on a 96-point scale (mean 36.3 points). Sibships with up to four members were considered „smaller" while those of five or more were regarded as „larger". When paternal occupation was controlled, men from smaller sibships had a positive deviation from the mean and men from larger sibships a negative one. In both sibship categories, middle sons (being biased for larger sibship size) had lower status than oldest and youngest sons. Apart from these sibship size effects, birth order effects were negligible. In large sibships lastborn sons (who, under the hypothesis that sibship size has been declining, were overrepresented among the older sample members) held the highest occupational position (a deviation of +2 from the sample mean). In smaller sibships lastborn sons had a deviation of +3.8 and oldest a deviation of +3.3 points from the sample mean. Probably due to the fact that the authors included sibships of up to four in their category of smaller sibships, the usual advantage of firstborns of younger, middle-class parents did not appear. (The youngest sample members were born in 1942.) When, besides paternal occupation, the education of the subject was held constant, differences in occupational level between sons in smaller and larger sibships became insignificant: Sibship size affected occupation mainly through education. The authors had a tendency to consider the position of oldest and youngest as the most advantageous. They admitted, however, that in their categories of smaller and larger sibships, sibship size was not completely controlled and that middle sons have a bias for larger sibships.

When paternal education and occupation was held constant, sibship size and birth order explained 2.77% of the variance in education. When education was controlled as well, sibship size and birth order explained 0.52% of the variance in first jobs. Jencks (1979) reports that birth order contributes 0.2% to the explained vairance when sibship size is controlled.

6.3 Occupational Status Among Sibs

Olneck et al. (1979) studied the occupational status of 346 pairs of brothers (see p. 47) by regression analysis. With control of age and family size it was independent of birth order. Strudler (1976) interviewed parents of high school students about their own and their siblings occupation. There were sex differences in occupational achievement but none by birth order.

6.4 Sibship Size, Fertility, and Social Mobility

There is some evidence that, within social class, upward social mobility is higher for persons from small sibships. Svalastoga (1959) examined a sample of 3,756 subjects representative of all Danish inhabitants over 21 years of age. In each social class, men from sibships of five and more had less upward and more downward mobility – in comparison to the occupation of their father – than those from smaller sibships. In the whole sample, middleborns (being biased for larger sibships) were less upwardly mobile than only children, first-, and lastborns. When sibship size was held constant, this difference disappeared.

Lipset et al. (1959) reported mobility studies from six Western European countries relating upward mobility in children from low social classes to small sibships.

Blau et al. (1967), in their census sample, studied 6,000 older couples with terminated fertility. Upward *and* downward mobile men had a slightly but consistently reduced fertility.

6.5 Conclusions

There is only one methodologically adequate study of nonsibs: Blau et al. (1967) found birth order to be a negligible factor. The many investigations in which birth order is the independent variable are methodologically inadequate. By neglecting social variables, they have contributed to a mythology of the firstborn. Though this kind of research is unfit to refute the hypothesis of equidistribution of occupation by birth order when background factors are controlled, it was still alive in the 1970s. Surprisingly, occupational status of sibs has rarely been investigated. The two studies that have come to our notice are not in favor of higher occupational status in firstborns. As education and IQ are the main factors influencing occupation (Jencks 1972), and there is no evidence for birth order influencing achievement, the independence of occupation from birth order does not come as a surprise.

Chapter 7 Birth Order Differences in Socialization and Personality

7.1 Introductory Remarks

In industrialized countries laws of heritage today no longer grant privilege to first- or lastborns. Sibling status has lost its former importance for the distribution of property or power. Reports from non-Western cultures, on the other hand, point to considerable differences in status and responsibilities between first- and laterborns. Firstborns may wield power over their younger sibs even as adults (Rin 1965; Rosenblatt et al. 1974). Avoidance rites of parents against firstborns have been observed and interpreted as a consequence of firstborns being the representatives of the following generation, destined to bury the preceding one (Fortes 1974).

Vestiges of the historical importance of birth order can still be found within Western culture. In a questionnaire given to over 1,000 unmarried USA students on the desired size and sex composition of their future families, a consistent preference for male firstborns resulted (Gray et al. 1976). Firstborns are more often named after kin than laterborns (Rossi 1965). We do not know whether, during the times when birth order was related to generally recognized assets and duties, being a first- (or last- or middle-)born contributed significantly to variance in personality variables. Even today children of different birth order might experience different treatment leading to variations in personality formation. On the following pages the evidence for such associations will be discussed.

7.2 Social Class, Sibship Size, and Personality

Studies of the effects of birth order on personality are mostly concerned with the difference between first- and laterborns, disregarding other background variables. It has been demonstrated (see p. 6ff) that birth order distribution varies with demographic change and that the latter varies with age, social class, religious denomination, and habitation. Since large sibships are more frequently found in the lower class, the question of whether personality varies with social class and sibship size must be answered before the influence of birth order on personality is discussed. If social class and sibship size do affect personality, it would follow that firstborn-laterborn comparisons are contaminated by between-group differences.

7.2.1 Social Class and Personality

There is extensive literature on associations between social class and personality that is impossible to survey here. Differential IQ and school-related achievement have already been discussed (see pp. 29, 50). There is good evidence for differential language behavior by social class (Lukesch 1976, p. 151), working-class mothers being less able than middle-class mothers to give verbal structure to problem situations. The former also report themselves as more restrictive and punitive than middle-class controls (Sears et al. 1957; Lukesch 1976, p. 131). Middle-class parents seem to be more concerned with misdemeanors as indicators of character formation and lower-class parents more with their actual consequences (Clausen et al. 1963; Trasler 1973; Lawson et al. 1974). There is evidence that lower-class parents describe themselves as more authoritarian and less achievement-oriented than middle-class parents (Sears et al. 1957; Bronfenbrenner 1958; Zuckerman et al. 1960; Gildea et al. 1961; Trudewind 1975; Caldwell 1964). Middle-class rather than lower-class children report positive relations with parents (Lukesch 1976, p. 127). Personality differences by social class were found in achievement motivation, acitivity, creativity, self-esteem, tolerance, parent-orientation (all directly related to status), in conformity (negatively related to status) (Becker 1964; Kohn et al. 1969; Kreutz 1975 a, b; Trudewind 1975; Singer 1971), and in behavior disorders (negatively related to status) (Steuber 1973).

These findings cannot be discussed and qualified here. They may be due merely to different ideas on social desirability, which lead to differential reporting of parental behavior in different social strata. On the other hand, as unwanted births increase in frequency from middle to lower class (Rainwater 1965), background differences may not only be caused by reporting. However, the studies mentioned here make it evident that social class should be controlled in birth order research on socialization and personality.

7.2.2 Sibship Size and Personality

7.2.2.1 Differential Socialization in Families by Size

When subjects from small and large sibships are compared, the groups may be different in many other variables besides sibship size, e.g., in social class, ethnicity or race, religious denomination, parental cohort, and urban or rural habitation. Bossard et al. (1954, 1960), comparing large and small family systems, did not control for social class. According to these authors, parents of small families plan the birth of their children and are emotionally dependent on them. They have great expectations for their children's future. The small family unit is, however, quickly destabilized by tensions. Parents of large families, on the other hand, have unplanned children who are the objects of parental emotions and wishes to a much lesser degree. In order to function, the large family unit needs more conformity and more role specialization than the small family.

These observations remind one strongly of differences not only between families of different size, but also between families of different social class, educational level, and cultural background. In research on the influence of sibship size on personality, these variables ought to be controlled. Clausen et al. (1973) rightly draw attention to the lack of methodologically sound studies and to the scarcity of convincing results.

Research Not Controlling for Social Class

Family Size and Unwanted Pregnancies and Births. In a national sample of American women in unbroken marriages who were questioned on the incidence of unwanted births during a 5-year period, fourth births were unwanted in 28%, fifth in 41%, and sixth and later births in 43% (Bumpass et al. 1970). A similar result was found in a longitudinal study of 7,500 pregnant West German women, who were considered somewhat above the level of the general population. Of the women with a third or later pregnancy, 55% reported it as unwanted (Deutsche Forschungsgemeinschaft 1977).

Relations Between Children and Parents. More rules for the children and increasingly authoritative power structures, as well as more hostile and less-accepting behavior, were related to increasing sibship size (Bossard et al. 1954, 1955; Hawkes et al. 1958; Bartow 1961; Templeton 1962). Parental interest in school was weaker in large families (Eysenck et al. 1969), but behavior fostering dependency was more frequent (Cicirelli 1976 b). Relations in large families seem more negative than in small ones. It remains to be seen how much of this effect is not due to family size in itself, but to other variables related to it.

Research Controlling for Social Class

Health in Children and Parents. In a national sample of British children followed up since birth (Douglas et al. 1958, 1964), care of infants, assessed according to ratings of visiting health workers and reported use of tax-free medical services, decreased in quality with family size in the working class. In the middle class, level of care became significantly lower only in families with four or more children.

A random 10% sample of families living in two lower-class areas in London (Hare et al. 1965) was studied with the help of practitioners' records and interviews of parents. Indices of ill health and indices of neurosis became more frequent in parents with increasing family size. In children both indices were lower in sibships of four or more than in smaller sibships. The authors believe that with increasing family size, parents become less attentive to symptoms of ill health in their children.

Parental Interest in School and Achievement Expectations. Elder (1962 a) studied a representative sample of all North Carolina and Ohio high school students for parental plans to send them to college. In students in the final three grades, sex and social class being controlled, there was a trend – described by the author as "by no means consistent and linear" – for parental college plans to decrease with increasing sibship size. Lower-class and male subjects were more affected than middle-class and female subjects.

In a British national sample (Douglas 1964) (see p. 31), parental interest in school progress decreased linearly and regularly with sibship size in the middle- as well as in the working class. On a questionnaire on parental encouragement to continue education given to almost 3,000 male, 11th grade high school students in six middle-sized Pennsylvania cities, there was a negative relationship of parental encouragement to continue education with sibship size when social class was controlled on five levels. In the managerial and professional class, however, the variable was not related to sibship size (Rehberg et al. 1967).

Quality of Emotional Relations. Among about 2,000 employed mothers from the Washington D.C. area, satisfaction with the relationship to their children was negatively related to family size when income was controlled. In the same study 600 high school students given a questionnaire on parental attitudes reported, within social class, increasing neglect and rejection by parents as sibship size increased. Unfortunately, very few methodological details were given (Nye et al. 1970). Nuttall et al. (1970, 1971) factor-analyzed scores on a parental behavior inventory given to 5,300 Puerto Rican high school students (80% of those attending school in one district). Higher social class was associated with reporting higher acceptance by parents and number of children in the sibship with lower acceptance. On the other hand, in a sample of middle-class high school students in Catholic schools in the USA, Puerto Rico, and Mexico, no decline of parental support with sibship size was found (Thomas 1972a).

Restriction and Punishment. The Elder (1962b) sample (see p. 76) was also given a questionnaire on parental authoritarianism. There was a slight positive correlation to family size. In the Elder et al. (1963) study of 1,200 white, Protestant seventh-graders from urban areas, lower-class girls reported moderately more frequent corporal punishment and less frequent praise with increasing sibship size. The 600 high school students of Nye et al. (1970) reported, within social class, less frequent discussions between parents and children and more frequent physical punishment with increasing sibship size.

Acceptance of Parental Authority. A questionnaire on orientation towards parents (e.g., quality of feelings, similarity of values) was given to over 4,000 high school students (Singer 1971). Sex and social class being controlled, orientation towards parents declined with increasing sibship size, but not significantly so. There were sex and social class differences, females and middle-class subjects scoring higher. In a sample of male and female high school students and university freshmen consistent results for acceptance of authority, when sex and social class were controlled, appeared only in high school males. Acceptance was higher in middle-class than in lower-class subjects and higher in subjects from small sibships than from large ones (Smith 1971).

Educational Involvement of Father. Interviews with a probability sample of white women in the Detroit area showed that the number of children had very little impact on parental role differentiation when income, education, religious affiliation, and length of marriage were held constant. Husbands were reported to take more decisions in the area of education as family size increased (Campbell 1970). Elder et al. (1963) studied a large random sample of white Protestant seventh-graders in urban areas of central North Carolina. When sex and social class were controlled, sibship size had a modest influence on the likelihood of lower-class girls' reporting their father as prominent in child-rearing decisions. The same was also true for middle-class boys. The authors were surprised by the relatively small importance of sibship size.

Parental Attitudes and Family Atmosphere Perceived by Parents and Children. Schneewind (1978) compared 569 West German families, controlling for social class, with varying numbers of 9- to 14-year-old children. With increasing family size, parents reported themselves to keep more "distance" and to be more authoritarian. Children in larger families similarly reported more distance to and less help from parents. The family atmosphere tended towards more conflict and more regulations. Family size explained merely 2%–3% of the variance in attitudes and atmosphere. The direction was, however, consistently negative.

Conclusions

Certainly none of the studies quoted here support the Bossard et al. (1954) theory that large subships are associated with a particularly favorable socialization (Parsons 1977). Nearly all research relates larger sibships to unwanted births, ill health, lack of interest in school achievement, deteriorating parent-child relations, authoritarianism, and punitiveness. The association is, however, often extremely weak, particularly in the studies where socially homogeneous samples are investigated or where more social variables than just a summary division of subjects into lower and middle-class are introduced. Sibship size alone appears of little importance as a direct influence upon socialization; it may mainly be an indicator for biological and cultural differences between families.

There is, on the other hand, a consistent tendency for socialization influences to be less favorable in the lower class. Coming as an unexpected by-product of results concerning sibship size, this finding is quite impressive.

7.2.2.2 Sibship Size and Personality Measures

As increasing sibship size is, however tenuously, related to less achievement involvement and more punitiveness in parents and to deteriorating parent-child relations, in children from large sibships less achievement motivation, less adjustment, and more conformity might be expected.

Sibship Size and Achievement Motivation

Social Class Not Controlled. In a British national sample (See p. 31) tested at 11 and 15 years of age, children in large rather than small sibships were rated by teachers to be poor workers and to lack discipline. Also, at each level of an ability-achievement test score, children with three or more sibs were less likely to stay at school after statutory school-leaving age (Douglas 1964, Douglas et al. 1968).

Social Class Controlled. In the Elder (1962) large high school sample (see p. 76), five questionnaire measures of academic motivation showed a trend to decline with sibship size within social class, though the decrease was not regular. By restricting the sample to Protestant high-achieving 10th–12th graders, a consistent and significant decrease of college expectations with growing sibship size became visible when sex and social class (on two levels) were controlled.

A similar study (Turner 1962) was carried out with a large representative sample of Los Angeles high school seniors. A questionnaire was given on expected level of schooling, occupation, and income. Scores were combined to a "mean ambition index." For boys, a small, significant negative correlation of this index with sibship size remained when eight levels of background were controlled. Sibship size, however, explained merely 1%–2% of the variance in ambition. In the Rehberg et al. sample (1967) (see p. 77) the percentage of students expecting at least 4 years of college decreased with sibship size when social class, education of father, and parental encouragement were held constant. Family size contributed less than 2% to the explained variance. Falbo et al. (1979) studied 1,041 undergraduates from two universities using regression analysis. The variance contributed by sibship size to need-achievement scores on the Edward's Personal Preference Schedule (EPPS) was less than 0.5% when social class was controlled.

In a sample of USA college freshmen, academic achievement motivation was measured with a study habit checklist controlling for social class. A regression analysis indicated that sex but not family size had an influence on study habits (Keetz 1979).

Rosen (1961) used individually obtained Thematic Apperception Test (TAT) scores to measure achievement motivation in a stratified sample of 11-year-old boys in four American states. Six ethnic groups and five social classes were represented. Social class and sibship size were both independently related to achievement motivation, lower-class and larger sibships depressing it. In a second similar study only the influence of social class was confirmed.

Conclusions. The decline of achievement motivation with increasing sibship size, which appears when social class is not controlled, is very much reduced when social variables are held constant.

Sibship Size and Adjustment

Social Class Not Controlled. Adjustment was not related to family size in a sample of Indian high school students up to subships of eight. However, children from still larger sibships and low-income families scored lower (Prakash et al. 1963). Similarly, no association between sibship size and adjustment was found in a stratified sample of rural fifth graders (Hawkes et al. 1958).

Social Class Controlled. Among a random sample of 1,000 first graders, race and education of the mother predicted almost 30% of the variance in teachers' ratings of school adjustment, but sibship size at birth was a negligible predictor (Ramey et al. 1978). The preadolescent school children studied with the California Test of

Personality (CTP) by Lessing et al. (1967a) showed that high adjustment scores were related to high social class and to small sibships. In a more homogeneous middle-class sample of the same age, the authors (Lessing et al. 1972) found no major effect of sibship size. In this sample girls in large sibships scored higher on adjustment than those in small sibships. In 4,000 English 11-year-old school children Eysenck et al. (1969) found a negligible correlation of sibship size with neuroticism when six levels of occupational status were controlled. Altus (1959a, b) studied adjustment scores of 15,000 illiterate soldiers. Adjustment was highest in soldiers from sibships of up to five and again in those having 11 or more sibs.

The British nationally representative study of 6,055 7-year-olds controlled sex, social class, age of mother, and a number of biological factors such as birth weight and gestation length. On a standardized rating scale filled out by teachers the number of older sibs contributed 1.7% and the number of younger sibs 0.5% to the explained variance. Adjustment was negatively correlated to sibship size (Davie et al. 1972).

Conclusions. The Indian, the rural, and the illiterate military samples (the latter involving soldiers born in the 1920s or earlier) suggest that at times and places where birth control does not discriminate between families of different social backgrounds, large sibships are not related to low adjustment. Control for social variables leads to sibship size by itself appearing as a negligible influence.

Sibship Size and Self-Esteem

Social Class Not Controlled. Sears (1970) studied his sample of kindergarten children (see p. 87) again at 12 years of age. Self-esteem was measured with five scales and the total score was negatively related to sibship size. In freshmen from a small Southern college a measure of self-esteem was not related to sibship size in blacks whereas it was positively related to it in whites (Natsis 1975).

Social Class Controlled. In a homogeneous middle-class sample of public school children in Connecticut who were given a self-esteem inventory and rated by their teachers for self-esteem, no association of self-esteem with sibship size was found (Coopersmith 1967). The same was true in the samples from Catholic schools in the USA, Puerto Rico, and Mexico (Thomas 1972b) (see p. 77) for results on a self-esteem rating scale. Scores on a personality questionnaire given to junior high school children were studied by Dielman et al. (1974). When race and paternal education were controlled, associations of sibship size with self-esteem appeared only in interaction with sex and sex of sib and did not make sense.

One of the rare studies on adults was conducted by Kaplan (1970). A ten-item self-derogation scale was given to a probability sample of 500 adults in Texas by a marketing research firm. Within five social classes, self-derogation was not associated with sibship size.

Conclusions. As has been found for the variables discussed earlier, self-esteem becomes independent of sibship size when background variables are controlled.

Sibship Size, Extraversion, and Popularity

In a representative sample of 4,000 English 11-year-old school children, Eysenck et al. (1969) found a negligible correlation of extraversion with sibship size when social class was controlled on five levels. In black and white elementary school children from a homogeneous farming background in the South, sociometric popularity decreased with sibship size in subjects with five or more sibs (Baughman et al. 1968). Exactly the same result was found by Damrin (1949) in a small sample of high school girls. Murray (1971), on the other hand, found no association of popularity with sibship size among students from 12 English secondary modern schools.

Sibship Size, Conformity, Dependency, Anxiety, and Femininity

In a sample of 44 2.5-year-old nursery school boys, Waldrop et al. (1964), in a much-quoted study, found that coming from a large, densely spaced sibship correlated strongly with seeking contact with the female teacher, but also with two measures of lethargy given to the same children as newborns (Waldrop et al. 1966). A connection between postnatal lethargy and later dependency was established, which led the authors to the conclusion that the latter trait might be due not to sibship size as a psychological factor, but to biological influences associated with sibship size.

In the Catholic parochial sample (Thomas 1972b) (see p. 77, 80) a measure of conformity was not correlated with sibship size. The "embedded figure" test, which is at the same time a measure of field independence and perceptional flexibility, was given to a sample representative of all American men in civilian occupations. Larger sibship was weakly associated with less independence (−0.11) when age, religious denomination, region, paternal education, and locus of habitation were controlled (Schooler 1972b).

The mean of seven masculinity-femininity scales taken from well-known personality tests showed that in female university students femininity scores tended to decrease with increasing sibship size. In males there was no significant difference (Gormly 1968). On the other hand, in his famous study on birth order, anxiety, and affiliation Schachter (1959) found that among his 100 female university subjects those from large sibships were less easily frightened than those from small ones (see p. 115).

Sibship Size, Chronic Pain, and Reporting Pain

A small sample of inpatients who complained of chronic pain were compared with a representative sample of neurology patients (Button 1953). Sex, age, social class, and religious denomination were comparable in the two samples, but those who complained came from significantly larger sibships. Gonda (1962) compared consecutive patients whose chief complaint was pain with controls who did not report pain. The complainers over 35 years of age came from larger sibships than the non-complainers; there was no such difference in younger patients. In an experiment testing endurance in soldiers, on the other hand, subjects from small sibships reported pain more readily than those from large ones (Sweeney et al. 1970).

Sibship Size and Personality in General

A representative sample of American male adolescents were given a direct and a projective questionnaire. Within two social classes, personalities in small sibships appeared more active, more identified with, and yet more independent of their parents (Douvan et al. 1966). This result was not reproduced by Klockars (1968), who, in a personality inventory given to college and university students, found no variance explained by sibship size. Of particular importance is the Schooler study (1972a, b, c), which was based on interviews with a representative sample of American males in civilian occupations. When social background variables were not controlled, subjects from large sibships described themselves as more fatalistic and self-deprecatory and as less self-confident. When age, father's education, religious denomination, and coming from a broken home were controlled, associations of sibship size with personality traits became negligible.

7.2.2.3 **Conclusions** (Table 13)

Table 13. Sibship size and personality measures

	N	Social class controlled	Decrease with sibship size
Achievement motivation			
Douglas (1964) Douglas et al. (1968)	4,195 (males, females)	–	+
Elder (1962)	7,274 (males, females)	+	+
	890 (males, females)	+	+
Turner (1962)	2,175 (males, females)	+	(Explained variance 1%–2%)
Rehberg et al. (1967)	2,852 (males)	+	(Explained variance <2%)
Falbo (1979)	1,041 (males, females)	+	(Explained variance <0.5%)
Rosen (1961)	427 (males)	+	+
	367 (males)	+	–
Keetz (1979)	182 (males, females)	+	–
Adjustment			
Prakash et al. (1963)	200 (males, females)	–	–
Hawkes et al. (1958)	256 (males, females)	–	–
Ramey et al. (1978)	1,000 (males, females)	+	–
Lessing et al. (1967a)	855 (males, females)	+	–
Lessing et al. (1972)	599 (males, females)	+	–

Table 13. (continued)

	N	Social class controlled	Decrease with sibship size
Eysenk et al. (1969)	4,000 (males, females)	+	(Explained variance 1%)
Altus (1959 a, b)	15,000 (males)	+	(U-relationship)
Davie et al. (1972)	6,055 (males, females)	+	(Explained variance 0.5%–1.7%)
Self-esteem			
Sears (1970)	160 (males, females)	–	+
Natsis (1975)	272 (males, females)	–	–
Coopersmith (1967)	1,748 (males, females)	+	–
Thomas (1972 b)	? (males, females)	+	–
Dielman et al. (1974)	298 (males, females)	+	–
Kaplan (1970)	500 (males, females)	+	–
Extraversion and popularity			
Eysenck et al. (1969)	4,000 (males, females)	+	(Explained variance <1%)
Baughman et al. (1968)	1,000 (males, females)	+	+ (Sibship size 5+)
Damrin (1949)	156 females)	–	+ (Sibship size 5+)
Murray (1971)	709 (males)	–	–
Conformity, dependency, anxiety, and feminitiy			*Increase with sibship size*
Thomas (1972 b)	? (males, females)	+	–
Schooler (1972 b)	3,101 (males)	+	(Explained variance 1%)
Gormly (1968)	358 (males, females)	–	–
Schachter (1959)	100 females)	–	–
Chronic pain and reporting pain			
Button (1953)	27 (males, females)	+	+
Gonda (1962)	129 (males, females)	+	+
Sweeney et al. (1970)	52 (males)	–	–
Personality in general			*Associated with sibship size*
Douvan et al. (1966)	1,045 (males)	+	+
Klockars (1968)	? (males, females)	–	–
Schooler (1972 a, b, c)	3,101 (males)	+	(Explained variance <1%)

Corresponding to the negative socialization influences associated with larger sibship, the latter appears related to lower achievement motivation, lower self-esteem, higher dependency, less popularity, and, in general, to reporting a less favorable personality. The picture, however, is quite different if background variables are accounted for. *Differences in personality variables then disappear or become so small as to be negligible*. This is confirmed by the finding that personality variables are unrelated to, or even positively associated with having many sibs in an Indian sample, a rural sample, a Catholic sample, middle-class samples, and a sample of illiterate soldiers with extremely large sibships (and presumably older parents, see p. 12). In subjects born at times and places and into social groups where birth control does not discriminate between parents of different backgrounds, personality appears unrelated to sibship size. Investigations on personality variables confirm the conclusion drawn in relation to differential socialization by family size: The latter variable appears much more an indicator of biological and cultural differences between groups than a socialization influence in itself. It is impressive to see that just as socialization influences tend to appear less favorable with lower social class, this is also found for personality variables.

The importance of controlling for background variables will be discussed by means of two investigations that found personality traits to vary with sibship size. In two small studies the finding that complainers of chronic pain are from larger sibships deserves special attention for methodological reasons. The complaining and the noncomplaining groups have not been compared for rural or urban background and ethnicity. In Switzerland, immigrants from Southern European countries have the reputation of complaining more often of chronic pain than members of the native working class, and in their countries birth control is less popular than in Switzerland. A group of Southern complainers of chronic pain compared with Swiss patients of the same age, denomination, and social class would be different for sibship size – but for many other culturally and biologically relevant variables as well.

College and university girls of large sibships tend towards less anxiety and femininity than those of small sibships. Supposing that large sibships are overrepresented among the less wealthy but more rural and traditional segments of the population, girls finding their way to college and university from such backgrounds may be selected for fearlessness and unconventionality. Perhaps they are also more intelligent than the average upper-middle class girl who goes to college as a matter of course, even when moderately gifted. Different mechanisms of selection rather than sibship size itself would explain this difference between girls of large and small sibships.

In our example comparing Swiss and Southern European workers, the concept of „social class" is, of course, insufficient to size up the background variables differentiating these two groups. It ought to be replaced by other concepts describing smaller units of socialization influence. Classifying variations in socialization into two large compartments, as when subjects are divided into „middle" and „working" class, and then believing that differences within these compartments are differences between families is inappropriate (Lukesch 1976, p. 100) and may lead to fallacious results. West et al. (1973, pp. 30, 43) describe several studies where the use of the British Registrar General's social class subdivision veiled differences between groups of subjects which were discovered when other subdivisions were used.

7.3 Hypotheses on Socialization and Personality Differences by Birth Order

The following survey reports opinions based partially on speculation or clinical and personal uncontrolled experience and partially on research which has proved fertile for hypothesis formation (Table 14).

Psychoanalytical hypothesis formation has rather neglected relations between sibs. According to Freud (Dechêne 1967), these are dominated by aggression for same-sex and libidinal impulses for different-sex sibs. Sibs are mere appendices of the same-sex parent, and the Oedipus complex dominates sibling as well as parent-child relations. Freud did not attempt to delineate different personalities by birth order.

Adler (1927, 1928, 1958; see Dreikurs 1950; Ansbacher et al. 1956; Dechêne 1967) postulated an indelible, everlasting influence of birth order upon lifestyle. His interest concentrated on first-, second-, and lastborns, and other birth ranks were hardly discussed. According to this author, firstborns, having been „spoilt," are suddenly dethroned by the birth of a second child. This dethronement is particularly harmful when occurring before the age of 3 years. If it is successfully overcome, firstborns develop a striving to imitate their parents, to feel responsible for their sibs, and to protect others. They may develop a talent for organization. Firstborns' loss of status gives them a particular understanding of power and authority, and an admiration for the past. They may exaggerate the importance of law and order and become power-hungry conservatives. On the other hand, by fighting for the lost love of their mother they may become high-tempered, critical, and rebellious, or resigned, hopeless, and peevish (Adler 1958, pp. 144–148).

Table 14. Traits ascribed to first- and laterborns

Firstborns	Laterborns
Protector and leader, creative	Ready to cooperate
Strong need to achieve	Extremely ambitious
Power-hungry conservative	Inclined to new ideas
Introspective	Extraverted
Adult-oriented	Peer-oriented, empathizing, popular
Interested in abstract thought	Interested in practical problems
Rebellious	
Resigned	
Vulnerable and uncertain	Harmonious and leisurely
Low self-esteem	
Fearful, dependent, affiliative	
Indirect expression of aggression	Direct expression of aggression
Strongly sex-typed	

From birth, second children share parental attention with another child. This makes them more cooperative than firstborns. They have a „pacemaker“ in the first child and are continuously stimulated to catch up. They are rivals par excellence. Second children often prove more talented and successful than firstborns because they exert themselves more (Adler 1958, pp. 148–150).

Youngest children are spared dethronement. They are pampered and may become misfits. They may be lazy because of discouraged ambition and suffer from inferiority feelings because everybody around them is older and stronger. On the other hand, stimulated by their manifold chances for competition, they may overcome all their older sibs (Adler 1958, pp. 151–152).

Only children are spoiled by the mother and compete against the father. They want to be the center of attention forever and suffer from the loss of this position in adult life. Growing up in an atmosphere of anxiety (pessimism having prevented their parents from having more children), they are almost predestined for faulty development (Adler 1958, pp. 152–154).

While some authors have amplified Adler's descriptions (Montagu 1948; Takuma 1971; Sonstegard 1973), new traits were added by others. Dethronement is believed to make first-borns vulnerable and uncertain (Dittes 1961). According to some authors it is more parental inexperience than dethronement that is most important in firstborn childrens' personality development. Parents' supposedly being more anxious and at the same time more permissive and more frustrating with first- than laterborns is believed to make firstborns more fearful and dependent (Sears et al. 1957; Lasko 1954). A particularly fruitful hypothesis was proposed by Schachter (1959, p. 43): Mothers respond more quickly to the distress of their first child, while with later children they are less easily alarmed. This associates, in the firstborn's mind, anxiety with affiliation, i.e., seeking the company of others.

Another line of reasoning starts with parents' supposed overestimation of firstborns' capacities. The consequences are twofold: a stronger need to achieve in first- than laterborns and, through an insight that parental models are unattainable, low self-esteem in firstborns. Laterborns, on the other hand, are believed to have more attainable models in their older sibs and less-impaired self-esteem (Sampson 1965; De Avila 1971). Having to take over the role of parent-substitute at an early period, firstborns become serious, conforming, and inclined to introspection and self-examination (Harris 1964). Being more exposed to the socialization influence of their parents, they are more strongly sex-typed than their younger sibs (Edwards et al. 1973). For the same reason, they tend towards indirect and younger sibs towards direct expression of aggression (Herrman 1969; Feshbach 1970).

Hypotheses on laterborns' personalities are less often brought forward. Second children are supposed to be harmonious and leisurely, and youngest, pensive and withdrawn (König 1963). While firstborns are inclined to abstract thinking, secondborns are extraverted, pragmatic, and given to solving practical problems (Harris 1964). In contrast to eldest children's conservatism, laterborns like new ideas (Forer 1969). Being peer-oriented while firstborns are more adult-oriented, they will empathize more readily than firstborns and consequently be more popular (McArthur 1956; Stotland et al. 1963).

A third line of research was started by Galton (1874, 1887) who found an overrepresentation of firstborns among men of genius. Since then, greater creativity in firstborns has been claimed many times.

Conflicting Hypotheses. According to Adler, firstborns can be conservatives as well as rebels, power-hungry as well as resigned. The obvious contradictions between these terms are avoided by postulating differential environmental influences on firstborns' development. Other hypotheses are opposed to Adler's or to each other. Firstborns being leaders and protectors and having a strong need to achieve excludes their being fearful, uncertain, dependent, or affiliative. There is also incompatibility between creativity, conservatism, and conformity in firstborns, between their being affiliative and (in the case of males) strongly sex-typed, and between their being rebellious and their indirect expression of aggression. Secondborns' leisureliness and good nature does not agree with their extreme ambition.

As personality differences by birth order must necessarily be caused by differential socialization, evidence for differential treatment of children by birth rank is considered here first.

7.4 Birth Order and Familial Socialization

7.4.1 Differential Treatment of Children by Birth Order: Investigated in Parents

7.4.1.1 Questionnaires

When parents' reminiscences were compared with data based on direct observation, their validity was found wanting (Robbins 1963; Yarrow et al. 1964; Price 1969). Consequently the results reported here (Table 15) need confirmation by other sources. Sears et al. (1957) interviewed mothers of New England kindergarten children in unbroken families stratified for size. Results are given separately for sibship size of two on the one hand, and of three and four on the other. In comparison with the second child, the first is more often taken care of by persons other than the mother; the father takes more part in education; the first child is toilet trained earlier than the second. The delight over pregnancy is greater, weaning less severe, and education in some aspects more permissive for firstborns. They are, however, more often deprived of privileges than laterborns. In larger sibships the first child is significantly more frequently punished physically than laterborns and there is more disagreement between parents about his training than for middle and younger children. Delight over pregnancy decreases sharply from first to last child, but demonstrations of affection are lowest for first- and highest for lastborns. Duration of breast feeding decreases from first- to lastborns and toilet-training is started increasingly later.

Besides probably having a younger mother, a child who at 5 years is the oldest of four (extremely narrow spacing) will live in a familial situation quite different, from that of a child who at 5 years is the youngest of four. Differences in maternal age, social class, and spacing interfere in this study with birth order differences. They contribute to the fact that a firstborn with one sib fares considerably better than a firstborn of three or four children.

More tolerance for laterborns than for firstborns was also found by questioning parents of Harvard students (McArthur 1956), of preschool children

(Vernon et al. 1967; Schramm 1978) and in a longitudinal study of 70 children over an 18-year span (Stout 1960).

Three studies concern independence training. The mothers of 11-year-old sons reported earlier independence training in firstborns and only children than in middle and youngest children (Rosen 1964). The same result was found in a small sample of mothers of private-school boys (Bartlett et al. 1966) and in parents of 185 Canadian middle- and lowerclass school boys (Marjoribanks et al. 1975a).

A somewhat special investigation (Biber 1974) was concerned with a small sample of parents expecting either their first or second child. Attitudes were measured with a check list. In prospective parents of a second child, idealistic expectations were fewer and feelings of anger and hostility were more accepted than in prospective parents of a first child.

Conclusions (Table 15)

It has to be remembered that these studies do not concern sibs. Parental reports on educational practice almost unanimously point to greater demands being placed upon firstborns than upon laterborns. Firstborns are biased for smaller sibship size and younger parents and, according to demographic findings (see p. 10), may be biased for higher social class. This is confirmed by the only investigation controlling for sibship size (Sears et al. 1957): Firstborns in sibships of two are more often punished by withdrawal of love than secondborns, but they have more freedom for aggression. Both parental behaviors were found more often in middle- than in lower-class mothers (Lukesch 1976, p. 131). The much harsher treatment of first- than laterborns in sibships of three and four may be due to between-family differences associated with differential spacing. The conclusion that greater demands are placed upon firstborns will be taken up later with the help of studies in which background variables are better accounted for (see p. 90).

Table 15. Birth order and self-reported parental behavior

Author	*N*	Report by	Tolerance highest for
Sears et al. (1957)	379	Mother	Firstborns in sibships of two, laterborns in sibships of three and four
Vernon et al. (1967)	32	Mother	Laterborns
Schramm (1978)	138	Mother	Laterborns males, firstborns females
McArthur (1956)	336	Parents, father	Laterborns
Stout (1960)	70	Parents	Laterborns
			Independence training earliest in
Rosen (1964)	122	Mother	Firstborns
Bartlett et al. (1966)	31	Mother	Firstborns
Marjoribanks et al. (1975a)	185	Parents	Firstborns
			Differences in attitudes
Biber (1974)	84	Parents	More hostility, less idealism for 2nd child

7.4.1.2 Observation of Parental Behavior in Natural Settings

For obvious reasons, studies using this method mainly concern infants who are followed up by a natal clinic. Roberts et al. (1972) studied 90% of all live births ($N=$ 197) in a Welsh administrative area during an 18-month period. A health visitor who saw each baby once a month rated variables of child care. Some variables were highest for firstborns, lowest for secondborns, and increased again slightly for third and subsequent births. In the middle and lower classes this was true for mother-child contact, maternal competence, and physical freedom given to the child. Independence training decreased linearly for the lower class and was U-shaped for the middle class. Differences between first and second children were significant at the 1% level. In general, care given to firstborns was of a higher quality than that given to laterborns.

Health visitors' ratings at 2 and 4 years of age were also used by Douglas et al. (1958) in their British national representative sample of 5,368 children. In all social groups firstborns were taken more often to welfare centers than laterborns. There were no significant differences in the date of starting toilet training. At the follow-up of the sample at age 11 (Douglas 1964), health care differences by birth order were small. Middle-class mothers of firstborns tended to worry more about the health of the child, though it was better than that of laterborns.

In several other studies using smaller nonrepresentative samples the same trend was found in that mothers gave better care to firstborns than to laterborns, spent more time playing with and talking to them, and worried more about them. Fathers were also more involved with first- than laterborns (Gewirtz et al. 1969; Thoman et al. 1970, 1972; Cohen et al. 1976, 1977; Lewis et al. 1979).

Conclusions

While parents report demanding more of firstborns, the observational data unanimously point to firstborns being better cared for than laterborns at the infant age. Here again, as in the studies mentioned before, it is not possible to differentiate as to how far the impairment of maternal care from the first to the second child is due to firstborns' mothers being younger and possibly more modern in their ideas about health care, independence training, physical freedom, and so on. As, however, the quality of care improves again with the third child, some of the variance in care cannot be explained by cohort differences.

7.4.1.3 Observation of Parents in Experimental Situations

Just as observation in the home is restricted to infants, experimental studies of parent-child interactions usually concern children of kindergarten age: Parents (mostly mothers) and child solve a problem together. Samples are usually small.

A sample of children from same-sex sibships and equidistributed for being firstborn, laterborn, or single was studied by Hilton (1967). The subjects did puzzles, presented as intelligence tests, in the presence of their mothers. Only children and firstborns were rated significantly higher on dependent behavior (more running to mother, more asking for help). Their mothers, on the other hand, interfered more and expressed more concern at successes and failures than mothers of laterborns. The same setting was used by Rothbart (1971) in a sample of children with one sib. Mothers of firstborns interfered more, pressed more for achievement, and gave more complex explanations than mothers of laterborns. In another study middle-class parents were separately observed doing puzzles with their 5-year-old first- or lastborn daughter. Fathers interfered with and spoke to their firstborn child more than to their lastborn, while in mothers there was no difference (Osofsky et al. 1971).

In a similar study with adolescents there were no clear-cut birth order differences (Thomas 1976).

Conclusions (Table 16)

Table 16. Birth order and observed parental behavior

Author	*N*	Parent	Press for achievement highest for
Hilton (1967)	60	Mother	Firstborns
Rotbart (1971)	56	Mother	Firstborns
Osofsky et al. (1971)	42	Parents	Firstborns (father)
Thomas (1976)	?	Parents	–

The majority of studies (Table 16) show that firstborns at kindergarten age are more interfered with and more pressed for achievement than laterborns. Just as for results of parental self-reports and observation in natural settings, the objection can be raised (the subjects not being sibs) that firstborns' mothers may be younger, better educated, and more ambitious for their offspring. The decisive evidence of differential treatment by birth order will be furnished by the comparison of sibs within the same family

7.4.1.4 Comparison of Parental Treatment of Sibs Within the Same Family

This was possible during longitudinal studies of child development. Lasko (1954) compared 46 pairs of first and second children who were observed twice a year from 15 months to 10 years of age by trained raters. Their parents were above the national average for income and education. Sib comparisons were made longitudinally and cross-sectionally: 40 pairs matched for age were compared, first versus second child, in 21 variables.

The groups differed at the 0.05 level of confidence on only two variables, a result that may have been due to chance. There was, however, a consistent though nonsignificant direction of difference indicating that in comparison with first children, second children were (1) treated with more acceptance and affection, (2) with less restrictiveness and coerciveness, (3) with more protectiveness and babying. Due to small numbers it was not possible to find consistent results for differential sex composition and age spacing of the pairs.

A longitudinal analysis was done comparing the first and the second child at different points in time at the same age. While at the age of about 2 years the first child had a more highly child-centered environment and was exposed to more language and toilet training than the second child, at 3 and 4 years he appeared less warmly treated than the latter at the same age. When both children had reached school age, however, parental behavior towards both children became very similar. The most striking difference in favor of the second child at preschool age was his being treated with more warmth and approval. For the first child there was more disciplinary friction, but also more acceleration. Though the data at different age levels are not based on independent sampling, it may be said with some certainty that the first child has a less-stable preschool environment than the second child, who starts at a lower level of parental interest.

Jacobs et al. (1976) observed 32 sib pairs in middle-class families once when the older and once when the younger child was 3 months old. There was a significant change in 20 of 41 rated variables. In Comparison with firstborns, secondborns received less affectionate care-taking activities and were less often spoken to, while feeding remained unchanged. There were no significant differences in infant behavior between the two groups. In order to eliminate the maternal age variable, behavior of secondborns' mothers (being older) was compared with the behavior of a control group of the same age consisting in mothers of first children. The behavioral differences did not depend on maternal age.

Lawson et al. (1974) collected reports of the 24-h period preceding interviews from 54 English mothers of two children in working- and middle-class families. The first interview took place when the second child was expected, the second when the child was about 3 months old, and the third when the child was 14 months old. In 17 cases, there were data for the first and the second child at 14 months. Firstborns experienced more attention, more linguistic stimulation, more toilet training, more basic care, and more time with the father. On the other hand, they were more often subject to adult intervention and spent more time in prams and playpens than their younger sib.

7.4.1.5 The Evidence of Dethronement

Dunn and her group (Dunn et al. 1980; Kendrick et al. 1980; Dunn et al. 1981) studied 40 mainly working class families at Cambridge (England) with an excellent method. Observations at home and interviews with the mother were conducted 1–3 months before the birth of a second child and again in the 2nd and 3rd weeks after birth. Attention centered on the changes in interaction between the mother and her first child (mean age at birth of the second child: 25 months) and on the first child's reactions.

In comparison with prebirth *observations*, those conducted after the birth of the younger child showed a significant decrease in maternal attention toward the older child: there was less initiating of conversation and less interest in and help for child activities, while, on the other hand, confrontations between mother and child became more frequent (Dunn et al. 1980), in particular when the age difference between the sibs was small (Kendrick et al. 1980). These changes in interactions were independent of the distance between pre- and postbirth observations and thus probably not due to developmental change in the older child.

Using rank correlations the authors assessed to what extent mother and child behavior, though changing in frequency, retained rank order consistency. While maternal measures remained relatively stable, individual differences in child behavior increased over observation time. Children seemed to react in an individual way to a general lowering of maternal attention.

Pre- and postbirth *interviews* with the mother made possible the study of reports on behavioral changes in the older child (Dunn et al. 1981). They were quite impressive: 13 of the 40 children observed had become at least moderately more tearful, 24 more demanding, and 23 more negative toward the mother. Eight children lost previously acquired toilet habits and four showed severe sleep problems, while feeding problems were practically absent. Eight older sibs frequently irritated the baby and three were plainly hostile. On the other hand, two-thirds showed affectionate behavior toward their new sib and 25 were reported to be more independent in some area of behavior or to have made rapid progress in language ability. The intercorrelations between the various aspects of negative behavior were weak. Male sex and younger age in firstborns, depression and fatigue in mothers, and a postbirth increase in confrontation were associated to a varying extent with the incidence of the negative firstborn reactions described above. Thus signs of disturbance in the mother-child relationship and in the child's behavior are evident 2 or 3 weeks after the birth of a second child. The families were followed up until the younger child was 14 months of age. The results have not yet been published, but the authors (Dunn et al. 1981) indicate that the prognostic implications of the various firstborn reactions – as may be anticipated from their low intercorrelations – are quite different.

Powers (1980) assessed adjustment in small children 3 months before and 3 months after the birth of a sibling by means of an extensive interview with the mother. A control group was studied in the same way. The subjects had significantly more adjustment problems at the second point in time than before their sib was born. Controls, on the other hand, did not change.

There is, as yet, only preliminary evidence that the negative reactions of the firstborn could usually be transient. A longitudinal study on 110 middle-class children (Thomas et al. 1961) reports on 18 children whose mother gave birth to a second child during the observation period. Nine of them showed behavior disturbance, though in six cases it was mild and transient. Five children, on the other hand, reacted in the long run with improved relations with parents. In a survey of literature on reactions to a new sib (consisting mostly of unsystematic observations on small numbers of subjects), Legg et al. (1974) that disturbed behavior was associated with younger age and lower social class and was usually transient.

Conclusions

The results of studies comparing parental attitudes toward sibs within the same family agree with observations in non-sibs that firstborns receive better care than secondborns in infancy and that firstborns receive more verbal stimulation and earlier toilet training. The only investigation going beyond preschool age agrees with experimental studies in finding more acceleration, coerciveness, and confrontation in the treatment of firstborns.

There is also well-supported evidence that firstborns suffer a kind of "dethronement" at the birth of a sib. They are subsequently treated less attentively by their mother and there is more friction. Two or three weeks after the birth of a second child, firstborns are still decidedly upset and after 3 months the older child is still less well adjusted than before the birth of the younger child. We do not yet know from longitudinal studies of representative samples whether, when, and under what conditions this crisis is overcome or whether as a rule it leaves indelible traces. Nor do we know how second and third children react to the birth of a new sib; they could be dethroned as well. There is at present only very preliminary and restricted evidence that the negative reactions of the older child could be transient.

7.4.2 Differential Treatment of Children by Birth Order: Investigated in Children

7.4.2.1 Perception of Differential Treatment by Parents

Authority and Control. While a small sample of kindergarten children questioned about the perception of parental dominance did not give results varying by birth order (Laosa et al. 1972), in lower-class fourthgraders and in male college students firstborns were more aware of parental authority or more often considered their parents as "strict" than laterborns (Corsello 1973; Zimbardo et al. 1963). In a large sample of Swedish schoolchildren, perceived control decreased from first to last child in sibships of three and more. Sex and social class were not controlled and birth order contributed less than 1% to the explained variance in perceived control (Schaller 1972).

Affection. Koch (1960b) studied 360 6-year-old middle class school beginners with one sib, matched for sex, sex of sib, birth order, spacing and father's occupation (see p. 44 for IQ). Hers is the only study where firstborns felt less favored by the mother than the other sib. In more representative and in part much larger samples of school children, adolescents, and young adults, differences in perceived parental affection or appreciation did not appear (Corsello 1973; Robertson et al. 1962; Singer 1971) or were in favor of firstborns (Schwab 1978).

Perception of Differential Treatment in Sibs. Bartelt (1973) studied 129 pairs of first and second sibs at the same age and attending a New Jersey high school. Background was socially homogeneous and sibship size was two to four in 70%. Firstborns did not perceive parental discipline as stricter than secondborns.

7.4.2.2 Perception of Differential Relationship with Parents

In this area the dependent variables are concepts that merge into each other. If all were studied in one sample they could be highly correlated. Accordingly the results must be considered with reservation.

Acceptance of Parental Authority. A large population of male and female public school and university students was questioned on acceptance of parental authority (Smith 1971). Controlling for sex, large and small sibship, working or middle-class background, and level of school, it was found that among high school males firstborns accepted parental authority more readily than laterborns. This result was not reproduced in the other groups.

Orientation to Parents. A questionnaire on orientation to parents was given to a large population of New Jersey 10th and 11th graders, family background being controlled. Firstborn girls in small families of any class and firstborn boys in middle-class families of two children reported having more communication with and being more influenced by parents (Singer 1971). Also firstborn female students in a private Middle East college reported greater parental influence on their occupational aspirations (in interaction with the education of the father). Other measures of family orientation did not vary by birth order, and frequency of extrafamilial contacts was lowest in youngest children (Tomeh 1969, 1970, 1971, 1972).

In three smaller samples the Bene-Anthony family relation test was used to measure involvement with parents versus involvement with sibs. In two of them, which included subjects of elementary age in well-matched sibships of two, no difference was found (Frankel 1968; Sutton-Smith et al. 1970). In the third, which compared high school students with one or two sibs, stronger involvement of firstborns with parents and of laterborns with sibs appeared (Laitman 1975).

Perceived Identification with Parents. In the studies presented here small samples were used. In a questionnaire given to Harvard males, firstborns scored higher on perceived similarity with the father in half of the measures, social class being controlled (Palmer 1966). In college females with one sib tested with the Gough adjective checklist, firstborns tended to perceive themselves as more similar to adults than secondborns. The authors concluded that this finding indicates stronger identification with parents (Sutton-Smith et al. 1970, pp. 113–114). The results of a Q-sort (Roost 1976) given to college students without control of sibship size showed that firstborns identified more closely with their fathers than laterborns. Hypotheses on parental identification of laterborns were not supported.

The following investigations used larger samples. In a parent-role questionnaire given to a male high school sample with social class controlled across groups, firstborns identified more closely with parents than laterborns (Purpura 1971). Oldest daughters reported more similarity to their mothers on an identification scale (while males did not differ by birthrank for identification with their fathers) in a college population of students visiting a counseling center (Heilbrun et al. 1965). On a semantic differential, on the other hand, firstborns among a male college sample did not rate themselves as more similar to their fathers than laterborns (Nash 1970). Singer (1971) also found no differences in perceived similarity of values by birth order in his large high school population described above.

Intrafamilial Comparisons. Eleven-year-old boys and their mothers were given a nine-statement scale on values. There was a decrease of value similarity between mother and son with decreasing social class. Within two classes, however, value similarity was not significantly associated with birth order (Rosen 1964). Biegelsen (1976) studied a large sample of university freshmen to assess the association between their probable vocational choice and the occupation of their parents, expecting higher identification of firstborns with their parents. The hypothesis was not supported.

Bartelt (1973) gave 129 pairs of first and second children of the same sibship selected from high schools in a New Jersey town a questionnaire on parent-peer orientation. Firstborns were not different from secondborns.

7.4.2.3 **Conclusions** (Table 17)

Table 17. Birth order and perception of differential treatment by parents (A) and birth order and differential relations to parents (B)

	Author	*N*	Age, sex	Social class controlled	Sibship size controlled	Highest score
A	*Authority and control*					
	Laosa et al. (1972)	93	Kindergarten (males, females)	–	–	–
	Corsello (1973)	201	Fourth grade (males, females)	+	–	Firstborn males
	Zimbardo et al. (1963)	99	college males	–	–	Firstborns
	Schaller (1972)	822	10-14 years (males, females)	–	+	Firstborn > middle > youngest (size three or more) Explained variance 1%
	Affection					
	Koch (1960 b)	360	5 years (males, females)	+	+	Secondborn
	Corsello (1973)	201	Fourth grade (males, females)	+	–	–
	Robertson et al. (1972)	1,009	High school (males, females)	–	–	–
	Singer (1971)	4,400	11th grade (males, females)	+	+	–
	Schwab (1978)	308	College (males, females)	–	–	Firstborn (females)
	Comparison of sibs (discipline)					
	Bartelt (1973)	129	pairs (males, females)			–
B	*Acceptance of parental authority*					
	Smith (1971)	1,415	Public school, university (males, females)	+	+	Male firstborns (public school)
	Orientation to parents					
	Singer (1971)	4,440	10th, 11th grades (males, females)	+	+	Firstborn girls in small sibships

Table 17. (continued)

Author	N	Age, sex	Social class controlled	Sibship size controlled	Highest score
Tomeh (1971) (Middle East)	523	College females	+	–	Firstborns and youngest
Frankel (1968)	113	Sixth grade	+	+	–
Sutton-Smith et al. (1970)	40	8–11 years (males)	+	+	–
Laitman (1975)	89	Junior high school	–	+	Firstborns
Identification with parents					
Palmer (1966)	55	University males	+	–	Firstborns
Sutton-Smith et al. (1971)	80	College females	–	+	Firstborns (more similar to adults)
Roost (1976)	120	College (males, females)	–	–	Firstborns
Purpura (1971)	311	High school males	+	–	Firstborns
Heilbrun et al. (1965)	346	College (males, females)	–	–	Firstborns (females)
Nash (1970)	201	College males	–	–	–
Singer (1971)	4,400	10th, 11th grades (males, females)	+	+	–
Intrafamilias comparisons (values, occupations, parent-orientation)					
Bartelt (1973)	258	High school sibs (males, females)			–
Rosen (1964)	122	11 years (males)			–
Biegelsen (1976)	1,883	College (males, females)			–

Of the four studies shown in Table 17 concerning *perception of authority and control*, two found it to be highest in firstborns (being biased for small sibship size) while a third, controlling for sibship size, found a minimal decrease in perception of control with birth rank. In a study of sibs there was no evidence that firstborns perceive more parental control than laterborns. Koch's finding that firstborns feel less secure of their mothers' *affection* was not reproduced in samples of older subjects.

The case is different for *acceptance of parental authority* and *orientation to parents* as reported by children. Since better emotional relations with parents were associated with higher social class and smaller sibship size (see p. 77), higher scores could have been expected in firstborns in studies in which sibship size and social class were not controlled. However, also one large well-controlled study found greater acceptance of parental authority in male firstborns at high school age, and another, involving adolescents of the same age, found parent orientation to be higher in firstborn females in small sibships (Smith 1971; Singer 1971). Of three small-scale studies employing the Bene-Anthony test, on the other hand, only one found stronger involvement of firstborns with parents.

The evidence for *greater identification* with parents in first- than in laterborns is less convincing, as most studies do not control background. While a small well-controlled study found firstborn girls to be more similar to adults than secondborns (which is not necessarily indicative of higher parent orientation), a very large and similarly well-controlled investigation found no difference by birth order in the similarity between subjects' values and those they reported for their parents. This negative finding is confirmed by the fact that three intrafamilial comparisons between subjects and their parents and between sibs were negative both for parent identification and parent orientation. This finding raises some doubts as to whether the firstborn lead in parent orientation and acceptance of authority is due to between-group differences. We conclude, however, that there is evidence that firstborns in small families report themselves as more oriented toward their parents and, when male, are more ready to accept their authority. Because of the haziness of the concepts this only signifies that firstborns may have a somewhat better relationship with their parents than laterborns.

7.4.3 Differential Interactions of Siblings by Birth Order

7.4.3.1 Nonsibs

Koch (1960) interviewed her well-matched sample of 360 middle-class 6-year-old children in sibships of two (see p. 93) on sibling interactions. Secondborns wanted to play with their older sib more than firstborns with their younger one. They also reported being verbally and physically attacked by their sib more often than firstborns. In an interview with 140 third- to fifth-grade boys and girls on the means used to make a sib do something, Sutton-Smith et al. (1970, pp. 45–53) found – in addition to sex differences – that firstborns used more aggressive techniques than laterborns, who tended to plead and reason. The results, however, were not analyzed for significance. A questionnaire on the same subject was given by the same authors to 95 middle-class fifth and sixth graders selected for being first- or secondborns in sibships of unspecified size. Firstborns reported themselves as, and were reported by secondborns to be, more bossy and more given to using physical power. Secondborns reported themselves, and were reported by firstborns, to whine, tell tales, and induce guilty feelings more often ($P<0.05$). These findings were confirmed in a sample of 120 male and female college students (Sutton-Smith et al. 1970, pp. 57–61).

Bigner (1974a) made an extensive study of 578 male and female children from kindergarten to grade eight. The subjects were secondborn or single children from unbroken middle-class homes. Age spacing to the oldest sib was either less than 20 months or 28–48 months. The children were tested individually with drawings representing sibs of different ages and sex. They had to assign sentences to these figures connotating high or low power to interfere or to help. There was a consistent and significant difference between secondborns and only children in attributing power to the older sib on the drawing and in differentiating power attribution by sex. Secondborns with the smaller age difference attributed more power to the older sib than those with larger spacing.

In another study the same author (1974b) found that 120 secondborns at five age levels (kindergarten to eighth grade) similarly gave more detailed descriptions of their older sib when age difference was small.

Schachter et al. (1976) studied the opinion of being different from one's sibling with a questionnaire and a semantic differential in 383 undergraduates with one or two sibs. Firstborns described their secondborn sibs and secondborns their first-born sibs as more different from themselves than was the case for firstborns describing their thirdborn sibs and vice versa.

7.4.3.2 Sibs Within the Same Sibship

Verger (1968) studied the three oldest sibs of the same sex in 70 sibships with the Luder vocational preference record at adolescence. First- and secondborns were more dissimilar in interests than first- and thirdborns. This was confirmed in a sample of 140 middle class mothers of two or three children (mean age 6 years): On a questionnaire and with a semantic differential they described more dissimilarity between the first and the second than between the first and the third child (Schachter et al. 1978), thus confirming the former Schachter (1976) study. The results obtained by Hayden (1973), on the other hand, do not show any dramatic differences between first- and secondborns at adult age. With the 16 PF (Personality Factor Questionnaire), which consists of 16 scales, the author studied 90 university students and their sibs, all in unbroken two-child families and representing all combinations of sex of subject and sex of sib within a spacing of 5 years. Oppositeness of traits was defined as a score difference between sibs of more than 33 percentiles. Only the subgroup spaced less than 3 years differed to this degree: within this subgroup male sibships did so on two scales and mixed sibships on one, but female sibships did so on none.

Birth Order Difference or Age Difference? Do firstborns behave more aggressively toward secondborns because of their birth rank or because they are older and stronger? Bragg et al. (1973) tried to answer this question in an experimental study: 27 firstborn and the same number of lastborn boys had to persuade an older, same age, or younger person to do a task. The major differences in approach were due to the age of the target person and not to birth order of subjects. Thus behavior directed at sibs does not seem to be automatically transferred to persons outside the family.

7.4.3.3 Conclusions

Studies of sibs and nonsibs are in good agreement: the older – and thus usually stronger – firstborns are more directly aggressive toward their younger sibs than vice versa. The latter are more aware of the oldest sib's power to interfere or help than only children. Positive and negative relationships with and interest in the older sib are stronger when spacing is small. In childhood and adolescence first- and secondborns describe themselves and are perceived as more different from each other than first- and thirdborns: Rival sibs tend to retire to an area of their own. On the other hand, when oppositeness of traits is measured in young adults, it appears quite unspectacular. On the evidence presented here the influence of sib rivalry on personality formation seems to have been overrated.

7.5 Summary of the Evidence on Differential Familial Socialization by Birth Order

Observation of parents and retrospective data are generally restricted to infants and preschool children. Both point to firstborn children being given better care in infancy and having greater demands put upon them at preschool age, particularly for independence. These findings are confirmed by studies of sibs within the same family. Better care for firstborns in infancy is confirmed by several of these: Their being treated less affectionately and more coercively and their being given more language and toilet training has found support in one well-conducted longitudinal investigation. The finding that firstborns are under more pressure to achieve is again confirmed by experimental observations of parent-child interactions at preschool age, since mothers of firstborns interfere more and overrate success more than those of laterborns. There is, however, preliminary evidence that differential treatment is not any more present at school age.

Studies covering a time span of up to 3 months show that shortly after the birth of a second sib the firstborn's relationship with his mother has deteriorated and that some children are considerably disturbed. There is very preliminary evidence that the sequela of this "dethronement" are transitory and that to consider it generally a dramatic and disruptive event may be unwarranted, Though the birth of a sib is usually considered an important event in a young child's life, research in this field is merely starting. The view that possibly differential parent-child relations by birth order could be of little consequence is supported by questionnaires given to elementary, high school, and university students, which are lacking however, in clarity of concept. Firstborns' apparently greater awareness of parental authority and control may be due to a between-group difference. *There is some preliminary evidence that male firstborns at high school age accept parental authority more readily than laterborns and that firstborns of both sexes in small sibships at high school age are more strongly oriented toward parents.* There is no evidence, however, for stronger parent identification in firstborns, and the few studies conducted within families find no difference in orientation or identification by birth order. This is a strong argument for some of the variance in parent relatedness found in nonsibs being due to between-group differences.

On the other hand there is good evidence for power relations between older and younger sibs (firstborns appearing more directly aggressive than secondborns) and, accordingly, for greater attraction between the less competitive nonadjacent than between adjacent pairs. There is, however, very little evidence for a sizeable and lasting oppositeness in personality traits in adjacent sibs.

Though transfer of interpersonal techniques typical for older and younger sibs to situations outside the family is the basis of birth order typologies, very little research has been done in this field. On the basis of the extremely tenuous evidence there is, as yet, no support for this transfer.

7.6 Birth Order and Personality

7.6.1 Introductory Remarks

The following review of studies is ordered according to method. Each hypothesis is discussed first on the base of experiments, then of paper-pencil tests (personality questionnaires ratings by self and others or projective tests), and lastly of observations of real-life behavior.

The subjects in the following studies are mainly students from kindergarten to college or university, the latter with a strong bias for those taking psychology classes. Firstborns as a rule are opposed to laterborns without consideration of other birth ranks, sibship size, or background.

7.6.2 Birth Order, Anxiety, Sensitivity to Pain, and Risk Taking

In this section the hypothesis that anxious and inconsistent treatment by inexperienced parents makes firstborns more anxious, fearful, and consequently more sensitive to pain and less inclined to take risks than laterborns (see p. 86) is examined. In the experimental investigations and those relying on observations in natural settings, fear of bodily harm rather than anxiety is the dependent variable.

7.6.2.1 Experimental Studies

Waiting for an Electrical Shock. In his classical experiment, which brought about a revival of interest in birth order studies, Schachter (1959) announced to 62 female psychology students the delivery of either a painful or a painless electrical shock. Arousal of anxiety was measured with two self-rating scales. Under the pain condition, firstborns indicated a higher level of anxiety than laterborns and were willing to withdraw from the experiment in greater numbers. The experiment was repeated by Darley (1966), Willems et al. (1972), and Weller (1962) with female college or university students. There was no association of being firstborn with reported anxiety or, in the Willems' Dutch sample, with avoidance. In this study middle children were less frightened than first- or lastborns. Two mixed-sex samples did not report differential anxiety or differential wish to withdraw by birth order (McDonald 1969, 1970).

The experimental setting was modified by Eisenmann (1965) and by Staples et al. (1961). In the former study a small sample of female students was given the choice between painless and painful shocks. Firstborns decided in greater number for painless ones. In the latter study first- and laterborn female students had to choose between participating in or refusing an experiment including shock. The decision to participate was independent of birth rank.

In a further study a different measure of anxiety was introduced. A sample of high school males, while waiting for shock, had to report on perceived anxiety and do a tracking task. While the former measure was not related to birth rank, tracking errors were more frequent in firstborns in two of three trials (Landers et al. 1971).

Weiss (1970) modified both setting and measure of anxiety. He tried to put a small sample of high school males under stress with arithmetic problems, sounds, and shocks. Change in heart rate, serving as a measure for anxiety, was independent of birth rank.

Waiting for Sensory Deprivation. A pilot study by Dohrenwend et al. (1967) was taken up by Suedfeld (1968, 1969) and Zuckerman et al. (1968), who gave a stress scale and an anxiety checklist to male student volunteers waiting for sensory deprivation. There was no difference for birth rank in scores on arrival and after the experiment.

Pretest and Test Anxiety. A sample of female high school students under the impression of having to pass an important test indicated their anxiety on a scale. There was no significant association of anxiety with birth rank (Yaryan et al. 1961). The same result was found in male and female volunteers expecting to undergo an experiment unknown to them (Jacoby 1968).

First- and laterborn male college students with varying scores for previously measured test anxiety learned a series of words under the impression of taking an intelligence test. Among those with high test anxiety, firstborns did more poorly than laterborns (Sarason 1969).

Sensitivity to Pain. Schachter (1959) reports that when shocks of increasing intensity were given to female students, firstborns told the experimenter to stop before maximum intensity was reached significantly more often than laterborns. The same result is reported for a similar sample by Nisbett et al. (1966) and Nisbett (1968). On the other hand, no difference in pain sensitivity by birth order was found in female nursing students tested with an ultrasonic apparatus (Gelfand 1962).

Readiness to Take Risks. Alberts et al. (1977) found in a very small sample of 6- to 7-year-old children that secondborns were more ready to jump from heights of up to 1.8 m than firstborns. A larger sample of 10- to 12-year-old school children were tested with games of hazard. First-, middle-, and lastborns were matched across groups for sex, age, and social class. Risk taking was not associated with birth order but increased with sibship size (Jamieson 1969). No association of birth order with risk taking was found in college students who chose whether to solve a difficult problem for more or an easier problem for less money (Hartnett 1971). A similar situation was presented to male and female Israeli adolescents. In those who had grown up in a kibbutz risk taking was not associated with birth rank. In a city group, however, firstborns and only children were more cautious than laterborns (Weller et al. 1976 a).

Conclusions (Table 18)

There is no evidence that in experimental settings supposed to arouse fear, firstborns are more anxious. There is, on the other hand, some evidence that sensitivity to pain is higher and inclination to take risks lower in first- than in laterborns. This could well be a spurious finding due to the firstborn bias for smaller sibships and the differences in family background this represents (see p. 12).

In previously reported studies it was found that in college and university women, fear decreased with sibship size (see p. 81). In the Willem et al. (1972) study middle children, biased for larger sibships, were the least anxious. In addition, reporting pain in an experimental setting was related to smaller sibships (see p. 81), while, on the other hand, Jamieson (1969) reports an association of risk-taking with large sibship size.

Table 18. Experimental studies on fear, sensitivity to pain, and readiness to take risks

Author	*N*	Sex	Firstborns more anxious
Waiting for or readiness to undergo electrical shock			
Schachter (1959)	62	Females	+
Weller (1962)	234	Females	–
Darley (1966)	78	Females	–
Willems et al. (1972)	118	Females	–
Eisenmann (1965)	38	Females	+
Staples et al. (1961)	64	Females	–
McDonald (1969, 1970)	70	Males, females	–
	149	Males, females	–
Performance and heart rate under stress			
Landers et al. (1971)	122	Males	+ (two of five trials)
Weiss (1970)	29	Males	–
Pretest and preexperimental anxiety			
Suedfeld (1968, 1969)	40	Males	–
Zuckerman et al. (1968)	40	Males	–
Yaryan et al. (1968)	60	Females	–
Jacoby (1968)	120	Males, females	–
Sarason (1969)	80	Males	+ (interaction with test anxiety)
Sensitivity to pain			
Schachter (1959)	115	Females	+
Gelfand (1962)	62	Females	–
Nisbett et al. (1966) Nisbett (1968)	59	?	+
Readiness to take risks			
Alberts et al. (1977)	24	Males, females	+
Jamieson (1969)	84	Males, females	–
Hartnett (1971)	240	Males, females	–
Weller et al. (1976a)	375	Males, females	+ (city youths only)

Schachter (1959, p. 55) describes laterborns within his rather small female student sample as follows: "There is good evidence that subjects from large families are more frequently from rural background than subjects from small families... It is conceivable that subjects from rural and relatively poor homes are simply tougher and more impervious to the brand of threat implied in the experimental manipulation." Also, the author found that laterborns reported more experience with electrical current than firstborns.

By summarily comparing first- with laterborns, differences between families are lost. The results of these experiments cannot be accepted as pointing to an association of more fear under threat, higher sensitivity to pain, and lower risk taking with birth order.

7.6.2.2 Paper-Pencil Tests

Child Samples. A checklist of fears was given to a population of third and sixth graders in Florida. Higher social class was associated with a greater number of political fears. Accordingly first- and last borns (biased for smaller sibship size) held more political fears than middleborns (Catlin 1972). On a death anxiety scale given to ninth graders from various schools in Florida, oldest and youngest children reported more anxiety than intermediates (Iammarino 1975).

In the following four samples sibship size was controlled. In a large population of first graders (Miller et al. 1976) two anxiety scales were not related to birth rank when sibship size, sex, and race were controlled. A sample of male and female fourth to sixth graders with one or two sibs from 14 schools in Ohio gave inconsistent results for birth rank on an anxiety scale (Rosenberg et al. 1964b). In a sample of 251 male and female high school students with one sib, differences between first- and secondborns on a similar scale were not significant (Sampson 1962; Sampson et al. 1967).

Two authors controlled for social class. A sample of 10- to 11-year-old Edinburgh school boys answered a personality questionnaire. Among middle-class boys, laterborns were higher on an anxiety factor than firstborns. In the skilled and the unskilled working class, first- and laterborns were not significantly different, but only children were highest (Robertson 1971). An increase of test anxiety with birth rank was found in a small sample of middle-class 8- to 10-year-old schoolboys (Bartlett et al. 1966). Sibship size was not controlled.

Koch (1957a) gives *teachers' ratings* for fear and shyness of 5- to 6-year-old boys with one sib. Differences were inconsistent and related to sex of sib and spacing.

College and University Samples. The following studies found no difference in anxiety as measured with questionnaires and rating scales in samples of, in most cases, several hundred subjects and controlling for sex: Schachter (1957, p. 65), Sampson (1962), Rosenfeld (1966), Farley (1967), Karabenikc (1971), Bronzaft (1972), Longstreth (1970), and Wudel et al. (1979). Mealiea et al. (1973) gave Wolpe's fear survey to female students. Total fear was not associated with birth order. In sibships of two, however, firstborns indicated extreme fear concerning more items than secondborns. In opposition to Iammarino's result (see p. 103), Eckstein et al. (1979) found less conscious concern about death in firstborns than in other birth ranks.

Nonstudent Adult Samples. No association of anxiety with birth rank was found in 184 teachers tested with the MMPI anxiety scale (Witchell 1966), and 205 adults studied with a manifest anxiety scale (Eisenmann 1968a). In 160 outpatients, the scores of first- and laterborns on an anxiety inventory did not differ (Baar 1977).

Indian Samples. In 80 secondary school students of both sexes, firstborns scored higher on an anxiety scale (George et al. 1971). The same result was found in 200 college students (Prasad Singh 1972) but was not confirmed in a sample of 144 secondary school girls (Jawa 1973) or in 135 7- to 8-year-olds (Bharathi et al. 1976).

Conclusions (Table 19)

Table 19. Birth order an anxiety measured by questionnaires and scales

Author	*N*	Age	Social class controlled	Sibship size controlled	Highest anxiety
Child samples					
Catlin (1972)	1,176	Third, sixth grades	+	–	Firstborns, lastborns
Iammarino (1975)	249	Ninth grade (males, females)	–	–	Firstborns, lastborns
Miller et al. (1976)	1,750	First grade (males, females)	–	+	–
Rosenberg et al. (1964)	352	Fourth to sixth grades (males, females)	–	+	–
Sampson (1962) Sampson et al. (1967)	251	High school (males, females)	–	+	–
Bartlett et al. (1968)	31	8–10 years (males)	+	–	Laterborns
Robertson (1971)	297	10–11 years (males)	+	–	Laterborns (interaction with social class)
Koch (1957)	192	5–6 years	–	+	(teacher's ratings)
College and university student samples					
Schachter (1957) Sampson (1962) Rosenfeld (1966) Farley (1967) Karabenick (1971) Bronzaft (1972) Longstreth (1970) Wudel et al. (1979)	Several	hundred	–	–	–

Table 19. (continued)

Author	N	Age	Social class controlled	Sibship size controlled	Highest anxiety
Mealia et al. (1973)	148	College (females)	–	+	Firstborns (extreme fear)
Eckstein et al.	118	Undergraduates	–	–	Middle-lastborns
Adult samples Witchell (1966) Eisenman (1968 a) Baar (1977)					–
Four Indian samples		6 years to college age			Firstborns (two samples)

The evidence (Table 19) is against firstborns reporting themselves as more anxious than laterborns.

7.6.2.3 Behavior in Real-Life Situations

As in the experimental studies, fear of bodily harm is investigated.

Children in Medical Settings. In four studies small groups of preschool and elementary school children being left by their mother or having to undergo frightening procedures in hospital were observed. Collard (1968) found that 9- to 12-month-old firstborns cried more when being left by the mother than laterborns of the same age. Vernon et al. (1967) studied the reaction of 2- to 5-year-old children to admission procedures and anesthesia induction: First- and laterborns did not differ, regardless of whether they were in company of their mother or alone. Observing 4- to 9-year-olds being given injections, Vernon (1974) found firstborns to be slightly more upset before, but not after, the injection.

In a much quoted study De Fee et al. (1969) had 146 5- to 10-year-old children of sibships sizes 1–3 rated for anxiety during treatment by three dentists, to whom the aim of the investigation was unknown. First and only children appeared very significantly more frightened and uncooperative than laterborns. The selection of the sample is unknown. Age and sex of the children and the treatments they were subjected to were not controlled, though these variables may influence the presence and expression of fear.

University Students' Participation in Dangerous Sports, Behavior of Pilots and Divers. There are several – also very well known – studies that, using the Greenwood-Yule method, found and overrepresentation of laterborns among male university students who participate in dangerous sports, such as American football, soccer, and rugby, and interpret this finding as a consequence of higher fear in firstborns. Yiannakis (1976) did not control for sibship size, while Nisbet (1968) found an increase in participation with sibship size and an overrepresentation of secondborns in comparison with firstborns over all sibship sizes. Casher (1977) found an overrepresentation of thirdborns in a much smaller upper middle class sample. Participation in dangerous sports increases with sibship size and is more frequent among lower class subjects (Nisbett 1968, McPherson 1978). Though the birth order distribution varies with social class, none of these studies used a control group comparable for background.

Among a very small sample of successful war pilots, Torrance (1954) found a smaller number of firstborns than among less successful ones. Helmreich (1968) measured diving time outside a capsule in a group of divers: firstborns stayed outside for less time than laterborns. Though these results are methodically more than questionable and have never been reproduced, they are still influential. They are in opposition to the Reinhardt (1970) result, where Firstborns prevailed among outstanding jet pilots and astronauts.

Reaction to a Catastrophe. Passersby on the morning after the 1965 New York blackout were questioned on perceived anxiety. Firstborns reported slightly more fear than laterborns (Zucker et al. 1968). A similar study was carried out with a larger sample of undergraduates after the Los Angeles earthquake of 1971. Firstborn females and laterborn males reported more fear than laterborn females and firstborn males (Hoyt et al. 1973.

Conclusions (Table 20)

Table 20. Birth order and fear in real-life situations

Author	*N*	Age	Control for social class	Control for sibship size	Greatest fear
Children					
Collard (1948)	18	9–12 months	–	–	Firstborns
Vernon et al. (1967)	?	2–5 years	–	–	–
Vernon (1974)	20	4–9 years	–	–	Firstborns (one situation in two)
De Fee et al. (1969)	146	5–10 years	–	–	Firstborns (only children included)
Nisbett (1968)	2,410	(males)	–	+	Firstborns
	494	(males)	–	+	Firstborns
Yiannakis (1976)	166	(males)	–	–	Firstborns
Casher (1977)	127	(university males)	+	+	Firstborns, secondborns
Hoyt et al. (1973)	428	(males, females)	–	–	Firstborn females, laterborn males
Reinhardt (1970)	23	(astronauts)	–	–	Laterborns
	105	(jetpilots)	–	–	Laterborns
Torrance (1954)	31	(pilots)	–	–	Firstborns
Helmreich (1968)	28	(divers)	–	–	Firstborns
Zucker et al. (1968)	100		–	–	Firstborns

There is some evidence (see pp. 81, 102) that fearlessness and daring behavior are positively correlated with sibship size. On the other hand, the ability and readiness to express the anxiety that was felt during a catastrophe may be higher in persons from smaller families, and smaller and larger families represent different backgrounds. The studies cited here suffer from a conspicuous lack of methodological sophistication. Either they ignore possible between-group differences or, when birth order is the dependent variable, they do not use control groups. Thus they cannot be taken as evidence for greater fear or anxiety in firstborns. Greater anxiety in firstborns up to 2 years of age fits well with the formerly presented data on their dethronement, but the samples are very small.

7.6.2.4 Birth Order and Guilt Feelings

In their study of 379 5- to 6-year-old children (see p. 87), Sears et al. (1957) reported that firstborns, according to their mothers, more readily admitted to faults than laterborns. When, however, 166 of these children were followed-up at age 12 (Sears 1970) and completed scales of self-criticism, self-aggression, and ideas of reference, self-criticism was significantly lower in first- than in laterborns in both sexes, while there were no differences on the two other scales. Sixty female college students were given a guilt inventory (Ray et al. 1973): First- and only-borns were overrepresented among high guilt subjects, who also reported higher grades and going to church more often than low-guilt subjects. On the other hand, on three guilt scales given to a sample of 126 college students, laterborns were found highest in one, while scores on the others were not correlated to birth rank (Welch 1977).

The evidence is inconsistent. Expressed guilt feelings may depend on religious denomination and other background variables, which should be controlled when birth order differences in guilt feelings are investigated.

7.6.2.5 Summary of Research on Birth Order and Anxiety

Experimental studies and paper-pencil tests give no consistent evidence for greater fear or anxiety in firstborns. The studies based on real-life behavior that find firstborns to be more fearful of bodily harm are methodologically inadequate.

7.6.3 Birth Order and the Disposition to Associate

The hypotheses discussed here stem from Schachter's (1959) theory that because firstborns are closer to the mother in early childhood than laterborns, they will, when anxious or fearful, tend to reduce fear by affiliation, i.e., by seeking out the companionship of others. Further, because of inconsistent treatment and strong adult-relatedness, firstborns' dependency and conformity are believed to be enhanced (see p. 86). Thus in this section, constructs such as dependency, conformity, ease of influence, and suggestibility are discussed. Few authors have taken pains to define clearly, separate, and contrast these concepts (De Avila 1971). Therefore, the neutral expression "disposition to associate" is used to include all of them. As in the previous section, investigations are classified according to method.

7.6.3.1 Experimental Studies

These are discussed according to the pressure put on the subjects, which should make firstborns seek contact with other persons. The survey begins with observations of spontaneous play and ends with studies of affiliation while waiting for an elctrical shock. Several of these studies have been analyzed and criticized for statistical reasons by De Avila (1971).

Ratings of Play Behavior

Seeking Contact with Adults. According to two unpublished theses (Gewirtz 1948; Beller 1948), among a small sample of kindergarten children, firstborns and only children were rated somewhat higher on seeking help and contact from adults than laterborns (Schachter 1959, p. 85; Sutton-Smith et al. 1970, pp. 97–98). In a similar experimental setting (McGurk et al. 1972) among kindergarten children, secondborns were higher than first- or laterborns on seeking help, approval, and affection from adults. In an experimental study involving a larger sample of 8–24-month-old children from seven Israeli kibbutzim, firstborns protested more than laterborns at any departure of their mothers or of other known and unknown persons. The sample was stratified for age, sex, and social class (Fox 1976).

Solitary Play. There are four studies on this subject. One (Clark et al. 1969) found firstborn kindergarten children spending more time alone than laterborns. In two other samples this was true only for boys (Laosa et al. 1970, 1972). In a third investigation no such difference was found between first- and laterborns, and firstborns did not seek out adults more often (Moore et al. 1974).

Various Experimental Measures of the Tendency to Associate

Attraction to Others. The following studies were each carried out with 100–200 psychology students. One male and female sample had to chose between doing an experiment in company or alone. Choice was not related to birth rank (Brock et al. 1965). Other male and female subjects were presented faked measures of social desirability in supposed strangers and each subject scored his or her attraction to this stranger. There were sex differences, but no consistent differences for birth rank in attraction (Nowicky 1971). Among male and female students who wrote down their most recent dream, firstborn males reported more positive interaction than laterborn males. There was no difference among females (Ward et al. 1973).

Associating Under Conditions of Intellectual Incertitude. In the four following studies the hypothesis was tested that under the stress of uncertitude firstborns will rather seek information (i.e. associate) more frequently than laterborns.

In an influential investigation, Radloff (1961) used a large sample of female students, who discussed a problem in groups under differential conditions of supplementary information. The difference in wishing for more discussion was larger for firstborns than for laterborns when both birth ranks were confronted either with no information or with information by an expert. Three other studies with similarly sophisticated experimental situations did not find significant differences between first- and laterborns in information-seeking (Singer et al. 1965, Gordon 1966, Hamilton 1950).

Conformity to Rules in a Moral Dilemma. These studies test the hypothesis that under the pressure of a moral dilemma firstborns will associate in the sense of conforming to the general moral law.

A large sample of Canadian boys from kindergarten to third grade were presented with two toys, one to play with and one not to be touched. Subjects then saw a boy playing with either the forbidden or the allowed toy on television. A control group saw no television. The subjects were then left alone and watched through a one-way screen. Firstborns and only children were significantly more influenced by the conforming model than laterborns, while behavior without a model or in the "nonconforming model situation" was not associated with birth rank (Finley et al. 1976).

Three studies investigated cheating at school. No birth order differences were found in a group of ghetto fifth graders (David 1973), while more cheating was found in firstborns than in laterborns among male and female college students (Hetherington et al. 1964). In a small sample of college females, firstborns cheated less than laterborns when expecting a control, but more so when feeling safe (Singer et al. 1966).

A group of male student volunteers were pledged not to discuss an experiment they had participated in. After 1 week a questionnaire was given as to how many persons subjects had spoken to about the experiment: Firstborns indicated fewer than laterborns (Wuebben 1967).

Effectiveness of Reinforcement. Here the hypothesis is examined that firstborns, given their stronger need to associate, will be more susceptible to reinforcement.

Three authors used a "marble-in-the-hole" game to study reinforcement effectiveness in 5- to 8-year-old children. In two studies (Gilmore et al. 1964; Unruh et al. 1971) firstborns played longer when not reinforced, and laterborns when reinforced. In a third study, using a sample of 144 subjects homogeneous for sex, social class, and sibship size (Yando et al. 1975), there was no birth order difference for effectiveness of reinforcement. A study investigating effectiveness of aversive stimuli in 80 14- to 16-year-old boys indicated that firstborns are more easily conditioned (La Voie 1973).

Interviews were conducted with university students under conditions of either reinforcement by nodding at positive or negative statements or nodding at random. The same design was used for 40 subjects who each came for six interviews. In both settings reinforcement effectiveness was independent of birth order (Babladelis 1972). When male students were given a learning task with reinforcement consisting either in approval or in being shown the correctly guessed card, firstborns gave better results than laterborns under social reinforcement (Hines 1973).

Conclusions (Table 21)

There is no evidence that the experimental settings described elicit a higher tendency to associate in firstborns. At kindergarten age they seek adult

Table 21. Birth order and various experimental measures of the disposition to associate

Author	*N*	Age	Social class controlled	Sibship size controlled	Highest score
Seeking contact with adults					
Gerwirtz (1968) Beller (1948)	42	Kindergarten	–	–	Firstborns, only children
McGurk et al. (1972)	52	Kindergarten	–	–	Secondborns
Fox (1976) (mother)	122	8–24 months	+	–	Firstborns
Solitary play					
Clark et al. (1969)	40	Kindergarten	–	–	Laterborns
Laosa et al. (1970)	96	Kindergarten	–	–	Laterborns (males)
Laosa et al. (1972)	93	Kindergarten	–	–	Laterborns (males)
Moore et al. (1974)	116	Kindergarten	–	–	–
Attraction to others					
Brock et al. (1965)	110	College (males, females)	–	–	–
Nowicky (1971)	202	College (males, females)	–	–	–
Ward et al. (1973)	179	College (males, females)	–	–	Firstborns (males)
Associating under intellectual incertitude					
Radloff (1961)	480	College (females)	–	–	Firstborns
Singer et al. (1965)	37	College (females)	–	–	–
Gordon (1966)	79	College (males, females)	–	–	–
Hamilton (1950)	192	College	–	–	–
Conformity in moral dilemma					
Finley et al. (1976)	390	Kindergarten	–	–	Firstborns, only children
David (1973)	79	Fifth grade (males, females)	+	–	–
Singer et al. (1966)	39	College (females)	–	–	Laterborns
Wuebben (1967)	113	University (males)	–	–	Firstborns
Hetherington et al. (1964)	78	College (males)	–	–	Laterborns

Table 21 (continued)

Author	N	Age	Social class controlled	Sibship size controlled	Highest score
Effectiveness of reinforcement					
Gilmore et al. (1964)	40	5–8 years	–	–	Laterborns
Unruh et al. (1971)	144	5–8 years	–	–	Laterborns
Yando et al. (1975)	144	5–8 years	+	+	–
La Voie (1973)	80	14–16 years (males)	–	–	Firstborns
Babladelis (1972)	124	College	–	–	–
	40	College	–	–	–
Hines (1973)	40	College (males)	–	–	Firstborns (only under social reinforcement)

contact more frequently, but they also play alone more often than laterborns. For all other settings and for later ages there is no difference by birth rank in the tendency to associate.

Asch-Type Situation and Modifications

Seeking the Company of Others When Apparently Wrong (Conformity). The Asch-Type Situation

The Asch-Type Situation

In the classical Asch-type experiment (Ruch 1975) subjects in groups compare lines of different lengths to a standard line. The task is so conceived, that under normal conditions no more than about 1% of the comparisons are erroneous. In the Asch-Type situation all group members except one are instructed to give wrong answers. In this situation usually 30% of the noninstructed group members are influenced by the opinion of the group and make mistakes. More of females tend to be influenced by group opinion than males. The following studies test the hypothesis that firstborns will be more open to group influences than laterborns.

Child Samples. Becker et al. (1962, 1964, 1966) studied small samples of elementary- and high-school boys with the classical Asch setting. Firstborns yielded more to group pressure than laterborns, even when motivation was enhanced by the introduction of monetary rewards for guessing correctly. When, however, lines were compared retrospectively by memory, firstborns yielded less.

Another Asch situation was created for sixth graders, who selected stories to fit a given picture. Under this condition firstborn males conformed more than laterborns, while there was no difference for females (Carrigan et al. 1966). When first- and secondborn male fifth and sixth graders (sibship size and number of subjects not specified) rated the number of concentric circles on posters while an adult encouraged or discouraged conformity to false peer norms, yielding was independent of birth rank (Katz 1973). In a German sample of male sixth, seventh, and eighth graders, estimating dots on tablets was most influenced by replies of other subjects in middle children (Langenmayr 1976), while firstborns were least influenced. Among male high school juniors firstborns yielded more than laterborns to group pressure (kind of experiment not specified) (Purpura 1971).

In three studies there was some control of background variables. A population of first graders did not differ in yielding to peer pressure by birth rank when sex and race were controlled (Miller et al. 1976). Rhine (1968, 1969, 1974) gave female firth and sixth graders the task of counting metronome clicks under group pressure, in one condition as a game and in the other as an achievement test. In the game condition, but not in the achievement condition, middle-class firstborns yielded more than laterborns. Among lower-class subjects there was no difference by birth rank. One study controlled for sibship size: Sampson et al. (1967) and Hancock (1967) studied all students from one high school with one sib. Firstborn males yielded more to group norms in estimating length of lines than laterborns, while females did not differ by birth order.

College Student Samples. A problem was given to male college students who chose a solution from a list. Each subject was then told that his solution was deviant and he was asked to consider the problem again. More firstborns than laterborns gave another solution after reconsideration (Ehrlich 1958). This experiment was reproduced with female undergraduates (Arrowood et al. 1965), and firstborns again changed their solution more often than laterborns. Among a small sample of male students who counted metronome clicks and heard prerecorded voices giving incorrect results, there was no difference in yielding for birth rank (Masling 1965). The same negative result was found by Moore (1964) in an Asch-type situation concerning judgements on case studies and in an autokinetic experiment with male students.

Resistance to a leader was measured by Sampson (1962). In one study female subjects discussed a political issue, while a hired assistant tried to influence the debate with assumed expertise. Resistance to the expert was measured by the difference in attraction felt for him before and after the experiment. Firstborns were, nonsignificantly, more resistant. In the same study recruits drew circles and performance was evaluated by a group leader who either fined them for not increasing production or gave them a reward for increasing it. Then the subject evaluated his production himself. Resistance to the leader was measured by the discrepancy between the leader's and the subject's evaluations. In the reward condition firstborns tended to deviate less from the leader than laterborns.

Resistance to an accomplice was measured by Steiner et al. (1966) in 61 male college students who answered multiple choice questions after hearing the (partially wrong) answers of a student accomplice. Firstborns tended to conform less than laterborns.

Adult Samples. A sample of adults (up to 50 years of age) taking college courses did not differ in yielding during an Asch-type situation by birth rank (Eisenmann 1968 a). A group of firemen solved some technical problems, discussed them in their firestation group, and then considered them again. Firstborns adapted their solution to the group opinion more often than laterborns. A greater number of the former were, however, in official leadership positions (Smith et al. 1963).

Conforming Under Fear to the Opinion of a Majority. In the following studies pressure on subjects in an Asch-type situation was heightened by threat. Staples et al. (1961) tested female college students in an autokinetic situation and found that firstborns responded more quickly than laterborns to the suggestion that a light was going to move. Subjects then had to judge the distance the light had moved. In the no-fear condition the experimenter gave a random correction to each answer. In the fear condition the experimenter did the same and added a threat of electrical shock for mistakes in further trials. Under the fear condition, firstborns adapted their judgement significantly more to the experimenters' suggestions than laterborns. Darley (1966) threatened female students with either painless or painful electrical shocks and then produced an Asch-type situation where subjects counted metronome clicks while hearing wrong answers. Readiness to change opinion was not related to birth rank.

A sample of naval recruits were given a questionnaire on a military problem. For half of the subjects a fear condition was created by announcing gas exercises after the experiment. After having filled out the questionnaire an expert opinion was given to the subjects, who then reconsidered their answers. Change of attitude was significantly more frequent in those subjected to the fear condition. Laterborns under fear tended to change their opinion more often than firstborns (Helmreich et al. 1968). A similar experiment was given to male and female college students. After answering a questionnaire on a scientific problem, two fear conditions were created by announcing either a painless or a painful experiment. Subjects then read an article on the problem and reconsidered their answers. Among males under the fear condition, laterborns changed their opinion more often than firstborns: Under the nonfear condition the correlation was reversed. In females there was no difference by birth rank (Hendrick et al. 1970).

Conclusions (Table 22)

There are ten samples of elementary and high school pupils, and in three of the six male samples, firstborns more readily changed their opinion under group pressure than laterborns. This is also true of the one female sample. In three mixed samples, male firstborns again changed their opinion more readily than laterborns in two instances, while there was no difference for females. In five male college student samples, firstborns yielded more in two instances, and so did female firstborns in one of two female samples.

Table 22. Birth order and reaction to an Asch-type situation (A) and birth order and conforming under fear (B)

Author	*N*	Firstborns more conforming
A *Children*		
Male samples		
Becker et al. (1962)	30	+
Becker et al. (1964)	36	+
Becker et al. (1966)	48	– (Laterborns higher)
Purpura (1971)	311	+
Katz (1973)	?	–
Langenmayr (1976)	286	– (Middle children higher)
Female sample		
Rhine (1968, 1969, 1974)	128	+ (Interaction with condition and social class)
Mixed samples		
Carrigan et al. (1966)	96	+ (Males only)
Miller et al. (1976)	1,750	–
Sampson (1967)	251	+ (Males only)
College students		
Male samples		
Ehrlich (1958)	134	+
Sampson et al. (1962)	116	+ (Interaction with condition)
Masling (1968)	44	–
Steiner et al. (1966)	61	–
Moore (1964)	80	–
Female sample		
Arrowood et al. (1965)	92	+
Sampson et al. (1962)	68	–
Adults		
Male samples		
Smith et al. (1963)	153	+ (Inequality in leadership position)
Eisenmann (1968 a)	205	–
B *College students*		
Female samples		
Staples et al. (1961)	64	+
Darley (1966)	64	–
Mixed sample		
Hendrich et al. (1970)	48	– (Laterborn males higher)
Recruits		
Helmreich et al. (1964)	258	– (Laterborns higher)

Among two adult samples yielding was higher in firstborn males in one instance, but this finding should be considered with reserve. In by far the largest sample, no birth rank differences in yielding were found (Miller et al.).

Since Table 22 shows the experiments according to the age of subjects, it becomes apparent that greater conformity of firstborn males is only found in children and is missing in the one large sample where at least race was controlled. However, when conformity under threat of bodily pain is measured, there is no evidence that firstborns conform more than laterborns. This corresponds to the fact that the evidence for their greater fear of bodily harm is also insufficient (see p. 106 f.).

There are no data on Asch-type conforming and sibship size. We will accept the evidence that, in this particular situation, *males at elementary and high school age conform more when firstborn*, keeping in mind that this result may be due to failure to control background variables.

Seeking the Company of Others when in a State of Fear (Affiliation)

Schachter's Classical Experiment

Schachter (1959) has been extremely influential in birth order research with the following experimental setting: In 108 female psychology students a high-anxiety condition was created by announcing painful electrical shocks and a low-anxiety condition by announcing painless shocks. As measured by an anxiety scale and refusal to continue, there were 76 truly anxious subjects. All subjects chose between waiting alone or with others for the shock treatment. Among the 76 truly anxious subjects firstborns wanted to wait with others highly significantly more often than laterborns. There was no difference in subjects with low anxiety. Schachter did not consider sibship size an important variable in this context, though the proportion of anxious subjects decreased with growing sibship size, as did the proportion of anxious subjects who wanted to wait together. The study had other failings (besides using very small subgroups) that were discussed by Doren (1972). For example, subjects who answered "don't care" to the question of whether they wished to wait alone were united with the subjects who wanted to wait alone (Gerard et al. 1961).

Replications of the Schachter Experiment

The replications and modifications have almost exclusively used subjects from college and university: either psychology students or volunteers. In one study (Gerard et al. 1961) anxiety was measured by skin conductance. Firstborns females were more afraid than laterborns and, when afraid, wanted to wait with others significantly more often. As there were very few males, results were not significant. Two other replications with male (Zimbardo et al. 1963) and female (Darley et al. 1966) subjects confirmed Schachter's results. Then a series of studies with negative results followed: Haywood (1969); Barthell (1971); and Willems et al. (1972) with female and MacDonald (1970) with male subjects.

Modifications of Schachter's Experiment

Various Procedures for Anxiety Arousal. Two authors tried to differentiate anxiety (with situations connotating shame or embarrassment) from fear (with situations of potential danger). Sarnoff et al. (1961) announced to male subjects either painful or painless shocks or having to suck pacifiers or neutral objects. Firstborns wanted to wait more often with others than did laterborns only under the fear condition.

Navar et al. (1971) substituted looking at pictures of nudes for sucking pacifiers and found no difference by birth order for waiting alone or with others in female subjects.

In two studies induced fear was combined with negative or positive faked personality diagnoses (an ethically questionable procedure). In a high school sample wanting to wait with others was independent of sex, faked diagnosis, and birth rank (Miller et al. 1966), while in a naval recruit sample subjects with a negative diagnosis in combination with a low score on a self-esteem measure more often chose to wait in company rather than alone for a "stress test" if firstborn (Sterner 1973).

Various Procedures for Measuring Affiliation. Weller (1964) and Latane et al. (1966) studied the expressed liking for a companion among college females threatened with painful or painless shocks. Results were inconsistent. Ring et al. (1965) exposed female college students to contact with an associate either mimicking fear of a forthcoming experiment or remaining silent. Firstborns perceived themselves as reacting more strongly to the associate than laterborns, but as growing more anxious when waiting in a group. Thus they appeared at the same time easier to influence but less able to overcome stress through affiliation.

Choise of Working Condition Under Anxiety. A sample of psychology students (Becker 1967) chose whether to participate in an experiment on pain tolerance alone or with another subject: Decision was related to sex, but not to birth rank. In two samples of male high school students, three conditions of anxiety were created by announcing painful or painless shock or no shock. First- and laterborns did not differ in wanting to solve problems during waiting alone or in groups (Helmreich et al. 1968).

Effect of Waiting Condition on Reported Fear. An anxiety scale was given to male and female students who were made to believe that they were going to receive an intravenous injection; the subjects were then assigned to wait in a small group or alone. After a few minutes of waiting, anxiety was measured again. Firstborns but not laterborns experienced a greater decrease in anxiety when waiting in groups than when waiting alone (Wrightsman 1960).

Other Experimental Settings. Subjects of the following experiment were the student populations of two high schools. They worked on unsolvable arithmetic problems and then completed an anxiety scale. Birth rank, anxiety level, and number of extracurricular school organizations the students belonged to were correlated. Firstborns who were anxious tended less often to be members of organizations than laterborns who expressed equal anxiety (Robertson et al. 1969).

A sample of male and female college students placed sets of two and three felt figures on a felt background. During the intervals between placing the figures, they either did subtraction at the highest possible speed or were just waiting. Sets of two figures were placed nearer together by firstborns than by laterborns under both conditions. Under the stress condition firstborns placed sets of three figures nearer together than laterborns (Jackson et al. 1977).

In male and female college students made to believe that they were waiting for no shock or for a painless or painful shock, scales for dogmatism and authoritarianism (understood to be measures of conformity) did not vary in either group by birth rank within sex (Jacoby 1967).

Dauphinais et al. (1978) considered readiness to join an encounter group as an indicator of affiliation under anxiety. In a sample of college seniors laterborn males in large sibship most frequently reported readiness.

Two studies were done on children's affiliative tendencies under fear. An anxiety or a nonanxiety condition was created for 6- to 8-year-old boys by having them led to an experiment either by an unknown silent man or by a well-known friendly woman. The effectiveness of reinforcement to continue monotonous play was dependent on the anxiety condition, but not on birth rank (Walters et al. 1960). On the evening before entering a hospital for minor surgery, 4- to 9-year-old children were shown a movie with either a child reacting with some displeasure to an injection or a child reacting indifferently to it. On the next day the child's mood was rated during an injection. Firstborns were not more influenced by the movie than laterborns (Vernon 1974).

Conclusions (Table 23)

Table 23. Classical Schachter-Type experiments and modifications

Author	*N*	Sex	Firstborns higher in affiliation
Gerard et al. (1961)	100	Females, males	+ (Females only)
Zimbardo et al. (1963)	99	Males	+
Darley et al. (1966)	78	Females	+
Haywood (1969)	80	Females	–
MacDonald (1970)	149	Females, males	–
Barthell (1971)	?	Females	–
Willems et al. (1972)	118	Females	–
Modifications			
Sarnoff et al. (1961)	72	Males	+ (Fear only, not anxiety)
Navar et al. (1971)	101	Females	–
Miller et al. (1966)	132	Females, males	–
Sterner (1973)	101	Males	+ (Interactions with two conditions)
Weller (1964)	234	Females	– (Laterborns higher)
Latane et al. (1966)	58	Females	+
Ring et al. (1965)	96	Females	+ (Increasing fear in company)
Becker (1967)	821	Females, males	–
Helmreich et al. (1968)	61	Males	–
	122	Males	–
Wrightsman (1960)	204	Females, males	+
Robertson et al. (1969)	1,009	Females, males	–
Jackson et al. (1977)	96	Females, males	+ (Interaction with number of figures)
Jacoby (1967)	120	Females, males	–
Dauphinais et al. (1978)	83	Females, males	– (Male laterborns higher)
Walters et al. (1960)	40	Males	–
Vernon (1974)	30	Females, males	–

These 23 studies involved 24 samples varying in size from 30 to 1,009 subjects. Seven were based on Schachter's classical experiment. His result (stronger need to associate in firstborns when under fear) was reproduced in three. Seventeen experiments were modifications of the Schachter setting; Schachter's result was reproduced in three. In another two Schachter's result was found only in interaction with highly specified conditions, i.e., concurrence of low self-esteem and a negative personality diagnosis (Sterner) and when a three-figure set rather than a two-figure set was used (Jackson et al. 1977). A sixth study gave a contradictory result. On the other hand, among the 11 experiments failing to support the hypothesis, there were three studies in which laterborns appeared more affiliative when afraid than firstborns (Weller; Ring et al.; Robertson et al.). We may conclude that there is no evidence that firstborns affiliate more than laterborns when in a state of fear.

7.6.3.2 Summary of the Experimental Studies on the Tendency to Associate

There is slight evidence (mainly found without control of sibship size) that male firstborns at elementary and high school age more readily change their opinion in an Asch-type situation than laterborns, but not so when afraid. On the other hand, firstborns do not differ in terms of conformity to moral rules, in conditionability, and in conforming to or associating with others when under conditions of fear. While firstborns seek more adult contact at an early age, they also play more often alone.

7.6.3.3 Experiments on Visual Field Independence

The following two experimental settings measure the ability to ignore distracting visual cues as a measure of field independence. The rod and frame test consist in having the subject place an illuminated rod vertically within a frame in a darkened room. Scores are positively correlated to nonverbal IQ and to resistance to persuasion by others and negatively to scores on social desirability (Roodin et al. 1974). Males score higher on field independence than females (Maccoby et al. 1975). In the embedded figure test the subject has to recognize a hidden "gestalt," ignoring the visual field it is presented in. Scores are positively related to IQ (Buros 1972, p. 54). The following studies tested the hypothesis that firstborns, because of their supposed insecurity caused by inconsistent parental treatment, are also more field dependent.

Rod and Frame Test

Six studies have come to our notice where visual field dependency of subjects of different birth rank was measured with the rod and frame test. In three of them no difference was found between first- and laterborns (Culver et al. 1969; Sherman 1974; Roodin et al. 1974). Two studies compared only children with firstborns

(Kinsolving et al. 1971; Andrews et al. 1974) and obtained divergent results. Another study included 673 consecutive psychiatric inpatient admissions up to 65 years of age. Firstborns were found to be less dependent than laterborns and only children. This finding is not surprising when one considers the correlation of field independence with nonverbal IQ and the latter's association with sibship size, age, and social class (Reighard et al. 1973).

The Embedded Figure Test

Child Samples. In four studies on elementary and high school students which involved samples of varying size – one, an entire population of first graders – no birth rank differences in scores were found (Miller et al. 1976; Finley et al. 1975; McDonagh 1971; Roach 1980); on the other hand, visual field dependence was associated with being female, having a lower IQ, and a lower level of paternal education.

Adult Samples. Three of four studies on college students did not demonstrate a firstborn-laterborn difference (Culver et al. 1969; Simon et al. 1971 b; Andrews et al. 1974). One found firstborn middle-class males with at least two sibs to be more field dependent than comparable lastborns (Stewart 1967). In his nationally representative sample of 3,101 American men in civilian occupations, Schooler (1972 a, b, c) found that sibship size had a very slight, but significant, positive correlation with field dependence when seven psychosocial variables were controlled. However, effects of birth order on field dependence were negligible (see p. 82).

Conclusions

There is no evidence that firstborns are more field-dependent than laterborns.

7.6.3.4 Paper-Pencil Tests

The Marlowe-Crowne Test for Social Desirability

Measures of social desirability consist in saying "true" or "false" to culturally approved statements which are untrue for virtually all people (e.g., "Before voting I investigate carefully the qualifications of all candidates"). Tests for social desirability measure socially recognized attitudes. According to the hypothesis (see p. 86), firstborns would be expected to be more conforming and conservative than laterborns.

College Student Samples. The following studies summarily compared scores of first- and laterborns. Higher scores in both male and female firstborns were found by Olson (1969) and Johnson (1973) and in female firstborns of a mixed sample by Moran (1967). Walker et al. (1967), Karabenick (1971), Becker (1970) in four samples, MacDonald (1971 b) in two samples, and Macbeth (1975) in two samples found either no difference in social desirability by birth rank, higher scores in laterborns or nonreproducible results.

One author differentiated between first-, middle-, and lastborns and found that among females first- and middleborns scored highest, while among males there were no differences (Nowicki 1971). In three studies there was control for sibship size. Owyang (1971) compared a small sample of males and females with one sib and found no difference between first- and secondborns within sex. Two authors controlled sibship size in larger samples (Masterson 1971; Boor 1972). In the Masterson sample higher social desirability scores were merely found in firstborn females with two sibs. This result does not make sense and was not reproduced in the Boor sample.

Affiliative Needs Measured by the Edward's Personal Preference Schedule (EPPS)

Child Samples. A very slight birth order effect on one of three factors relating to affiliation that were extracted from the EPPS and two other tests was found in a middle-class sample of sixth graders, sex and sibship size being controlled (De Avila 1970). No significant association of birth order with EPPS scores appeared in a large sample of high school students with no or one sib (Hancock 1967; Sampson et al. 1967). In a small and socially in homogeneous sample of male high school students, firstborns expressed stronger affiliative needs on the EPPS than laterborns (Query et al. 1973).

Adult Samples. In two large college populations (Waters et al. 1967; Payne 1971) with control for sibship size no birth order effects on results were found. Krinsky (1963) studied EPPS scores of male graduates who were contacted by mail. Results on four scales connotating affiliation were unrelated to birth order (return rate 50%). In a sample of Antarctic volunteers, birth rank explained 2% of the variance in affiliation needs (Gunderson 1969).

Affiliative Need Measured by the California Psychological Inventory (CPI) and Combinations of Tests (Marlowe Crowne, EPS, CPI)

In two large college and university entrant populations, scores on the CPI scales measuring independence, tolerance, and self-control (Weiss 1966) and socialization, good impression and femininity (Marquette 1972) were not influenced by birth rank.

Macbeth (1975) investigated an annual set of undergraduates in psychology with three measures of affiliative need, two measures of conformity, and four measures of dependency taken from various scales, and tested results on a second large undergraduate sample. With control of sex and sibship size measures of dependency and affiliative need were not influenced by birth order. With regard to conformity, lastborns had the highest and firstborns the lowest scores.

Various Tests and Scales

Of the 11 studies listed in Table 24, three need some explanation. Getzels et al. (1958) studied "socialization" of subjects, scoring differences in the answers given on political and racial issues when the questions were first presented as a verbal speed test and some time later as opinion research. Higher scores were related to being older, female, and upper-middle class. The result was obtained without controlling for age, sex, sibship size, or social class. In the Koenig (1969) study the question "Who am I?" was answered 20 times. Answers of the type "I am a student" were given highly significantly more often by firstborns than by laterborns, as opposed to answers like "I am tall." (One would like to know to what degree giving more general, or, as the author stipulates, more "highly socialized" answers is related to education, social class, and/or IQ.)

Solomon (1977) studied a sample of students coming to a college student mental health clinic. Dependency needs expressed on a questionnaire on patient expectations were less frequent in first- than in laterborns in large sibships. In small sibships the inverse was true.

Affiliative Needs Measured With the TAT (Thematic Apperception Test) and Other Projective Tests)

Among a small sample of volunteers, 16–60 years of age (selection not described), firstborns were highest on affiliative need as measured by the TAT (Dember 1963, 1964). This result was not confirmed by Conners (1963) in a sample of male college students (only children and firstborns were nonsignificantly higher than laterborns) or by Rosenfeld (1966) in five student samples totaling 513 subjects.

Two authors used the Rorschach test to measure oral dependency, which they expected to be higher in firstborns (Masling et al. 1968; McDonagh 1971). The findings did not support the hypothesis. Two authors controlled for sibship size, testing female subjects in sibship of two: In one study (Schmuck 1963) compliance and defiance were measured with pictures similar to the TAT; in the other (Brittain 1966), ninth and tenth graders were given stories to finish to measure compliance with parents and peers. Neither investigation found a difference in scores by birth rank. Nonspecified projective measures were used with 10- and 14-year-old male and female subjects from two cultures and two social classes. Affiliative needs were not related to birth rank (Stenning 1968).

Conclusions (Table 24)

Of 28 samples in which the tendency to associate was measured *with well-known tests and scales*, five indicated a higher social desirability score in firstborns and two more did so in interaction with sex, sibship size, or extracted factors. For one sample higher social desirability scores in laterborns was reported. The largest studies and one using several scales and validating results on a second sample

Table 24. Birth order and affiliation measured by Marlowe-Crowne, EPPS, CPI, and combinations (A) or various other tests and scales (B)

	Author	N	Age	Social class controlled	Sibship size controlled	highest score
A	*Marlowe-Crowne*					
	Moran (1967)	178	College (males, females)	–	–	Firstborn females
	Olson (1969)	320	College (males, females)	–	–	Firstborns
	Johnson (1973)	80	College (males, females)	–	–	Firstborns
	Karabenick (1971)	170	College (males) females)	–	–	–
	Walker et al. (1967)	142	College (males, females)	–	–	–
	MacDonald (1971 b)	768	College (males, females)	–	+	–
		476	College	–	+	–
	Becker (1970)	71	College (males, females)	–	–	–
		256		–	–	–
		100		–	–	Laterborn males
		97		–	–	–
	Macbeth (1975)	716	College (males, females)	–	+	–
		265		–	+	–
	Nowicki (1971)	202	College (males, females)	–	–	First- and middleborn females
	Owyang (1971)	82	College (males, females)	–	+	–
	Masterson (1971)	155	College (males, females)	–	+	Firstborn females (interaction sibship size)
	Boor (1972)	116	College (males, females)	–	+	–
	EPPS					
	De Avila (1970)	196	Sixth grade (males, females)	–	+	Firstborns (one factor in three)
	Sampson et al. (1967)	251	High school (males, females)	–	+	–
	Query et al. (1973)	50	High school (males)	–	–	Firstborns
	Waters et al. (1967)	564	College (males, females)	–	+	–
	Payne (1971)	1,023	College (males)	–	–	–
	Krinsky (1963)	159	Adult (males)	–	+	–
	Gunderson (1969)	219	Adult (males)	–	–	Firstborns (explained variance 2%)
	CPI					
	Weiss (1969)	864	College (males)	–	–	–

Table 24. (continued)

Author	N	Age	Social class controlled	Sibship size controlled	highest score
Marquette (1972)	2,407	College (males, females)	–	–	–
Combinations (Marlowe-Crowne, EPPS, CPI)					
Macbeth (1976)	716	College (males, females)	–	+	–
	265	College (males, females)	–	+	–

	Author	Test	Subjects	N	Highest scores
B	Getzels et al. (1958)	Paired direct and projective questionnaire	8–13-year-old children	913	Only children > firstborns > laterborns
	Delaney (1973)	Children's adult role test	7–8- and 11–12-year-old children	60	–
	Conners (1963)	Guttman scale of interpersonal orientation	College students (male), no or one sib	123	Laterborns > firstborns > only children (tendency)
	Moore (1964)	Stanford hypnotic susceptibility scale	College students (male)	80	Laterborns
	Wolkon (1968)	Sentence completion test for dependency	Consecutive psychiatric discharges	540	–
	Koenig (1969)	20-statement test	College students	212	Firstborns > laterborns (more general statements)
	Becker (1970)	McDavid's social reinforcement scale	College students (male, female)	118	Males: laterborns > firstborns; females: firstborns > laterborns
	Hartnett (1971)	Social responsibility scale	College students	97 230	– –
	McDonald (1971)	Social responsibility scale	College students	476	Only children > firstborns > laterborns ($P < 0.05$)
	Solomon (1977)	Patient request form	College students	196	Interaction of birth rank with sibship size
	Wudel et al. (1979)	Lie scale of the Eysenck Personality Inventory	Undergraduates (males, females)	103	–

(Weiss; Marquette; Macbeth) gave no evidence of firstborns being more affiliative, conforming, socialized, or dependent.

Among 11 samples in which affiliation was measured *by various methods*, higher scores in firstborns were reported in three, higher scores in laterborns in two, and no influence of birth rank or interaction of birth rank with sibship size or sex in seven. Projective tests (see p. 121) also failed to provide evidence for greater affiliation in firstborns.

Questionnaires on the Acceptance of Traditional Values

Accepting traditional values may be considered conforming to (associating with) the majority.

Moral Attitudes. Questionnaires on church attendance and religious preference (MacDonald 1969) and on extramarital sexual contacts (Touhey 1971) were given to college and university samples. Results were not consistent: Firstborns of either sex indicated both more church attendance and more extramarital contacts. The latter difference was not confirmed among underprivileged young black women experiencing their first pregnancy (Dixon 1980). Among a large sample of male seventh and eighth graders firstborns less often reported to have committed theft than middle and youngest children (Dentler et al. 1961). On a questionnaire of acceptance of conventional morality given to college subjects with control of sibship size, higher conformity of firstborns appeared only in males with one sib (Hess 1971). Among females secondborns were more conforming.

Attitudes Toward the Family. In a female college sample investigated by Murdoch 1966 firstborns indicated preference for an earlier marriage age than laterborns, which was considered to indicate their stronger affiliative tendency. In one of two other samples the result was not confirmed (Murdoch et al. 1969). Two authors (Joesting et al. 1973, 1975; Hendershot 1969) who questioned college women on the number of their prospective children found that firstborns indicated that they wanted smaller families than laterborns. This was interpreted as the consequence of a stronger sense of responsibility. This birth rank difference was not, however, reproduced in a lower-class sample from large families (McAllister et al. 1974). In a USA probability sample of several thousand women, firstborns' preference for small family size disappeared when race, duration of marriage, and size of family of origin were controlled (Stokes et al. 1977). In samples in which social background and sibship size are not controlled, firstborns are biased for smaller sibship size and the social variables that go with it and want families of a size that conforms to the norm of their background.

Attitude Toward Medical Authority. One author (Franklin 1973) assumed that firstborns would take the sick role more readily than laterborns, because inexperienced parents consult medical authorities more often. A sample of students were given a questionnaire on their readiness to adopt the sick role in three hypothetical situations and firstborns were more ready to do so. As there was no control for sex, sibship size, and social class (the latter variables are known to influence seeking of medical care) (Suchman 1965; Mechanic 1966), this study does not seem to constitute evidence for stronger affiliation in firstborns.

Rating for Dependency and Conformity

In a small sample of nursery school children, firstborn males, but not females, were rated higher by their teachers for dependency behavior (touching adults, attention seeking) than laterborn males (Haeberle 1958). More dependency was also found in firstborn school beginners of either sex when rated by their teachers (Hollinger 1976). Neither study controlled for background variables.

Blustein (1967) studied teachers' ratings for conformity at school of a large sample of fourth to sixth graders with one sib from seven public schools in Maryland. Firstborn boys appeared more conforming than secondborns, while there was no difference in females. In her well-matched sample of children with one sib (see p. 93) Koch (1955a, b), on the other hand, did not find clear-cut birth order differences in conformity, dependency and related traits as rated by teachers. Only interactions of birth order with sex of subject, sex of sib and spacing emerged, which led the author to warn against generalizations. There is only one study of adults: Among male and female college students rated by their dormitory counselors for cooperativeness, no association with birth rank appeared (Roodin 1971).

Conclusions (Table 25)

Table 25. Birth order and acceptance of traditional values (A) and birth order and ratings for dependency and conformity (B)

	Author	*N*	Age	Social class controlled	Sibship size controlled	Highest score
A	*Moral attitudes*					
	Dixon (1980)	419	young black women	+	–	–
	MacDonald (1969)	393	College (males, females)	–	–	Firstborns
	Touhey (1971)	174	College (males, females)	–	–	Laterborns
	Dentler et al. (1961)	912	Seventh, eighth grades (males)	–	–	Firstborns
	Hess (1971)	?	College (males, females)	–	+	Firstborn males, secondborn females
	Attitude toward family					
	Murdoch (1966)	71	College (females)	–	–	Firstborns
	Murdoch et al. (1969)	252	College (males, females)	–	–	Firstborn females
		233	College (males, females)	–	–	–
	Joesting et al. (1973, 1975)	44	College (females)	–	–	Firstborns
		139				
	Hendershot (1969)	389	College (females)	–	–	Firstborns
	McAllister et al. (1974)	635	Ninth grade	–	+	–
	Stokes et al. (1977)	6,752	Adult	+	+	–

Table 25. (continued)

	Author	N	Age	Social class controlled	Sibship size controlled	Highest score
	Attitude toward medical authority					
	Franklin (1973)	152	College (males, females)	–	–	Firstborns
B	Haeberle (1958)	36	3–6 years (males, females)	–	–	only children, firstborn (males)
	Koch (1955 a, b)	384	5 years (males, females)	+	+	–
	Hollinger (1976)	214	First grade (males, females)	–	–	Firstborns
	Blustein (1967)	341–83	Fourth to sixth grades (males, females)	–	+	Firstborn males
	Roodin (1971)	111	College (males, females)	–	–	–

Findings for traditionalism in moral attitudes are not consistent. The result that firstborn boys report committed theft less often is questionable because of failure to control social class and sibship size, as is the finding that firstborn students address themselves more often to medical authorities, where not even sex is controlled. That differences between first- and laterborns may be artifacts of missing control for background variables becomes apparent in studies on the relationship between size of sibship and number of prospective children.

Among ratings for dependency and conformity, mostly by teachers, one study in five is in favor of greater conformity in firstborns and two (one controlling for sibship size) in favor of greater conformity in firstborn males (Blustein). It will be remembered that better adaptation to school is associated with higher social class and smaller sibship size (see p. 50, 53). Since, however, Blustein's result was obtained in sibships of two and confirms the slight experimental evidence of higher conformity in males of school age (see p. 113 f.), it can be accepted.

7.6.3.5 Summary of Paper-Pencil Tests on the Tendency to Associate

In the Marlowe-Crowne test for social desirability, scales of the EPPS and the CPI, and various projective and other tests, the evidence for a stronger tendency to associate in firstborns is negative. On questionnaires concerning attitudes toward the family and the sick role, firstborns appear more traditional and conforming. That this difference may be due to lack of control of social background variables is made probable by a large representative sample where firstborn differences in attitudes toward the family disappear with some control of such variables (Stokes et al. 1977). The same objection holds for the finding that firstborn children are rated higher for school conformity by their teachers than laterborns.

However, on the basis of one study that controls sibship size, it can be accepted that firstborn males of elementary school age are more conforming than laterborns (Blustein 1967).

7.6.3.6 Association in Real-Life

Age at Marriage

Earlier age at marriage in male firstborns was found by Murdoch (1966) in faculty members and their wives. The result was not, however, reproduced in another sample of faculty members and in married college students (Murdoch et al. 1969) or in faculty women (Friedman et al. 1978).

Birth rank of all married students at one university did not differ from that of all students (Montgomery et al. 1975). In a representative sample of Dublin males Walsh (1973) found that in all-male sibships firstborns married earlier; the author, however, considered that economic reasons were responsible for this difference.

Seeking Out Company at College and University

As membership in clubs and fraternities/sororities can be strongly related to social background, taking this variable as an indicator of stronger affiliative tendencies without controlling for background variables seems particularly questionable. Two studies revealed greater participation in organizations by firstborn students (Smart 1965; Query et al. 1973), while one study showed greater participation by laterborns (Baker et al. 1969); nonreproducible results were obtained in two samples (Forbes 1970a). Firstborn college goers wanted to live in a campus residence more than laterborns (Fandrich 1976), but birth rank did not influence wanting a double or single room or participating in group sports (Masling 1965). When it was found that among college roommates laterborns' but not firstborns' abilities influenced their partners, the author ascribed the finding to chance and enumerated the many methodological pitfalls (Hall 1963). None of the studies attempted to control for social class, income, or grades at school. That in two large series of officer candidates of the Israeli army (Amir et al. 1968) firstborns were overrepresented is not surprising when the educational and cultural prerequisites of becoming an officer are considered. There is no reason to interpret this fact in the sense of stronger affiliative tendencies in firstborns. It may be due to differences between subjects in terms of sibship size, social class, and ethnicity.

Political Interests, Health Care, Violations, and Crime

That firstborns use health care facilities more than laterborns was found by the following authors: MacDonald (1967); Byrdy et al. (1962); Wolkon (1968); Baar (1977); and Hansson et al. (1978). No such difference was reported by Misovich (1973); Weiner (1973); Dale (1973); and Strickland et al. (1963). In these studies first- and laterborns were not equalized for variables relevant to treatment, such as age, sex, income, and education. The alternative hypothesis that differing behavior with regard to health care is a consequence of between-group differences cannot be excluded. The same objection is valid for the finding that firstborns are more interested in politics than are laterborns (Hansson et al. 1977).

Firstborn college students receive fewer traffic violation tickets than laterborns (Hansson et al. 1978). Among prisoners, firstborns were found to have committed violent crimes less often than laterborns (Herrell 1969, 1970, 1972). Neither study controlled for sibship size, social class, and race, though all these variables could be related to the behaviors in question. Four real life life observations concern affiliation under stress. When 1,500 male and female undergraduates in different-sized classrooms were given a questionnaire on their present feelings, crowding being considered a stress that might induce affiliation, answers were influenced by crowding and by sex, but not by sibship size or birth order (Schettino et al. 1976). Under the assumption that being hospitalized for schizophrenia would lead to stronger affiliation in first- than in laterborns (Schooler et al. 1962), 45 female chronic schizophrenics and their nurses were given a questionnaire on social attitudes. Firstborns scored higher on a sociability factor extracted from questionnaires and observation, but there was no control for age and length of hospitalization. In a sample of passersby, reported behavior during and observed behavior on the morning after New York's power failure was studied (Zucker et al. 1968). Affiliative behavior in females was independent of birth rank, while among males laterborns were more affiliative. A large sample of undergraduates reported on seeking contact with others after the Los Angeles earthquake in 1971. There was an interaction of birth order with sex and situation for contact behavior (Hoyt et al. 1973): The 24 firstborn females who were alone during the earthquake spoke more quickly to relative strangers than laterborn females ($n = 22$) in the same situation.

Conclusions

According to some, but not all, studies firstborns marry earlier, enter officer schools in greater number, make more use of health care facilities, are imprisoned for less violent crimes, and get fewer traffic tickets. As firstborns are biased for smaller sibships, and as sibship size is related to IQ, age, education, and social class, all these findings may be based on between-group differences and thus be irrelevant to birth order research. Studies trying to show more affiliative behavior in real-life stress either do not support the hypothesis or are not convincing because of methodological failings or are based on such small numbers that their considerable influence (e.g. Hoyt et al.) is quite surprising.

7.6.3.7 Three Special Cases of So-called Affiliative Tendencies: Need for Interpersonal Distance, Self-Disclosure, and Volunteering

Need for Interpersonal Distance

Under the hypothesis that firstborns have stronger affiliative tendencies, they may be expected to begin to feel uncomfortable at a closer interpersonal distance than laterborns when a person approaches. Interpersonal distance was studied in 170 male college students (Pedersen 1973) by bringing two subjects unknown to each other together in an experimental room. Closer proximity was associated with being either first- or lastborns (rather than a middle child) with higher scores on extraversion and higher IQ. The same variable was studied with a paper-pencil test (Hollender et al. 1973) where comfortable distance from certain persons was marked on a diagram. In small samples of elementary school children and college students there were no consistent results. While the experimental study points to a possible association of sibship size with interpersonal distance, there is no evidence for firstborns' tendencies for closer interpersonal distance.

Self-Disclosure

Having stronger affiliative needs than laterborns, firstborns might be expected to more readily disclose themselves. Dimond et al. (1968, 1969) studied a small sample of male and female high school students with a self-disclosure questionnaire. Laterborns reported themselves more ready for self-disclosure than firstborns. The result was confirmed with a population of 1985 high school students, for males and females separately. An attempt at replication (Lord et al. 1975) with college students led, however, to the result that self-disclosure was independent of birth rank for both sexes.

Testing 180 college students from divorce and nondivorce homes (Ohlson 1974) with a self-disclosure scale, it was found that among divorce subjects firstborns report more readiness to disclose themselves than laterborns. In nondivorce subjects the relation was reversed.

Conclusions (Table 26)

Table 26. Birth order and self-disclosure

Author	*N*	Age	Social class controlled	Sibship size controlled	Highest score
Dimond et al. (1968, 1969)	60	High school (males, females)	–	–	Laterborns
	1,985		–	–	Laterborns
Lord et al. (1975)	145	College (males, females)	–	–	–
Ohlson (1974)	180	College (males, females)	–	–	Firstborns, laterborns (interaction divorce)

The findings shown in Table 26 are not in favor of a stronger tendency to self-disclosure in firstborns. One might be inclined to take the result in subjects from divorce homes for evidence that firstborns affiliate more under stress, were it not that the author describes firstborns from divorce homes as less affected by their situation than laterborns. As laterborns are biased for larger sibship size, they may have suffered more disruption than firstborns, divorce in large families being less frequent than in families with one or two children. Comparing first- and laterborn subjects from divorce homes may result in between-group differences.

Volunteering for Tests and Experiments

Volunteering is considered to fulfil affiliative and dependency needs. Being believed to be more affiliative and dependent, firstborns are expected to volunteer in greater numbers than laterborns. Subjects are college or university students.

Volunteering for Group Experiments. Group experiments may be particularly apt for satisfying affiliative needs. Two studies found firstborns more ready to volunteer than laterborns (Capra et al. 1962; Varela 1964). Firstborn volunteers (number not specified) were found to choose group rather than individual experiments more often than laterborns (Weiss et al. 1963; Wolf et al. 1965). In a further sample of male and female undergraduates, however, no difference in volunteering by birth rank was found, but there was a significant difference for sex in that females were less willing to volunteer. Group experiments were also not preferred by firstborns (Wilson et al. 1966). The same negative result was found in three further studies with college students (Ward 1964; Brock 1965; Roodin et al. 1978).

Volunteering for Hypnosis Experiments. As hypnosis implies a high degree of dependency, firstborns might be more interested than laterborns in this kind of experiment. Volunteers and nonvolunteers for hypnosis were, however, not found to differ in birth rank among female undergraduates (Zuckerman et al. 1967) or among female nursing students (Lubin et al. 1962).

Volunteering for Sensory Deprivation Experiments. Sensory deprivation being the extreme form of isolation, firstborns, having strong affiliative tendencies, might be believed to abstain from participation. However, in one study with 29 volunteers, 23 firstborns were found (Suedfeld 1964). In another study with a small number of college women (Schultz 1967), there was equidistribution of birth rank between volunteers and nonvolunteers.

Volunteering for Extensive Interviews. Extensive interviews could be supposed to satisfy affiliative needs. In 394 student subjects, however, there was no difference in birth rank among those volunteering and those not volunteering. Subjects from the upper or upper-middle class volunteered more often than subjects with other backgrounds (Fischer et al. 1969).

Volunteering for Various Tests and Experiments. Negative results by birth rank were found by Diab et al. (1968); Waters et al. (1969); Olsen (1969); MacDonald (1972a, b); and Roodin et al. (1974b) in samples of 100–600 students. Schubert et al. (1977) found middleborn males most ready to volunteer, while there was no birth rank effect on female volunteering. Rosenthal et al. (1975) quote three unpublished studies on volunteering by birth rank (Poor 1967; Wolf 1966; Ebert 1973). In one of them, firstborns more readily volunteered, while in the others there was no difference between first- and laterborns. Among volunteers there was a significant difference by birth rank in keeping the scheduled appointment, firstborns failing to appear in lesser numbers (MacDonald 1969).

Conclusions (Table 27)

Among 24 studies done with college ans university students, seven reported firstborns to volunteer more readily than laterborns. Firstborns, on the other hand, were neither particularly attracted by hypnosis or extensive interview-

Table 27. Birth order and volunteering for tests and experim ents

Author	N	Social class controlled	Sibship size controlled	Highest frequency
Group experiments				
Capra et al. (1962)	100	–	–	Firstborns
Varela (1964)	65	–	–	Firstborns
Weiss et al. (1963)	?	–	–	Firstborns
Wolf et al. (1965)	?	–	–	Firstborns
Wilson et al. (1966)	109	–	–	–
Ward (1964)	520	–	–	–
Brock (1965)	110	–	–	–
Roodin et al. (1978)	286	–	+	–
Hypnosis				
Zuckerman et al. (1967)	127	–	–	–
Lubin et al. (1962)	38	–	–	–
Sensory deprivation				
Suedfeld (1964)	29	–	–	Firstborns
Schultz (1967)	59	–	–	–
Extensive interviews				
Fischer et al. (1969)	394	–	–	–
Various tests and experiments				
Diab et al. (1968)		–	–	–
Waters et al. (1969)		–	–	–
Olson (1969)		–	–	–
MacDonald (1972 a)		–	–	–
MacDonald (1972 b)		–	–	–
Roodin et al. (1974 b)		–	–	–
Schubert et al. (1977)	100–600	–	–	Middleborns
Rosenthal et al. (1975)				
(unpublished study;		–	–	Firstborns
two other		–	–	–
unpublished studies)		–	–	–
MacDonald (1969)		–	–	Firstborns (keeping appointments)

ing nor repelled by sensory deprivation. But whenever there was a difference in volunteering by birth order, firstborns prevailed. In no case, however, was sibship size controlled.

Rosnow et al. (1969) found that volunteers are more often male, better educated, and of higher social class than nonvolunteers. This fact is equally well-known for responders in opinion surveys. Firstborns' apparently greater readiness to volunteer may be due to between-group differences related to their bias for smaller sibship. The evidence presented here is inconclusive because of failure to control background variables.

7.6.3.8 Summary of Research on the Tendency to Associate (Affiliation, Conformity, Social Desirability, etc.))

In experimental studies, the slight evidence that firstborn males of school age conform more than laterborns in terms of agreement with the believed opinion of a majority (Asch-type situation) was obtained without control of sibship size. Otherwise there is no evidence for a stronger tendency of firstborns to associate with others in a multiplicity of experimental conditions.

With paper-pencil tests, in one study (controlling for sibship size) evidence was found that firstborn males are rated more highly for conformity by teachers at elementary school than laterborns. In a large number of other testing situations no consistent differences by birth order or birth rank appeared.

Concerning real-life situations, no methodologically adequate evidence that firstborns behave more conformingly exists. All results in this direction were obtained without control of sibship size and may be due to between-group differences.

7.6.4 Birth Order and Achievement Motivation

In Sect. 7.2.2.2, it was found that achievement motivation decreased with increasing sibship size when social background variables were not controlled. In well-controlled studies, however, sibship size alone explained only small amounts of the variance. This finding is an argument for the necessity of controlling background variables when studying a possible association between birth order and achievement motivation.

7.6.4.1 Experimental Studies

Adults participating in a research project were asked to predict their scores on a symbol substitution test (Wolkon et al. 1965). An aspiration score was derived from the difference between predicted and obtained score. It was not related to birth rank.

7.6.4.2 Paper-Pencil Tests

The Need-Achievement Scale in the EPPS. The EPPS and fantasy items were given to a socially homogeneous sample of sixth graders (De Avila 1978). A factor analysis performed on achievement motivation items led to three achievement factors; one was related to sex, birth order, and sibship size in a three-way interaction without clear-cut results. In high school students (single children or children in sibship of two), Sampson et al. (1967) found firstborns to score significantly higher. The study was, however, objected to because of the failure to conduct post hoc comparisons between cells (De Avila 1971). In a similar sample (Rosenblüh et al. 1970) male firstborns scored higher than laterborns, and there was no birth order-related difference in females. Hornbostel et al. (1980) gave the test to college students with one sib and found a three-way interaction of sex, sibsex, and birth order explaining 5.5% of the variance: firstborns scored higher than secondborns if their sib was of the same sex, but lower if their sib was of different sex. In Taiwan students, well-matched for age, social class, and locus of habitation (Yang et al. 1973) scores were not related to birth order. Two adult nonstudent samples also gave negative results: Gunderson (1969) with volunteers for Arctic service and Wolkon et al. (1965) with research subjects. No difference by birth rank was found in a population of Air Force Academy freshmen enrolled in the spring and autumn of the same year, where results found in the spring sample were not reproducible in the autumn sample (Payne 1971). A large sample was also studied by Falbo et al. (1978); investigating undergraduates of two universities, they found that with control of sex, sibship size, and background birth order did not contribute to the explained variance in need achievement.

Other Need-Achievement-Related Scales. Costello's need-achievement scale did not reveal any birth rank differences among college students (though there were sex differences) or in another sample limited to subjects with one or two sibs (Munz et al. 1968). When Rokeach's value survey was given to female students, negative findings for birth order in evaluating accomplishments resulted (Penn 1973). Among male and female freshmen, scores on a study habit check list (associated with need for intellectual achievement) were independent of birth order (see p. 79) (Keetz 1979).

Combined Scales. Macbeth (1975) gave 14 achievement scales to two large populations of undergraduates. Interactions of birth order with sex and sex of sib found in the first sample in subjects with one sib were not replicated in the second sample.

TAT and Other Projective Tests

Child Samples. In the following two studies background variables, particularly sibship size, were not controlled. A decrease of achievement motivation with increasing birth rank was found in Chinese high school boys studied with the TAT (Yang et al. 1973). When, on the other hand, Rosen (1961) tested a large number of 11-year-old males with the TAT, controlling ethnicity, social class, and sibship size, there were no differences in achievement motivation by birth rank. The author found the same negative result with the same method also in three elementary school populations. In a study on 10- to 14-year-old American and Mexican children in which three projective measure were used, firstborns in the upper-middle but lastborns in the upper-lower class scored highest (Stenning 1968). Though the author remarks upon the rigidity of sib roles in Mexican families, no consistent differences in need achievement by birth rank were found in the Mexican sample.

College and University Student Samples. These samples comprised 100–200 subjects. Fakouri (1974) used an achievement imagery scale with male and female undergraduates and found that firstborns scored higher. In a male sample studied with the TAT (Karabenick 1971), on the other hand, there were higher scores for laterborns. The study of five male and female samples with the same test led to no reproducible results (Rosenfeld 1966). The control of social class in a large Indian sample (Mukherjee 1968) examined by a sentence completion test led to divergent results: In the upper-class laterborns scored highest, in the middle-class firstborns and in lower-class subjects there was no difference by birth rank.

Adult Samples. Also with a sentence completion test, no differences by birth rank were found in discharged patients from a mental hospital (Wolkon et al. 1965).

Ratings for Academic Motivation

Teachers' ratings. None of the following studies controlled for both sibship size and social class; subjects were elementary school children. Firstborns were rated higher for academic motivation in a small Canadian school (Start et al. 1974), among a nonspecified number of elementary school children within three social classes (Adams 1967), and among fourth and fifth graders rated at four different points in time within three ethnic groups and two social classes (Adams et al. 1972). Firstborns were also rated higher in a sample of about 350 elementary school children in sibships of two from a variety of social classes (Blustein 1967).

Self-Ratings for Efforts and Educational and Vocational Goals

High School Students

Social Class and/or Sibship Size Not Controlled. In male students firstborns wanted to go to college in significantly greater numbers than laterborns (Purpura 1971). In another sample of middle-class high school seniors no such difference by birth rank was found (Rosenblüh et al. 1970).

Social Class and Sibship Size Controlled. Janisch (1973) studied three samples of 12th graders from an upper-middle-class suburban high school, a middle-class city school, and a black ghetto school. Educational goals (from dropping out to becoming a graduate student) were measured on a 5-point scale. When sex and six social classes within each sample were controlled, birth order did not contribute significantly to the variance in educational goals.

In an Indian sample of ninth graders from three schools, occupational expectations did not vary with birth rank when sex and social class were controlled (Mehta et al. 1969).

The following studies were made with large representative samples. Elder (1962 a, b) studied a questionnaire given to a random sample of the high school population of two American states. When sex, sibship size, and two social classes were controlled, self-reports on efforts for school and homework decreased by birth order within sibship size in middle-class subjects of both sexes while, in the lower class, youngest males and females in sibships of three and more demonstrated the upswing of scores found in large samples for both IQ and school achievement (see pp. 37ff., 55f.). The same tendency was found in the subjects expecting to go to college.

However, in a large sample of students from ten Los Angeles high schools selected to represent all social strata, subjects were questioned on level of schooling, occupation, and income they expected to attain. Sex, sibship size, and eight levels of paternal occupation being controlled, there was no difference in expectation by birth order (Turner 1962).

Glass et al. (1974) used a nationally representative sample of 2,523 10th and 12th graders (only children or children with one or two sibs) from Project Talent, giving them a questionnaire on educational expectations similar to Janisch's (1973), as previously mentioned. When sibship size and paternal education on two levels were controlled, birth order contributed less than 1% to the explained variance.

College and University Students

The following two studies were done without control of background variables. A sample of male and female students was asked whether they were interested in becoming a college professor. A firstborn-laterborn difference was apparent in females (Fischer et al. 1968). A sample of undergraduates indicated expectations for occupation and salary. Within sex, expectations were higher in first- than in laterborns (Platt et al. 1968).

On the other hand, in a mainly-class sample of South African students, first and second children were compared by self-ratings for achievement, sex and sibship size being controlled. Scores were not associated with birth order (Struempfer 1973). In two populations of university freshmen Biegelsen (1976) measured need-achievement by the level of academic aspiration, holding sex and sibship size constant. There was a sex difference, but no reproducible effect of birth order.

Nonstudent Adult Samples

A sample of 2,268 adults, mostly men, taking in US Armed Forces correspondences course at three levels, returned questionnaires on achievement motivation (76% of sample). As expected, in a sample of ages 18–52 years firstborns were more and lastborns least motivated. Age, social class, and sibship size were not controlled (Farley et al. 1974).

Academic Motivation in Sibs Within the Same Sibship

From one high school in a working-class neighborhood 205 sib pairs (excluding twins) were given a questionnaire on expected educational level. Aspirations decreased with social class and increasing sibship size, but were unrelated to birth order (Elliot et al. 1970). Controls for age and sex were not reported.

Ratings by Peers and Superiors for Occupational Achievement

If firstborns have higher motivation to achieve they might be expected to perform better in their occupations than laterborns. Evaluation by peers of performance of small samples of student teachers (Korte 1975) and by superiors of the performance of small groups of army-selected Antarctic researchers (Owens 1968) were independent of birth rank. Among a sample of Peace Corps volunteers working in underdeveloped countries, firstborns were rated higher than secondborns when teaching mathematics, but secondborns higher than firstborns when teaching languages (Exner et al. 1970). There is no evidence that forstborns generally perform better than laterborns.

7.6.4.3 **Conclusions** (Table 28)

In *various tests and scales* among 24 samples higher need-achievement of firstborns was found in three, an interaction with sex in one, interactions of birth rank with class in two, and a decrease by birth order in one. *In no case was a particular position for firstborns shown when there was control for both sibship size and social class.* No replicable results were found when 14 scales were given to entire college populations (Macbeth).

Two studies comprise populations of different cultural standards (Stenning; Mukherjee). In populations with presumably homogeneous large family sizes (Mexicans and lower-class Indians), no correlations of need-achievement scores with birth rank were found, while conflicting results were seen among Americans and middle-class Indians. We may conclude that positive findings in the studies mentioned here are at least partially due to failure to control of background variables.

Teachers at the elementary level rate firstborns higher in academic motivation. Since no study controlled for both sibship size and social class, it is not possible to differentiate between inter- and intrafamilial differences. Evidence for higher social class and smaller sibship size being related to higher acedemic achievement has been discussed (see p. 50ff.). However, Blustein's finding that firstborns in sibships of two at elementary school were rated higher for academic motivation by their teachers than secondborns can be accepted as evidence for higher motivation in firstborns. The same sample was also rated higher in school conformity (see p. 125). Of course, these two concepts are interrelated.

There are 13 samples in which *self-ratings* of educational and vocational goals were used as measures of the need for academic achievement. In none of these where a firstborn advantage appeared was there a sufficient control of background.

Elder's finding concerning the need for educational achievement corresponds to the decrease in IQ and achievement scores by birth order and the reversal of this trend in laterborns of large families, which was discussed earlier (see pp. 37, 55f.). The Glass study illustrates the amount of the variance explained by birth order.

One methodologically objectionable study of sib pairs and three investigations of ratings of occupational achievement (two done with small groups) do not support any particular position of firstborns.

We may conclude that there is insufficient evidence that firstborns rate themselves higher on questionnaires on need-achievement of on need for academic achievement, but that firstborn elementary school pupils are rated higher for academic motivation by their teachers.

Table 28. Birth order and need-achievement and birth order (A) and ratings of academic achievement (B)

Author	N	Age	Social class controlled	Sibship size controlled	Highest scores
A *EPPS*					
De Avila (1970)	196	Sixth grade (males, females)	–	+	Firstborns (interaction, sex, sibship size, one factor)
Sampson et al. (1967)	251	High school (males, females)	–	+	Firstborns
Rosenblüh et al. (1970	199	High school (males, females)	–	–	Firstborn males
Hornbostel et al. (1980)	120	College (males, females)	–	+	Firstborns/secondborns
Yang et al. (1973)	128	College (males)	+	–	–
Gunderson (1969)	219	Adults (males)	–	–	–
Wolkon et al. (1969)	219	Adults (males)	–	–	–
Payne (1971)	1,023	College (males)	–	–	–
Falbo et al. (1979)	1,041	University (males, females)	+	+	–
Various scales					
Munz et al. (1968)	200	College (males, females)	–	–	–
	180	College (males, females)	–	+	–
Penn (1973)	168	College (females)	–	–	–
Keetz (1979)	182	College (males, females)	+	+	–
TAT					
Rosen (1961)	427	11 years (males)	+	+	–
	367	Elementary school (males, females)	+	+	–
Yang et al. (1973)	98	High school (males)	–	–	Firstborns
Karabenick (1971)	170	College (males)	–	–	–
Rosenfeld (1966)	503	High school, college (five samples; males, females)	–	–	–
Other projective tests					
Stenning (1968)	?	10–14 years (USA; males, females)	+	–	First-, lastborns (interaction social class)
	?	10–14 years (Mexico; males,) females)	+	–	–
Fakouri (1974)	122	College (males, females)	–	–	Firstborns

Table 28. (continued)

	Author	N	Age	Social class controlled	Sibship size controlled	Highest scores
	Sentence completion test					
	Mukherjee (1968)	472	University (males, females)	+	–	First-, laterborns (interaction social class)
	Wolkon et al. (1965)	102	Adults	–	–	–
	Combination of scales					
	Macbeth (1975)	716	University (males, females)	–	+	–
		256	University (males, females)	–	+	–
B	*Teachers' ratings*					
	Start et al. (1970)	157	Elementary school	–	–	Firstborns
	Adams (1967)	?	Elementary school	+	–	Firstborns
	Adams et al. (1972)	371	Fourth, fifth grades	+	–	Firstborns
	Blustein (1967)	350	Elementary school	–	+	Firstborns
	Self-ratings					
	Purpura (1971)	311	High school (males)	–	–	Firstborns
	Rosenblüh et al. (1970)	199	High school (males, females)	+	–	–
	Janisch (1973)	300	12th grade (males, females)	+	+	–
	Turner (1962)	2,175	High school (males, females)	+	+	–
	Elder (1962 a, b)	7,274	High school (males, females)	+	+	Earlier-borns
	Glass et al. (1974)	2,523	10th, 12th grades (males, females)	+	+	Explained variance 1%
	Mehta et al. (1969)	283	Ninth grade	–	–	–
	Fischer et al. (1968)	496	College (males, females)	–	–	Firstborn females
	Platt et al. (1968)	235	College (males, females)	–	–	Firstborns
	Struempfer (1973)	318	University (males, females)	+	+	–
	Biegelsen (1976)	941 942	University (males, females)	– –	+ +	– –
	Farley et al. (1974)	2,268	Adult (males, females)	–	–	Firstborns
	Study of sibs					
	Elliot et al. (1970)	205 pairs	High school			–

7.6.5 Birth Order and Aggression

In this section the hypothesis that firstborns are less able to express aggression directly than laterborns (see p. 86) is discussed.

7.6.5.1 Experimental Studies

Doll Play Aggression. Sears (1951) observed 3- to 5-year-old day-care center children playing with a doll house. In total aggression firstborn girls were significantly lower than youngest girls. Boys did not differ by birth rank on a total aggression score, but firstborn boys inflicted fewer bodily injuries than laterborn boys. Though there was an aggression gradient for age, sibship size and age were not controlled. In a similar study, black preschool children were observed for aggression in doll play (Abramson 1973). Sibship size and birth order did not influence occurrence of violent versus nonviolent aggression. Among Hispanic 7- to 9-year-old males studied while assembling puzzles, greatest aggression was observed in lastborns from broken homes (Boone 1979).

Frustration Experiments. These experiments were performed on college and university students. In male subjects (Dittes 1961) it was found that experimental manipulation of peer acceptance led, in first- rather than in laterborns, to significantly higher aggression, e.g., impulsive closure of task or counterrejection of peers. Two studies investigated problem-solving under frustrating conditions: Among male subjects laterborns expressed a greater increase of annoyance than firstborns (measured by a questionnaire at the beginning and end of the experiment) (Glass et al. 1963). In subjects of both sexes, on the other hand, increase of aggression did not vary with birth rank (Owyang 1971).

7.6.5.2 Paper-Pencil Test

Projective Tests. Aggressive and sexual contents were more frequently projected into Rorschach cards and abstract paintings by first- than laterborns in a sample of psychology students of both sexes (Grossman 1974; Grossman et al. 1972). The authors take this to be proof that firstborns repress aggressive and sexual impulses more than laterborns, though this finding might equally well signify the reverse. When a projective "directness of anger scale" was given to fifth and sixth grade boys, scores of first- and laterborns were not significantly different (Katz 1973).

Inventories and Scales. From 14 schools in Ohio, fourth to sixth graders were selected for being single children or having one or two sibs. Scores on an impulsiveness scale were not related to birth order within sex (Rosenberg et al. 1964 a). Choynowsky et al. (1973) studied the 11- to 15-year-old population of two Swedish schools. The subjects were given a hostility inventory of eight scales. In one of these, birth rank accounted for 2% of the variance. The following studies used smaller college samples: Male laterborns scored higher than male firstborns in one of two aggression scales; in females there was no difference (Owyang 1971). A sample of 80 female subjects, 20 for each position of birth order and sex of sib in sibships of two, rated themselves for aggression by means of the Gough adjective checklist (Sutton-Smith et al. 1970). Secondborns gave higher ratings. Significances, however, were not given and differences were small.

Teachers' Ratings. In her sample (see p. 93), Koch (1955 a, 1957 a) reported higher anger ratings in first- than in laterborns. There were complicated interactions of birth order, sex of subject, sex of sib, and spacing for agression.

7.6.5.3 Conclusions (Table 29)

Table 29. Birth order and aggression

Author	*N*	Age	Social controlled class	Sibship controlled size	Highest scores
Experimental studies					
Sears (1951)	136	3–5 years (males, females)	–	–	Laterborns
Abramson (1973)	122	Preschool (males, females)	–	+	–
Boone (1979)	50	7–8 years (males)	–	–	Lastborns (interact. broken homes)
Dittes (1961)	?	College (males)	–	–	Firstborns
Glass et al. (1963)	108	College (males)	–	–	Laterborns
Owyang (1971)	82	College (males, females)	–	–	–
Projective tests					
Katz (1973)	?	Fifth, sixth grades (males)	–	–	–
Grossmann (1974) Grossmann et al. (1972)	239	University (males, females)	–	–	Firstborns
Inventories and scales					
Rosenberg et al. (1969 a)	352	Fifth, sixth grades (males, females)	–	+	–
Choynowsky et al. (1973)	715	11–15 years (males, females)			2% explained variance in 1 of 8 scales
Owyang (1971)	82	College (males, females)	–	–	Laterborns (males) (one scale in two)
Sutton-Smith et al. (1970)	80	College (females)	–	+	–
Teachers' ratings					
Koch (1955 a, 1957 a)	360	5–6 years (males, females)	+	+	Firstborns (anger)

As seen in Table 29, the *experimental studies* give conflicting results. In one of two studies using *projective tests* firstborns more readily projected aggressive contents, a fact which may indicate repressed aggression but may equally well indicate lesser inhibition. Results of *scales and inventories* are inconsistent for both female and male subjects.

Evidence that firstborns are less able to express aggression directly than laterborns is lacking. Studies suffer not only from failure to control background variables but also from insufficient operationalizing. This lack of evidence is in agreement with studies on relationships between sibs which found more direct aggression in firstborns (see p. 97 f.).

7.6.6 Birth order, Dominance, and Conservatism

Adler (1928) stipulated that firstborns, having lost their power by dethronement, like to take part in the exercise of authority, exaggerate the importance of rules and laws, and tend to believe that power should be preserved in the hands of those who are entitled to it (see p. 85). This greed for power would seem to be opposed to the presumed stronger affiliative tendencies of firstborns and their presumed inability to utter direct aggression, which have been discussed.

7.6.6.1 Dominance and Authoritarianism

Experimental Studies. Rothbarth et al. (1970) studied 80 female college students who were either first- or lastborns in sibships of three and had all male or all female sibs. Dominance was rated while the subjects discussed a problem and did a puzzle with either a male or a female partner. Firstborns with two male sibs were significantly lower on dominance than girls in other positions. This difference was restricted to the puzzle situation.

Paper-Pencil Tests. Three samples were studied with scales from the CPI. In the same sample referred to above, Rothbarth et al. (1970) found no birth order influences on the dominance scale. When Eisenmann et al. (1970) studied authoritarianism in college students with the femininity scale of the CPI, firstborn males, but not firstborn females, scored lower than laterborns. No birth rank differences appeared on the same scale in adults of a wide age range taking evening courses (Greenberg et al. 1963).

The dominance scale of the EPPS was given with negative results to small numbers of student couples (Pinsky 1974) and of clients of a family service (Levinger et al. 1965).

Two studies were restricted to subjects with one sib. Results were not influenced by birth order on an undescribed measure of authoritarianism (Frankel 1968) or on the dominance scales of both the CPI and the EEPS (Leventhal 1970) in an elementary and a college sample respectively. On a self-expression scale measuring assertiveness given to a college sample, female firstborns with one or two sibs scored higher than laterborns (Hall et al. 1977). In a matched sample of first- and secondborn male college students with one sib (see p. 143), factor analysis of an ad hoc questionnaire showed firstborns to be more inclined to organize and control (Hall 1963; Hall et al. 1964).

Real-Life Situations. In these studies vocational interests are brough into correlation with birth rank: Because of their tendency toward "law and order," firstborns are supposed to prefer occupations or major subjects that are highly structured.

Two studies tested this hypothesis on entire student populations. Altus (1967) found that at the University of California firstborn females majored more often in the less structured subjects of art and music than laterborns, while in the choice of other subjects there were no differences by birth rank. At the University of Edinburgh (Sheldrake et al. 1976) found a preference for studying arts in only children, but otherwise no difference in choice of subjects between first- and laterborns. Choice of major was also found to be independent of being first- or secondborn in a male and female college sample selected from an occupational counseling pool to represent all positions of birth order in sibships of two (Stenger 1975).

7.6.6.2 Conservatism and Dogmatism

Experimental Studies

Dogmatism was investigated in male and female college students by the degree to which they were able to differentiate the content of information from its source (Becker 1968). Within sex there was no significant difference between first- and laterborns.

Paper-Pencil Tests

Rokeach Dogmatism Scale. Kilpatrick et al. (1969), in college students, found firstborn males and lastborn females to score highest on dogmatism. The result was questioned by Swanson (1971) on statistical grounds: According to this author lastborns scored highest in both sexes. No difference by birth rank was found in male and female graduates or in male and female college students (Fakouri 1974; Wisdom et al. 1975; Marjoribanks 1979).

Various Measures of Conservatism. Altus (1963a) studied male and female college students by analyzing MMPI items for conservatism and found firstborns of both sexes to rate higher. Negative results were found with a conservatism scale in seminary students and participants in adult education (Boshien et al. 1971) and in female college students (Simon et al. 1972). In a questionnaire on conservatism given to college females, laterborns rated themselves higher (Roodin et al. 1972). In a matched sample of 104 first- and secondborn male college students in sibships of two, on the other hand (Hall 1963; Hall et al. 1964), firstborns scored higher on factors, deducted from an ad-hoc questionnaire on interest and activities, which implied conservatism and resistance to change (see p. 142).

Questionnaire on Political, Religious, and Sexual Attitudes. The following studies were carried out with college and university samples of, as a rule, several hundred subjects. In questionnaires and scales on political conservatism first- and laterborns did not differ in studies by Abramowitz et al. (1971), Looft (1971), Farley et al. (1974), and Macbeth (1975) (two samples). In an Indian male sample preference for democratic leadership was higher in first- and middleborns than in youngest children (Bhushan et al. 1972). In a sample of female undergraduates first- and laterborns equally often designated themselves as "religious" (Kammeyer 1966): In a sample of college males (Lewis 1976) laterborns scored higher on this variable. Reported church attendance was not associated with birth order among male and female college students (Lewis 1975). On a sexual liberality scale given to male and female subjects, firstborns of both sexes reported themselves as slightly less liberal than laterborns (Kilpatrick et al. 1969). The two latter findings are opposed to the result on a questionnaire on extramarital intercourse and religious preference (see p. 124) given in the context of measuring conventional morality.

Real-Life Behavior

Lemay (1968) compared 199 female college students against whom disciplinary action had been taken with a random sample of female students in the same college. In the disciplined group firstborns were underrepresented. Social background variables were not controlled.

7.6.6.3 **Conclusions** (Table 30)

In experimental studies, on various tests and scales, and in questionnaires on attitudes, firstborns do not appear as more authoritarian, dominant, dogmatic, or conservative than laterborns. They do not choose more structured studies than laterborns. The finding that firstborn college females are underrepresented in a group against whom disciplinary action had been taken is to be seen in the context of firstborns more highly "socialized" behaviour in real life as using more health care, getting fewer traffic tickets etc. The methodological objections against this kind of research have been presented on p. 128.

Table 30. Birth order, authoritarianism, and dominance (A) and birth order and dogmatism (B)

	Author	N	Age	Social class controlled	Sibship size controlled	Highest scores
A	*CPI dominance scale*					
	Rothbarth et al. (1970)	80	College (females)	–	–	–
	CPI femininity scale					
	Eisenmann et al. (1970)	263	College (males, females)	–	–	Laterborn males
	Greenberg et al. (1963)	264	Adult (males, females)	–	–	–
	EPPS dominance scale					
	Pinsky (1974)	80	College (males, females)	–	–	–
	Levinger et al. (1965)	120	Adult (males, females)	–	–	–
	CPI and EPPS dominance scales					
	Leventhal (1970)	145	College (males)	–	+	–
	Various scales and questionnaires					
	Frankel (1968)	169	Sixth grade (males, females)	–	+	–
	Hall (1963) Hall et al. (1964)	104	University (males)	+	+	Firstborns
	Hall et al. (1977)	140	College (males, females)	–	+	Firstborns, females (small sibships)
B	*Rokeach dogmatism scale*					
	Kilpatrick et al. (1969)	378	College (males, females)	–	–	Lastborns
	Fakouri (1974)	122	College (males, females)	–	–	–
	Wisdom et al. (1975)		College (males, females)	–	–	–
	Majoribanks (1979)	280	University (males, females)	+	+	–
	Various measures					
	Altus (1963 a)	584	University (males, females)	–	–	Firstborns
	Boshien et al. (1971)	253	Seminary (males)	–	–	–
		357	Adult (males, females)	–	–	–
	Simon et al. (1972)	176	College (females)	–	–	–
	Roodin et al. (1972)	107	College (females)	–	–	–
	Hall (1963) Hall et al. (1964)	104	University (males)	+	+	Firstborns

Table 30. (continued)

Author	N	Age	Social class controlled	Sibship size controlled	Highest scores
Questionnaires on attitudes					
Abramowitz et al. (1971)	51	College (males, females)	–	–	–
Looft (1971)	119	College (males, females)	–	–	–
Farley et al. (1974)	139	College (females)	–	–	–
Macbeth (1975)	716	University (males, females)	–	+	–
	265	University (males, females)	–	+	–
Bhushan et al. (1972)	110	College (males)	–	–	Lastborns (less "democratic")
Kammeyer et al.	209	College (females)	–	–	–
Lewis (1976)	99	College (males)	–	–	Laterborns (more "religious")
Lewis (1975)	137	College (males, females)	–	–	–
Kilpatrick et al. (1969)	378	College (males, females)	–	–	Firstborns (less "liberal")

7.6.7 Birth Order and Interest in Ideas or Persons

This section examines the hypothesis that firstborns are more interested in ideas and in leading others than in empathizing. These traits supposedly originate in a stronger interest in law and order among firstborns.

7.6.7.1 Questionnaires on Interests and Preferences

Strong Vocational Interest Blank. McArthur (1956) gave this test to a small sample of male Harvard students. First- and secondborns differed significantly on 17 of 40 items, secondborns appearing more group-oriented and approachable, more inclined to lend and borrow, and less sought after for advice. When, however, the same test was given to male and female college students in all positions of sex and sex of sib in sibships of two, there were no significant differences by birth order for interest in leading others versus interest in empathic behavior (Sutton-Smith et al. 1964). The same negative result was also obtained in male college students

(Gandy 1973), and in two large samples of undergraduates (Macbeth 1975). A difference in one scale was not reproducible in the other sample. Biegelsen (1976) studied two populations of university freshmen expecting stress on intellectual mastery and social service in firstborns and stress on competition in laterborns. Neither hypothesis was confirmed.

Kuder Preference Record. Oberlander et al. (1970) followed up 250 of the Koch (see p. 93) kindergarten children to the age of 18 and tested them with the Kuder Preference Record. Scores on one of five factors differed by birth order: Secondborns were more interested in group activities. Birth order contributed 2% to the explained variance.

Various Measures of Vocational Interest. A questionnaire on occupational interest given to Indian ninth graders revealed no differences by birth order when sex was controlled (Mehta et al. 1969). From a pool of college students seeking vocational counseling, subjects in sibships of two were asked to arrange items of work value according to importance. Several significant differences were based on interactions of sex of subject with sex of sib, but no rationale was found for the differences (Stenger 1975).

Role expectation and professional attitudes were studied in two teacher samples (Krumboltz et al. 1958; Witchell 1966). In neither sample were scores associated with birth rank.

Esteem for the Least Preferred Co-Workers. Fiedler's scores of "esteem for the least preferred co-workers" were given to college students. The test (a bipolar adjective checklist) is supposed to differentiate between emphasis on personal relations (the least preferred co-workers is favorably described) and on task effectiveness (he is negatively described). Firstborns appeared significantly more task-oriented than laterborns (Chemers 1970). The result was replicated with a smaller sample of undergraduates and with middle-class black fifth and sixth graders (Hardy et al. 1978). In one class of nursery school children the same author (1978) found firstborn girls (but not boys) to be more task-oriented. In none of these studies was there control of sibship size.

7.6.7.2 Value Surveys

Firstborns are expected to support traditional values, high morality, seriousness, and order.

College Student Samples. In the Koch sample, followed up at 18 years of age (see above Oberlander et al. (1971) found that firstborns wanted to meet men of science and writers, and secondborns movie and TV stars or persons eminent in social welfare. In their sample of first- and secondborn subjects (see p. 143) Hall (1963) and Hall et al. (1964) factor analyzed an ad hoc questionnaire on values and interests and found firstborns to be more serious and conservative and laterborns to be more adventurous and gregarious. The finding was not reproduced in a female college sample with the Rokeach value survey (Penn 1973) or with a male college sample given a moral judgement scale (Schwartz 1976). Similarly, the two Macbeth (1975) undergraduate samples did not differ by birth order on the Allport study of values.

Nonstudent Adult Samples. The Allport study of values (Greenberg et al. 1963) was not associated with birth rank in adults taking evening courses. In Navy volunteers for Antarctic service studied with the EPPS, firstborns were lower than laterborns on stressing organization, neatness, and endurance (Gunderson 1969).

Interests and Rated Values in Young Children. In her sample of kindergarten children (see p. 93), Koch (1956b) found that choice of playmates was mainly influenced by age and sex (older children and children of different sex being less available). The effect of subjects' birth order was negligible. The same author (Koch 1956c) found firstborns to be rated by their teachers more highly for planning their work than laterborns.

7.6.7.3 Leadership Orientation

Self-Report Scales. In one sample of college students, interest in leadership was highest in middle children when answers to a personality inventory were factor-analyzed (Klockars 1968). The result was not reproduced among university students with sex and sibship size controlled (*N* not given). Nurses were not different in preference for a trusting or a directive leadership style by birth rank (Dagenais 1979).

Teachers' and Peers' Ratings. In three samples of elementary school children rated by their teachers for leadership results were inconsistently associated with birth rank (Neetz 1974). When two annual sets of Air Force Academy freshmen were rated for leadership by their peers, only children were rated highest in one sample while in the other firstborns as well as only children surpassed middle- and lastborns (Payne 1971).

Real-Life Situations. In 295 members of a religious organization leadership positions were not related to birth order in males, while in females firstborns were more likely than laterborns to serve as organization officers (Sandler et al. 1975). This may be an artifact due to the lack of control of social class, sibship size, and age in females (the younger and better educated being more likely to take up leadership positions, while selection is less severe for men).

7.6.7.4 Conclusions (Table 31)

Table 31. Birth order, interest in ideas or persons, and leadership

Author	N	Age	Social class controlled	Sibship size controlled	Greatest interest in ideas
Strong vocational interest blank					
McArthur (1956)	38	University (males)	–	–	Firstborns
Sutton-Smith et al. (1964)	137	College (males, females)	–	+	–
Gandy (1973)	150	College (males)	–	–	–
Macbeth (1975)	716	University (males, females)	–	+	–
	265	University (males, females)	–	+	–
Biegelsen (1976)	941	University (males, females)	–	+	–
	942	University (males, females)	–	+	–
Kuder Preference Record					
Oberlander et al. (1970)	250	18 years (males, females)	+	–	Firstborns (less interested in group activities)
Various measures of vocational interest and attitudes					
Mehta et al. (1969)	219	Ninth grade (males, females)	–	–	–
Stenger (1975)	275	College (males, females)	–	+	–
Krumboltz et al. (1958)	426	Teachers	–	–	–
Witchell (1966)	184	Teachers	–	–	–
Esteem for the least preferred co-worker					*Lowest esteem*
Chemers (1970)	350	University	–	–	Firstborns
Hardy (1972)	106	Fifth, sixth grades	+	–	Firstborns
	66	College	–	–	Firstborns
Hardy et al. (1978)	36	Nursery school (males, females)	–	–	Firstborns (female)
Value surveys					*Greatest interest in ideas, conservatism, morality*
Oberlander et al. (1971)	250	18 years (males, females)	+	–	Firstborns
Hall (1963) Hall et al. (1964)	104	University (males)	+	+	Firstborns
Penn (1973)	168	College (females)	–	–	–
Schwartz (1976)	100	College (males)	–	+	–

Table 31. (continued)

Author	N	Age	Social class controlled	Sibship size controlled	Greatest interest in ideas
Macbeth (1975)	716	University (males, females)	–	+	–
	265	University (males, females)	–	+	–
Greenberg et al.	264	Adult (males, females)	–	–	–
Gunderson (1969)	291	Adult (males)	–	–	Laterborns
Ratings of values and interest					
Koch (1956b)	360	5–6 years (males, females)	+	+	–
Koch (1956c)	360	5–6 years (males, females)	+	+	Firstborns (more planning)
Questionnaires and ratings for leadership					*Greatest leadership*
Klockars (1968)	?	College (males, females)	–	–	Middle children
	?	University (males, females)	–	+	–
Dagenais (1979)	100	Nurses	–	–	–
Neetz (1974)	?	Elementary school	–	+	–
Payne (1971)	574	College (males)	–	–	Only children
	449	College (males)	–	–	First, only children

Questionnaires on interests and values do not give evidence for higher interest in ideas and leadership among first- than laterborns: Neither do ratings by others for leadership. Firstborns consistently describe persons who are difficult to work with more negatively than laterborns. According to the concept of the test this difference is caused by higher task-orientation in firstborns. No study, however, controlled sibship size and sex was controlled in only one.

Higher task-orientation may be a personality variable associated with smaller sibship. There is as yet no sufficient evidence that firstborns are more task-oriented than laterborns, but the measure of "esteem for the least preferred co-workers" may be a promising field for further, better controlled investigations. The question remains open how higher task-orientation could be reconciled with higher conformity of firstborns in Asch-type experiments, also mainly found without control of sibship size (see p. 113 ff.).

7.6.8 Birth Order, Autonomy, and Creativity

The opinion that firstborns are more creative than laterborns was first voiced by Galton (1874), who found firstborns to be overrepresented among English men of science (control groups were not used). Need for autonomy is supposedly higher in firstborns because of earlier independence training (Sampson 1962).

7.6.8.1 Need for Autonomy

Sampson et al. (1967) found in high school students (only children or from sibships of two) greater need for autonomy in firstborns as measured by the EPPS. With control of sex, however, the difference disappeared. Among scientists who answered the autonomy scale of the EPPS (see p. 120), only children and firstborns scored significantly higher than laterborns (Krinsky 1963).

7.6.8.2 Creativity

Paper-Pencil Tests

Studies Using the Barron-Welsh Art Scale and Modifications. The Barron-Welsh Art Scale consists of figures varying in complexity. Expressed liking for the more complex figures is reported to be positively related to originality and verbal fluency and negatively related to rigidity, conformity, and conservatism (Buros 1972, p. 41).

Eisenman (1965, 1967 a, b, 1968 a, b; Taylor et al. 1968; Eisenman et al. 1970 a, b) carried out seven studies with 38–450 male and female college subjects: In five laterborn females preferred more complex polygons than firstborn females, and in three firstborn men preferred more complex polygons than laterborn men. This was explained by stronger adult influence on first- than laterborns, resulting in stronger sex-typing (in males towards creativity, in females towards rigidity). The results, however, were not confirmed by other research.

Control for sibship size was introduced in an investigation comparing first- and lastborn male university students from sibships of three (Stewart 1967). There was no difference by birth order. Two further studies with university subjects (Looft et al. 1971; Macbeth 1975, with two samples) and one with a high school sample (Wiedl 1977) also failed to replicate Eisenman's results.

Unusual-Uses Test. This test consists of finding as many uses as possible for everyday objects (e.g., a brick). All studies referred to here used 100–450 college students. Results were inconsistent: One investigation resulted in firstborn males scoring higher than laterborns, while females did not differ by birth rank (Eisenman et al. 1970 a); another found equidistribution of scores by birth rank (Eisenman et al. 1970 b), and a third found laterborn females to score higher than firstborns, while among males there was no difference be birth rank (Staffieri 1970).

Various Measures of Creativity. In three studies creativity was studied mainly according to the use of language. In a sample of kindergarten children (Lichtenwalner 1969) firstborns scored higher on finding various designations for an object. Creativity was also higher in middle-class than in lower-class children. In a word association test given to male and female college students, firstborns of both sexes were more original (Staffieri 1970). A verbal creativity test given to 100 Indian college students, on the other hand, gave results which were negatively correlated to sibship size and independent of birth order (Shrivastava 1977).

Wilks et al. (1979) used the verbal part of the Torrance test of creative thinking, the Singer fantasy questionnaire and a picture story task with a small elementary sample from a large number of upper middle-class schools. With control of sibship size no birth order differences appeared. The Torrance test was also used by Farley (1978 a) with a sample of college women with one or two sibs. In sibships of two, secondborns were more creative, while in sibships of three differences by birth order were not significant.

One investigator controlled for IQ (Mothlagh 1968) and found sex, but not birth rank to be related to scores in creativity in an unreported test given to college students. When tolerance of ambiguity was measured among 450 college subjects, firstborn males scored higher than laterborns, while there was no difference for females (Eisenman et al. 1970 a).

Comparison of Sibs Within the Same Sibship. Sellwood (1975) gave ten measures of creativity (including the Barron-Welsh scale and the unusual-uses test) to 32 firstborn-laterborn male sib pairs from a suburban high school, with 32 laterborn-laterborn male sibpairs as a control group. None of the tests showed a significant difference by birth rank. Kaltsounis (1978) studied nine sets of four brothers, who were 1 year apart from each other, at elementary school age with the figural and verbal parts, of the Torrance test. On the figural part youngest sons were lower on one of four measures. On the verbal part the second son was higher than the first on two and than the last on one measure. Corneau (1980) used the figural part of the Torrance test with 36 volunteers who were first- and secondborn sibs of both sexes. Firstborns were higher on three of four measures of creativity.

Real-Life Situations

A large amount of research has been conducted on the birth rank of eminent men. In contrast to Bliss (1970), Bowerman (1947), Visher (1947, 1948), Jones (1954), Eiduson (1962), Roe (1953), Helson et al. (1970), and Schubert et al. (1977) regularly found with the Greenwood-Yule method an overrepresentation of firstborns of up to 60%. Datta (1967, 1968) rightly pointed out in criticism that these samples, based on data of registers and encyclopedias, were not compared to control groups of noneminent men within the same professions.

Using a control group leads to less consistent results. Craik (1961, see Datta 1968) compared a group of creative architects with a representative sample of architects and found firstborns to be overrepresented among the former. On the other hand, when creative psychologists and chemists were compared with noncreative members of the same profession, no overrepresentation of firstborns among creative men appeared (Chambers 1964). Paralleling creative and noncreative subjects outside the rangs of eminence led to the same result. According to a questionnaire sent to university graduates, the choice of a scientific career was not associated with birth rank (Krinsky 1963). Datta (1968) compared three groups of high school students rated differently for creativity. Within each group, whether creative or not, firstborns were overrepresented. When a group of creative faculty members who had been issued a patent were compared with unproductive members, there was no significant difference in the rate of firstborns between the groups (Cleland et al. 1975). A comparison of registered inventors with male controls at the same geographic location revealed the same distribution of birth rank in both groups (Albaum 1977).

7.6.8.3 **Conclusions** (Table 32)

Table 32. Birth order and tests of autonomy and creativity

Author	*N*	Age	Social class controlled	Sibship size controlled	Highest scores
EPPS autonomy scale					
Sampson et al. (1967)	251	High school (males, females)	–	+	–
Krinsky (1963)	182	Adult	+	–	Firstborns
Barron-Welsh art scale					
Eisenman (1965, 1967 a, b, 1968 a, b) Taylor et al. (1968) Eisenman et al. (1970 b)	Seven samples 38–450	College (males, females)	–	–	Laterborn females (five samples) Firstborn males (three samples)
Stewart (1967)	100	University (males)	–	+	–
Looft et al. (1971)	138	University (males, females)	–	–	–
Macbeth (1975)	716	University (males, females)	–	+	–
	265	University (males, females)	–	+	–
Wiedl (1977)	97	High school (males, females)	–	+	–
Unusual-uses test					
Eisenman et al. (1970 a)	450	College (males, females)	–	–	Firstborn males
Eisenman et al. (1970 b)	263	College (males, females)	–	–	–
Staffieri (1970)	100	College (males, females)	–	–	Laterborn females
Verbal creativity test					
Lichtenwalner (1969)	68	Kindergarten	–	–	Firstborns
Staffieri (1970)	100	College (males, females)	–	–	Firstborns
Shrivastava (1977)	100	College (males)	–	–	–

Table 32. (continued)

Author	N	Age	Social class controlled	Sibship size controlled	Highest scores
Various measures					
Wilks et al. (1979)	68	Elementary school	–	+	–
Farley (1978 a)	50	College (females)	–	+	Secondborns (interaction sibship size)
Motlagh (1968)	168	College (males, females)	–	–	–
Eisenman et al. (1970 a)	450	College (males, females)	–	–	Firstborns (males)
Study of sibs					
Sellwood (1975)	64 pairs	High school (males)			–
Kaltsounis (1978)	9 sets of four	Elementary school (males)			Secondborn (interaction measure)
Corneau (1980)	32 pairs	High school (males, females)			Firstborns

There is no evidence for higher *need for autonomy* in firstborns, and there is none for their higher creativity. Positive birth rank results in the preference for simple and complex drawings are restricted to one investigator and his co-workers. Among other creativity tests, those examining verbal creativity favor firstborns. As, however, background is not controlled and as language mastery is positively related to social class, the finding is not sufficient to conclude that firstborns are more creative. Sib studies do not give consistent results. Overrepresentation of firstborns among eminent men is a false inference due to the lack of adequate control groups.

7.6.9 Birth Order and Self-Esteem

Adler (1958, pp. 144–146) hypothesized that firstborns, because of their dethronement, may lose hope and imagine that they can never win affection. Another line of reasoning observes the more inconsistent treatment of firstborns by their mothers and considers this to be detrimental for building up a stable self-concept (Hilton 1967). A third hypothesis is based on the fact that firstborns are alone with their parents for some time. They supposedly feel that parents are unreachable ideals and, finally, consider themselves weak and vulnerable (McArthur 1956).

7.6.9.1 Experimental Studies

After a discussion of juvenile delinquency conducted with college females, subjects were made to rank each other and themselves for their ability to discuss the topic with authorities on television. Under the condition of having been made to believe that they deviated from group opinion, firstborns were slightly more ready than laterborns to reject themselves (Arrowood et al. 1965). Three hundred college males and females took part in a contest where half of the subjects were made to believe that their opponent was crippled, and half that he was normal. Both groups had to guess what would be their opponents' results in a second round. As hypothesized, the guesses were correlated to results on a self-esteem scale, but they were independent of birth rank (Eisenman 1970).

7.6.9.2 Paper-Pencil Tests

The Coopersmith Self-Esteem Inventory. Coopersmith (1967) studied a public school population with a 50-item self-esteem inventory. Firstborns' scores were somewhat higher. In three further studies, however, the birth rank difference was not reproducible. In an equally large population of first graders the Coopersmith inventory yielded racial and ethnic differences, but none for birth rank (Miller et al. 1976). The same was true for a small sample of high school students with one or two sibs (Laitman 1975) and for 11- to 13-year-old Filipino girls from large sibships (Watkins et al. 1980).

Self-Ratings. When a pictorial self-concept scale given to a small sample of kindergarten children (Irvin 1974), results showed no association with birth rank. Rosenberg (1965) studied self-esteem in high school students in ten New York public schools. With control of sex and sibship size, only males scored higher than other birth ranks while firstborns did not differ from laterborns. Sears (1970) in a 42% sample of his kindergarten children (see p. 87) followed up to the age of 12 years found that self-concept measured by four scales decreased with increasing sibship size. Firstborn scored higher than laterborns; youngest children were highest on self criticism. In high school juniors no difference by birth rank on a self-esteem scale was found (Purpura 1971).

Ratings by Others. In her well-matched sample of five 6-year-old kindergarten children (see p. 93), Koch (1955a, 1956d) obtained contradictory results. Firstborns were reported by teachers to react more strongly to defeat and to be more concerned about status than laterborns, but at the same time to have more self-confidence. Self-concept as rated by mothers and teachers in a small sample of kindergarten children was not related to birth rank, but to school readiness (Irvin 1974).

Various Measures. The following studies were conducted with college or university students (sample size 100–300). Hall (1963), Hall et al. (1964) compared a well-matched sample of first- and secondborn male subjects. Factor-analyzing a questionnaire on interests and activities, younger sibs were found to have greater self-confidence. Two studies used the semantic differential. In male and female subjects no association with birth rank was found (Nash 1970). Eisenman (1970) analyzed discrepancies between the real and the ideal self, interpreting large differences to signify low self-esteem. Laterborn females had significantly lower self-esteem than firstborn females. The result was, however, not reproducible in a second sample. No differences by birth rank were found in an investigation with the Tennessee self-concept scale in male and female subjects (Nystul 1974). Schwab et al. (1978) gave two male and female samples a rating scale of four personality traits. In both samples firstborn females rated themselves higher than laterborns. This was not the case among males.

Self-Rating for School Ability in School Children and University Students. A sample of fourth to sixth graders from sibships of two in seven public schools in Maryland rated themselves for school ability. Rates within sex were not associated with birth order (Blustein 1967). A different result was found by Altus (1967), i.e., among a university population, firstborns of both sexes were less inclined to declare themselves incompetent in their studies than laterborns.

Nonstudent Adult Samples. The K-scale of the MMPI was given to firemen as a measure of self-confidence. Firstborns tended to rate themselves lower (Smith et al. 1963). A very interesting study was done with the help of an opinion research firm on a representative sample of 500 adults in a county of Texas (Kaplan 1970). The questionnaire was taken from Rosenberg (1965) (see p. 154), whose finding of higher self-esteem in the only child was not confirmed. Sibship size and birth order did not influence self-esteem, though there was evidence of lower self-esteem in females.

Sibs Within the Same Sibship. Bartelt (1973) selected from one high school 129 pairs of first and second sibs from sibship sizes two to eight. A questionnaire revealed no differences in self-esteem by birth order.

7.6.9.3 Conclusions (Table 33)

Table 33. Birth order and self-esteem

Author	*N*	Age	Social class controlled	Sibship size controlled	Higher self-esteem in
Coopersmith self-esteem inventory					
Coopersmith (1967)	1,748	Public school	–	–	Firstborns
Miller et al. (1976)	1,750	First grade (males, females)	–	–	–
Laitman (1975)	89	High school (males, females)	–	+	–
Watkins et al. (1980)	204	High school (females)	–	+	–
Self-ratings					
Irvin (1974)	45	Kindergarten	–	–	–

Table 33. (continued)

Author	N	Age	Social class controlled	Sibship size controlled	Higher self-esteem in
Rosenberg (1965)	5,024	High school 15–18 years (males, females)	–	+	–
Sears (1970)	160	12 years (males, females)	–	–	Firstborns
Purpura (1971)	311	High school	–	–	–
Ratings by others					
Koch (1955 a, 1956 d)	360	5–6 years	+	+	–
Irvin (1974)	45	Kindergarten	–	–	–
Self-rating for school ability					
Blustein (1967)	350	Fourth to sixth grades (males, females)	–	+	–
Altus (1967)	5,664	University	–	–	Firstborns
Various measures					
Hall (1963) Hall et al. (1964)	104	College (males)	+	+	Secondborns
Nash (1970)	278	College (males, females)	–	–	–
Eisenmann (1970)	278	College (males, females)	–	–	Firstborn females
	300	College (males, females)	–	–	–
Nystul (1974)	131	College (males, females)	–	–	–
Schwab et al. (1978)	164	College (males, females)	–	–	Firstborn
	308	College (males, females)	–	–	Firstborn (females)
Smith et al. (1963)	165	Adult (males)	–	–	Laterborns
Kaplan (1970)	500	Adult (males)	+	–	–
Blustein (1967)	350	Fourth to sixth grades (males, females)	–	+	–
Altus (1967)	5,664	University	–	–	Firstborns
Study of sibs					
Bartelt (1973)	129 airs	High school			–

There is no evidence supporting the hypothesis that firstborns have lower self-esteem than laterborns (Table 33). Most studies do not demonstrate association of self-esteem with birth rank. Of those studies which do find differences, the majority show greater self-esteem among firstborns, which may be an artifact of not controlling sibship size. Opinion research in adults gives a negative result (Kaplan), as does the comparison of sibs within the same sibship.

7.6.10. Birth Order, Adjustment and Neuroticism

Adler (1958, p. 144) has ascribed disastrous consequences to dethronement: "The change always makes a great impression and we can often find in problem children, neurotics, criminals and drunkards that their difficulties began in such circumstances. They are oldest children...". Greater vulnerability and uncertainty are also attributed to firstborns because of their being harshly treated (Dittes 1961). The reason for firstborns prevailing in some psychiatric samples will be discussed elsewhere (see p. 222). Here, only adjustment in normal subjects will be considered.

7.6.10.1 Adjustment Scales

Child Samples. As a rule, these samples comprise several hundred subjects. No difference in scores on adjustment scales by birth rank was found by Damrin (1949) in high school girls or by Hawkes et al. (1958) in fifth graders. The Lessing et al. (1967 a) study of elementary and high school students resulted in the disappearance of adjustment differences by birth order on the CTP when social class, IQ, and sibship size were controlled. Lessing et al. (1972) studied two further samples from socially homogeneous suburban schools using the same test. They found firstborn girls to be better adjusted in one of the samples, but there was no such difference in the other sample and no differences were found in either sample when another well-known personality questionnaire was used. Birth order contributed not quite 3% to the explained variance. Better adjustment in male and female firstborns was found among fourth graders in Brooklyn with the CTP (Corsello 1973).

Krauthamer (1974) used the 16 Personality Factors (16-PF) questionnaire with a group of 8- to 18-year-old children whose mothers were undergoing private in- or outpatient psychiatric treatment. Youngest children appeared more disturbed than oldest children. Age of child was not controlled.

In two Indian samples of high school students ad hoc adjustment scales were used (Reddy 1967; Prakash et al. 1963): In the first study, with males, firstborns were least and secondborns most adjusted, while middle and last children were intermediate. In the second study, with males and females, first- and lastborns were less well-adjusted than middle children.

In the Koch sample (see p. 93) firstborn girls and secondborn males were rated by their teachers as having more nervous habits than secondborns girls and firstborn males (1956 d). When teachers rated school behavior of a population of male and female first graders, males and middle children received lower ratings than females, firstborns, and lastborns (Skovholt et al. 1973).

In the Douglas (1964) study of a British representative national sample of 11-year-old children, some adjustment data were collected by health visitors and school doctors. Lastborns were more often bed-wetters and thumb-suckers than children of other ranks. Teachers and mothers reported firstborns with one or two sibs, on the other hand, as having more difficulties with other children than lastborns. In the Davie et al. (1972) national British sample of 7-year-olds, teachers rated social adjustment with the help of a questionnaire; 7.5% of the variance was explained, the two most important variables being social class and sex. When these variables were controlled, earlierborn children were better adjusted than laterborns, and children having no younger sibs better than those having younger sibs. Unfortunately it is not possible to extricate from these data separate associations of adjustment with birth order within sibship size.

Student and Adult Samples. Two large samples of male and female undergraduates were tested by Swanson et al. (1972) and Macbeth (1975). The former author found adjustment, as measured using the Cornel Index and a questionnaire, to be independent of birth rank. The latter author tested a population of undergraduates with eight different adjustment scales. In two of them firstborns reported least maladjustment. Neither result was reproducible in a second sample.

With a facilitation-inhibition scale, Owyang (1971) found firstborns to be more inhibited than seconborns in a much smaller sample of college students with no or one sib. Among 101 women visiting a Swedish prenatal clinic, sexual adaptation was found to be higher in firstborns (Uddenberg 1974).

7.6.10.2 Measures of Neuroticism

Robertson (1971) stratified a sample of Edinburgh school boys for social class, and found neuroticism as measured with Cattell's high school personality questionnaire to be independent of birth rank. Five studies made use of the neuroticism measure in the Eysenck Personality Inventory (EPI). Eysenck et al. (1969) found negligible positive correlation of neuroticism with sibship size, and none with birth rank, in 4,000 English children investigated at the age of 11 years. Nonassociation of neuroticism with birth rank was also found in much smaller college samples (McCormick et al. 1975; Farley 1975a; Wudel et al. 1979). Sutton et al. (1977) investigated an adult male and female sample and found firstborn females to be overrepresented among subjects with a high neuroticism score.

7.6.10.3 Conclusions (Table 34)

Table 34. Birth order, adjustment, and neuroticism

Author	*N*	Age	Social class controlled	Sibship size controlled	Highest scores
Adjustment measures					
Damrin (1949)	159	High school (females)	–	–	–
Hawkes et al. (1958)	256	Fifth grade	–	–	–
Lessing et al. (1967a)	855	Elementary, high school (males, females)	+	+	–
Lessing et al. (1972)	321	Fourth to seventh grades (males, females)	+	+	–
	238	Sixth to eighth grades (males, females)	+	+	Firstborn females (one test in two, explained variance < 3%)

Table 34. (continued)

Author	N	Age	Social class controlled	Sibship size controlled	Highest scores
Corsello (1973)	201	Fourth grade (males, females)	–	–	Firstborns
Reddy (1967)	620	High school	–	–	Secondborns
Prakash et al. (1963)	200	High school (males, females)	–	–	Middle children
Krauthamer (1974)	120	8–12 years	–	–	Firstborns
Koch (1956 d)	350	5–6 years (males, females)	+	+	Secondborn females firstborn males
Douglas (1964)	5,362	11 years	–	–	Firstborns, lastborns
Davie et al. (1972)	1,548	7 years (males, females)	+	–	Earlierborns
Skovholt et al. (1973)	1,266	First grade	–	–	Firstborns, lastborns
Swanson et al. (1972)	704	College (males, females)	–	+	–
Macbeth (1975)	716	College (males, females)	–	+	Firstborns (two scales in eight)
	215		–	+	–
Owyang (1971)	120	College	–	+	Secondborns
Uddenberg (1974)	101	Adults (females)	–	–	Firstborns
Neuroticism					
Robertson (1971)	297	14 years (males)	+	+	–
Eysenck et al. (1969)	4,000	11 years	–	+	–
McCormick et al. (1975)	120	College (males, females)	–	–	–
Farley (1975 a)	141	College (females)	–	+	–
Wudel et al. (1979)	103	College males, females	–	–	–
Sutton et al. (1977)	353	Adults	–	–	Firstborn females

There is no evidence that firstborns are less well-adjusted or more neurotic than laterborns. In some studies they even appear better adjusted, which is in agreement with data on self-esteem (see p. 155).

7.6.11 Birth Order and Intro- and Extraversion

Being more adult-oriented and expected by parents to be a model for their sibs, firstborns supposedly develop more introspection and are more sensitive, serious, and conscientious than laterborns (McArthur 1956; Harris 1964). Middle-class parents characterize their firstborns in a way which coincides with Eysenck's concept of introversion (Price 1969) (see p. 168). Here we shall discuss the hypothesis that firstborns tend toward intro- and laterborns toward extraversion.

Personality Questionnaires. The EPI was used in four samples. Eysenck et al. (1969) tested 4,000 English 11-year-old children and, with sibship size controlled, extraversion was independent of birth order.

In two smaller undergraduate samples no difference in extraversion by birth rank was found (Farley 1975; Wudel et al. 1979), while in a third greater extraversion appeared in firstborn males and secondborn females (McCormick et al. 1975).

In a stratified sample of 14-year-old Edinburgh school boys tested with Cattel's high school personality questionnaire, only-children and firstborns were found significantly more introverted than laterborns only in the lower-working class. In the skilled working and the middle class birth rank was not associated with introversion (Robertson 1971). In male and female college students investigated with the Child test for intro- and extraversion no differences by birth order were found (Eisenman et al. 1970b).

Ratings. A sample of 87 male and female juvenile delinquents were questioned and rated on their preferred group interaction style. There were differences in conventionality and directness by sex and ethnicity, but none by birth rank (Bruff 1977).

A large sample of Austrian school children (11- to 14-year-olds) was rated by parents and teachers on an intro- and extraversion scale, results where the raters differed being excluded. Within sex, firstborns appeared more introverted than laterborns and only children (Hillinger 1958). MacFarlane et al. (1954) present mothers' ratings of problems from the age of 21 months to 14 years in first- and laterborn boys and girls (not sibs) from the California Growth Study. The sample diminished extremely (126 at birth, 41 at 14 years), middle-class parents tending to remain in the study. While firstborn girls scored higher on almost any problem behavior than laterborn girls, firstborn boys differed from laterborn boys by a more internalizing pattern (more fear and sensitivity, less destruction).

7.6.11.1 **Conclusions** (Table 35)

Table 35. Birth order and introversion

Author	*N*	Age	Social class controlled	Sibship size controlled	Highest scores
Personality questionnaires					
Eysenck et al. (1969)	4,000	11 years	–	+	–
Farley (1975)	141	College (females)	–	+	–
Wudel et al. (1979)	103	College (males, females)	–	–	–
McCormick et al. (1975)	120	College (males, females)	–	+	Firstborn females, secondborn males
Robertson (1971)	297	14 years (males)	+	–	Firstborns, only children (one social class in three)
Eisenman et al. (1970b)	263	College (males, females)	–	–	–
Questionnaires on social behavior					
Bruff (1977)	87	Adolescent (males, females)	–	–	–
Ratings by parents and teachers					
Hillinger (1958)	587	11–14 years (males, females)	–	–	Firstborns
MacFarlane et al. (1954)	126 41	21 months 14 years	+	–	Firstborns (males)

There is no evidence from personality scales that firstborns are more introverted, nor is there any such evidence when their social behavior is self-rated. Because of failure to control background variables (Hillinger 1958) and shrinking sample size (MacFarlane 1954) the result that parents and teachers consider firstborns more introverted can only be accepted as extremely preliminary evidence.

7.6.12 Birth Order and Empathy

Empathy is defined as the capacity of an observer to react emotionally because he perceives that another person is experiencing an emotion (Stotland et al. 1971). It is discussed here because of its kinship to the concept of extraversion. There are various hypotheses on the association of empathy with birth rank. According to one, in childhood firstborns model themselves after their parents, laterborns after their sibs: The latter, having many models, will become more socially flexible and more role-diffuse than firstborns and will be able to empathize more easily (Sutton-Smith et al. 1970). Another hypothesis postulates that laterborns, being sib-oriented, will most easily empathize with persons similar to themselves, while firstborns, being parent-oriented, will empathize with persons different from themselves (Stotland et al. 1971).

Studies of empathy are mainly experimental. Staffieri et al. (1970) investigated the ability to interpret facial expressions on pictures in 10- to 11-year-old children. Results were independent of sibship size and birth order. Sutton-Smith et al. (1970, pp. 111, 121) expected better histrionic ability in later- than in firstborns, which was not confirmed by ratings of the theatrical performance of school children. The same authors expected further that laterborns would be more able to interpret behavior of figures in line drawings than firstborns. This was seen among college subjects in male sibships of two, but not in mixed or female sibships.

A small sample of black and white adolescents had to predict the answers to a questionnaire that would be given by the other group members. There were differences in the predicting capacity by sex and race but not by birth rank (Parson 1978).

A large body of experimental studies on empathy with college subjects has been presented by Stotland et al. (1971), where the hypothesis that laterborns more readily empathize with persons similar to themselves than firstborns is tested. Similarity with a model was produced by reporting the model to have been working on the same task as the subjects, to have given similar results on a personality or values test, or to have the same status as the subjects. The modells emotion subjects were supposed to react to was produced by having the model succeed or fail in a task, or feel faked pain or faked pleasure. Empathy produced in the subjects was measured by standardized self-reports on feelings, by measuring palmar sweat, skin conductance, and vasoconstriction, and by their evaluating their own performance either in agreement or disagreement with the supposed performance of the model. According to the authors, results were not consistent. When differences by birth rank in the expected direction were found, they were not reproducible. The returns of these numerous and well-planned experiments are disappointing (see also Stotland et al. 1962 a, b; 1963 a, b).

One Investigation on empathic ability uses the EPPS. In rural white adolescents from the southern USA no relation of scores to birth order or sibship size was found (Ballante 1973).

Conclusions

There is no evidence that empathy is related to birth rank. Had it been found to be consistently higher in laterborns, this would have given some support to the hypothesis that they are more extraverted in the sense of being more affected by other persons' emotions than firstborns. As they stand, results of the experimental studies on empathy raise doubt about the validity of the results where firstborns were found to be more introverted by parents and teachers (see p. 159 ff.).

7.6.13 Birth Order and Responsibility

Stronger orientation towards their parents and delegated parental power over younger sibs supposedly develop in firstborns a more severe conscience than in laterborns. They will become "the responsible type" (Bossard et al. 1955), particularly if female. Several investigations examining this hypothesis have used "locus of control" scales. These are constructed to measure the degree to which a person attributes success or failure to him- or herself or to outside agents, i.e., the degree of perceived responsibility for the course of one's life. Perceived responsibility was found to be positively correlated with income and education by Husaini et al. (1981).

Locus of Control Scales. Crandall et al. (1965) studied a large number of elementary and high school students selected to represent schools in various communities. Among the younger children no association of responsibility with birth rank was found, while firstborns scored higher among the older. Scores were positively related to IQ and negatively related to sibship size. The Crandall scale was given to young black and white males at youth centers in ghetto and nonghetto areas of an American city. Smaller sibship size and higher work status of the father was correlated with higher responsibility. In nonghetto areas firstborns were more responsible (Hreshko 1977).

Similarly, higher responsibility of firstborns in a sample of black lower class adolescents was found by May (1978) with another scale. No association of locus of control with birth rank appeared in a sample of middle class sixth graders with one sib (Frankel 1968) or in 800 randomly selected fourth to sixth graders (Newhouse 1974), where, instead, sex differences were found.

Five studies make use of Rotter's internal-external control scale. In a sample of male and female college students there was no association of scores with birth rank in females. Firstborn males, however, felt more often externally controlled than laterborns (Eisenman et al. 1968). In none of the other samples (200–700 subjects) were differences by birth rank found (MacDonald 1971 b; Taylor et al. 1968; Roodin et al. 1974 a; Macbeth 1975 with two samples).

Various Measures of Responsibility. In her sample, Koch (1956c) (see p. 93) did not find responsibility as rated by teachers to vary with birth order. Girls, however, received higher scores than boys.

The following samples consist of college or university students and comprise 100–200 subjects. Hall (1963; Hall et al. 1964) factor-analyzed a questionnaire on interests and activities in a well-matched sample of first- and laterborn male university students in sibships of two. A factor of "inner-directedness of striving" was higher in older than younger sibs. A questionnaire on future-time perspective (correlating, according to the authors, highly with locus of control) was given to undergraduates (Platt et al. 1969). Only one scale in five differentiated between birth ranks: Only children and firstborns, particularly when female, scored higher for conceptualization of future-time span. In a value survey, on the other hand, there were no indications of firstborns valuing responsibility higher than laterborns in female subjects (Penn 1973). Reported responsibility for the environment was independent of birth rank in a population of undergraduates (Marks 1972).

A very large population of upper-middle class high school and professional school students was investigated by Harris (1964) and Harris et al. (1968) to test the hypothesis of stronger inner-directedness in firstborns. The subjects were given a questionnaire on the timing of rights and duties in childhood. Timing of duties was equalized with a responsibility score and timing of rights with a dependency score. Firstborns of *their sex*, but not firstborns in the conventional sense, preferred an earlier timing of duties than laterborns, while timing of rights was not related to birth order. The author observed that the high school students favored a later timing of responsibilities than more socially selected professional school students.

7.6.13.1 Conclusions (Table 36)

Table 36. Birth order and responsibility

Author	*N*	Age	Social class controlled	Sibship size controlled	Highest responsibility
Locus of control scales					
Crandall et al. (1965)	923	Elementary, high school	–	–	Firstborns (upper grades only)
Frankel (1968)	113	Sixth grade	–	+	–
Newhouse (1974)	800	Fourth to sixth grades (males, females)	–	–	–
Hreshko (1977)	120	Adolescent (males)	–	–	Firstborns (interaction with area)
May (1978)		Adolescents (males, females)	–	–	Firstborns
Eisenmann et al. (1968)	131	College (males, females)	–	–	Firstborn males

Table 36. (continued)

Author	N	Age	Social class con-trolled	Sibship size con-trolled	Highest responsibility
MacDonald (1971 b) Taylor et al. (1968) Roodin et al. (1974 a) Macbeth (1975) (two samples)	200–700 (five samples)	College and University (males, females)	–	–	–
Ratings					
Koch (1956 c)	360	5–6 years	+	+	–
Various measures					
Marks (1972)	662	College (males, females)	–	–	–
Hall (1963) Hall et al. (1964)	104	University (males)	+	+	Firstborns (one factor)
Platt et al. (1969)	235	College (males, females)	–	–	Firstborn females (one scale in five)
Penn (1973)	168	College (females)	–	–	–
Harris (1964) Harris et al. (1968)	1,200	High school, professional school (males, females)	+	–	–

There are 16 samples where responsibility scores in relation to birth order were studied (Table 36). Greater responsibility in firstborns was found in five (four times in interaction with grade, sex, area, scales). In only one of these studies was sibship size controlled, and in the Platt et al. (1969) and the Harris (1964) studies the operationalization seems questionable.

There is, on the other hand, evidence that measures of responsibility are connected with IQ, social class, sex, and sibship size, which points to the necessity of controlling these variables. There is not sufficient evidence that firstborns are more inner-directed and responsible than laterborns.

7.6.14 Birth Order and Personality in General

According to Adler (1958, p. 149), differences in birth order "leave their mark on all expressions of the personality." "Whenever I have studied adults I have found impressions left on them from their early childhood and lasting for ever. The position in the family leaves an indelible stamp upon the style of life" (Adler 1958, p. 154). According to this hypothesis, birth order differences may be expected on scales and inventories constructed to portray the whole personality, though the Stroup et al. (1965) survey, going back to the 1930 s, did not find consistent results.

7.6.14.1 Personality Scales

CPI, 16-PF. A study by Stroup et al. (1965), analyzing the scores of a population of middle-class college freshmen for birth rank with the 16-PF, yielded negative results for birth order differences in both sexes, as did the study of a much smaller college sample by McCutcheon (1974) with the CPI.

MMPI (Minnesota Multiphasic Personality Inventory). Most studies have investigated college and university student samples. In the Hall (1963) sample of 104 well-matched first- and secondborn male students (see p. 163) no significant difference by birth order was found. In a male and female sample (Olson 1973) on the other hand, firstborn males were higher on hypochondriasis than middle children, while there was no difference for females. Though in both sexes there were features distinguishing middle children from the other birth ranks, there was no control for sibship size. In this study, as well as in an investigation by Croake et al. (1977), first and youngest children scored higher on any scale than middle children. In a sample of both sexes from ten New England colleges, first- and laterborn males did not differ on any scale, while laterborn females were higher on hypochondriasis and hypomania (Dickson 1969).

In one study investigating nonstudent adult subjects, mental in- and outpatients' test results were not significantly correlated to birth rank (Eisenman et al. 1966).

EPPS. Ten scales of the EPPS were given to first- and secondborns in a sample of female undergraduates. Sibship size being controlled, there were no significant differences by birth order (McKeithen 1965).

Gordon Personal Profile. Among evening-session students, youngest children appeared more stable than only children and first- and middleborns. Though ages ranged from 18 to 62 years, there was no control for age and possibly increased stability with this variable (Greenberg et al. 1963).

Gough and Laforge Check Lists. Sutton-Smith et al. (1970, p. 113) gave the Gough adjective checklist to a small sample of female undergraduates in all positions of birth order and sex of sib in sibships of two. Firstborns were higher in nurturance, order, and self-control, and secondborns were higher in aggression and autonomy. Levels of significance were not given and differences seem small and inconsistent.

The Laforge interpersonal checklist was given to 100 male students, 80 of whom were first- or lastborns in sibships of three with same-sex sibs, while 20 were a control group not selected for birth order. Results were not correlated to birth order (Stewart 1967).

Scales Based on Birth Order Theories. Greene et al. (1970) constructed a scale based on Adler's and Schachter's hypotheses of birth order influences on personality. In Mexican male and female freshmen no association between birth rank and personality was found. Adler's hypothesis that birth order influences are stronger when sibs are born within 3 years was investigated in a subsample whose sibs were born within this space. Results were even weaker than for the whole sample. A similar scale was given to female college students. Differences were restricted to middle children. There was no control for sibship size (Peterson et al. 1972). In a scale constructed according to Toman's theories (Vockell et al. 1971) and given to female college students, results were equally negative.

Various Scales. From a pool of subjects in a university career counseling service subjects from sibships of two and comparable by social class were selected. The sample was equidistributed for sex of subject, sex of sib, and birth order. In two of five scales of a personality screening inventory there was a significant difference by birth rank: firstborns were higher on defensiveness, secondborns on social expression (Stenger 1975).

A sentence completion blank was given by Hall (1963; Hall et al. 1964) to the sample mentioned previously p. 163. Scores did not vary by birth order.

Personality variables derived by factor analysis from a new personality inventory given to a college sample (controlling for sibship size, sex, and sex of sibs) found middle children to score higher in leadership and status interest than youngest children. The finding was not, however, reproduced in a university population (Klockars 1968). Number of subjects is not given.

Combinations of Personality Scales

Mental Patient Samples. In a sample of schizophrenic patients, the MMPI, EPPS, and MPI (Maudsley Personality Inventory) showed middle children to differ from only children and first- and lastborns. Sibship size and age were not controlled (Novicki 1967). A sample of undergraduates and one of psychiatric patients was investigated with an hysteroid-obsessive questionnaire and a psychasthenia scale from the MMPI, testing the hypothesis that youngest children tend more toward hysteria and oldest toward obsession. An association with birth rank did not emerge (Ruff et al. 1975).

College or University Student Samples. Six personality scales were given to male and female undergraduates of sibship sizes one to three and were then factor-analyzed. Findings tended to demonstrate lower adjustment in laterborn males (Vaughn 1975). By far the largest sample was studied by Macbeth (1975): undergraduates were given eight personality measures, including CPI, MMPI, EPPS, and an adjective checklist. While the latter test and the EPPS did not result in significant differences by birth order, those obtained through the MMPI, the CPI, and other scales were not reproducible with a second sample of undergraduates. Controlling for sex, sibship size, sib sex, and in some instances social class did not lead to more consistent or reproducible results.

7.6.14.2 Personality Ratings

The largest and most carefully selected sample is Koch's (1955a, 1956d, 1957a), which consisted of 5- to 6-year-old children from unbroken, two-child suburban families (see p. 93). The subjects were rated by their teachers on two scales. Subgroups were formed according to sex, sex of sib, and spacing. Most birth order differences were based on an interaction with the latter two variables. From the large mass of data, no clear and consistent picture emerges. The traits that are attributed to a given birth position in some cases appear contradictory. Unfortunately the results are interpreted ad hoc and not used to examine previous hypotheses. The author herself (1957, p. 220) warned against using her results for broad generalizations concerning sib influence.

Her own ratings of children, based on interviews with them and their parents, were used by Vuyk (1959) with 125 8- to 12-year-old middle-class children from sibships of two who were selected from the control group of another investigation. While Koch found for example, older brothers with a sister to be particularly self-confident and popular, according to Vuyk having a younger sister leads to anxiety and seclusiveness in male children. "Typical" birth order differences were only found in same-sex pairs of small spacing; the oldest child appeared reticent, quiet, and introverted and the younger easy-going and extraverted.

7.6.14.3 Sibs Within the Same Sibship

Teacher's Ratings. Newbert (1969) studied 40 sibships of three. Subjects were in the first to the eighth grades and maximum age difference was 8 years. When rated on two scales by their teachers, middle children appeared at the same time more excitable and more phlegmatic, less fearful and more mature than first- and lastborns.

Parents Compare Their Children. A sample of 40 sibs, all below 7 years of age and all in sibships of two, were rated by their mothers (Dean 1947) with the help of a questionnaire. In comparison with second children, firstborns appeared more dependent, thoughtful, worried, sensitive, and helpless when faced with aggression. In the course of a follow-up of former Harvard students, 86 subjects who were fathers of two children gave a casual description of the childrens' personalities (McArthur 1956). In the descriptions of firstborns significantly more adjectives were used connotating seriousness, sensitivity, fondness of books, and adult-orientation. Secondborns instead were described by adjectives implying independence, cheerfulness, and rebelliousness. Age and sex of the children thus described are not given. A sample of 434 self-selected Dutch middle-class parents rated their two children with a list containing 135 adjectives (Vuyk 1961, 1963): The younger child was 6- to 12-years-old and firstborns were at most 4 years older. Adjectives like quiet, serious, sensitive, responsible, and thoughtful were significantly more often used in relation to first- than secondborns. Three years later the same parents were sent an abbreviated form of the former questionnaire and 60% answered: This time, differences between first and second children were mitigated in that secondborns were now more often described as nervous and sensitive. They did not appear more extraverted or popular than the older children.

A group of 40 couples rated peer relations of their three children (first to eighth graders). There was no association with birth order (Newbert 1969).

There is only one author who took care to control sex and age. Price (1969) collected by advertisement 723 middle-class parents with at least two children of the same sex above the age of 18 years. The subjects were sent a 100-item questionnaire for each child and 87% were returned: of 672 sib pairs 63 pairs were excluded because of being twins or chronically ill. In sibships of more than two children, the youngest same-sex children were compared. Parents were asked to compare the sibs at their present adult age. Three hundred and twelve pairs contained a firstborn. Reliability between parents was measured and found high. A deviation from expectation in item distribution was restricted to pairs containing a firstborn. In these descriptions 18 items differed at least at the 0.01 level, resulting in the following description of firstborns: They were earlier to talk and read, at school, tidier, more serious, and methodical, more law abiding, less impulsive, and less fond of cuddling. They were also more nervous, less happy, and less socially active. The author assumes the differences to connote greater introversion (in the sense of Eysenck) in firstborns. Among laterborns no significant differences were found, and "firstborns of their sex" were not distinguished in any particular way.

7.6.14.4 Conclusions (Table 37)

There are 26 samples that were given one or a combination of several personality scales or ratings. A difference for birth order or birth rank emerged in ten samples and in five of these, firstborns differed from laterborns (as personality differences between middle children and other ranks could be due to the former's bias for larger sibship size they are not discussed here):
MMPI: Firstborn females lower in hypochondriasis (Dickson)
MMPI: Firstborn males higher in hypochondriasis (Olson)
Personality screening inventory: Firstborn males more defensive, less expressive (Stenger)
Combination of six scales: Firstborns better adjusted (Vaughn)
Ratings: Firstborns more introverted (interaction with sex of sib and spacing) (Vuyk)

In no case was the same result reproduced by the same method in another sample. Also the largest samples and those where combinations of scales were used did not bring to light any difference between first- and laterborns. We may conclude that personality scales and ratings do not provide consistent evidence of a birth rank influence on personality.

Parental ratings of sibs, on the other hand, favor a "firstborn personality." Four of six parental ratings agree that firstborns appear more serious, methodical, problem-ridden, and introverted than the easy-going laterborns. One study finds this in preschool children, one in children of nonspecified age and sex, one in school children (where findings, however, did not prove reliable over 3 years), and one in young adults controlling for sex and social class. This latter is the largest and most carefully investigated sample (Price), though, being found through advertisements, it has no claim to representativity. Here, differences appear quite clear, consistent, and of appreciable size. They are indicative of a firstborn personality which in males and females has the same traits. The findings are in opposition to the much more tenuous results found by other methods both when sibs and nonsibs are com-

Table 37. Birth order and personality (A) and personality of sibs within the same sibship (B)

Author	*N*	Age	Social class con- trolled	Sibship size con- trolled	Differences
A *16-PF, CPI*					
McCutcheon (1974)	93	College (males, females)	–	–	–
Stroup et al. (1965)	1,560	College (males, females)	+	–	–
MMPI					
Hall (1963)	104	University (males)	+	+	–
Dickson (1969)	517	College (males, females)	–	–	Firstborns vs. laterborn (females)
Olson (1973)	261	College (males, females)	–	–	Firstborns vs. laterborn (males)
Croake et al. (1977)	216	College (males, females)	–	–	Middle vs. first- and lastborns
Eisenman et al. (1966)	127	Adult	–	–	–
EPPS					
McKeithen (1965)	495	College (females)	–	–	–
Gordon personal profile					
Greenberg et al. (1963)	262	Adult	–	–	Youngest vs. oldest, and middleborns
Gough and Laforge checklists					
Sutton-Smith et al. (1970)	80	College (females)	–	+	–
Stewart (1967)	100	College (males)	–	+	–
Scales based on birth order theories					
Greene et al. (1970)	471	University (males, females)	–	–	–
Peterson et al. (1972)	92	College (females)	–	–	Middle vs. oldest and youngest
Vockell et al. (1971)	102	College (females)	–	–	–
Various scales					
Stenger (1975)	240	University (males, females)	+	+	First- vs. secondborns
Hall (1963) Hall et al. (1964)	104	University (males)	+	+	–
Klockers (1968)	?	Colleges (males, females)	+	+	Middle vs. youngest (leadership)
	?	University (males, females)	+	+	–
Combinations of scales					
Novicki (1967)	200	Adult	–	–	Middle vs. first- and lastborns

Table 37. (continued)

Author	N	Age	Social class con-trolled	Sibship size con-trolled	Differences
Ruff et al. (1975)	55	College	–	–	–
	101	Adult	–	–	–
Vaughn (1975)	102	College (males, females)	–	+	First- vs. laterborns
Macbeth (1975)	716	University (males, females)	–	+	–
	265	University (males, females)	–	+	–
Ratings					
Koch (1955 a, 1956 d, 1957 a)	360	5–6 years (males, females)	+	+	Inconsistent
Vuyk (1959)	125	8–12 years (males, females)	+	+	Firstborns vs. secondborns (in interaction with sex of sib, spacing)

	Author	Method	N	Con-trolled sex	Con-trolled age	Result
B	Newbert (1969)	Teachers' ratings	120	–	–	Middle child different
	Dean (1947)	Parents' ratings	40	–	–	Firstborns more worried, dependent
	McArthur (1956)	Parents' ratings	172	–	–	Firstborns more serious, sensitive
	Vuyk (1961, 1963)	Parents' ratings	868	–	–	Firstborns more quiet, serious, sensitive
			520	–	–	–
	Newbert (1969)	Parents' ratings	120	–	–	–
	Price (1969)	Parents' ratings	612	+	+	Firstborns more introverted, nervous, precocious, conforming

pared. The discrepancy between results found by tests and experiments on the one hand, and those found in parental ratings on the other, can be explained in several different ways:

1. Parents' ratings are not reliable and of unproven validity. In fact only one of the investigations discusses the qualities of the measuring instrument: Price (1969) finds strong agreement between the father's and mother's ratings. The raters however, are anything but independent.

2. Parents compare their adult children at different ages, and introversion increases with age. To this explanation it may be objected that in the Price study a significant difference between sibs was found only when one member of the pair was a firstborn and that an effort was made to compare sibs at the same age.

3. Being self-selected, those parents participated who were worried about their oldest child's development. This objection, however, does not explain why, in four investigations, the description of the oldest child is quite congruous.

4. Self-selected middle-class parents are influenced in their description by existing popular views on birth order differences in personality and describe their children accordingly.

5. First- and laterborns have specific parent-related behaviors because the attitude acquired toward them is different, without their personality being profoundly affected by the experiences which have led to these attitudes. The firstborn personality may be *parent-specific*.

On the basis of existing studies it is impossible to refute the last two hypotheses. The difference between results of objective methods and the consistency of parental ratings is at the moment unexplainable. Similar studies on representative samples of parents might be as worthwhile as the study of the personality of sibs at the same age.

7.6.15 Birth Order and Sex Role

The hypothesis discussed in this paragraph is based on some research findings that firstborn women are less creative but firstborn men more so than laterborns of the same sex (see p. 150). It has been assumed by various authors that the difference in creativity between first- and laterborns is caused by firstborns being more exposed to the socialization influences of their parents, which would lead to their accepting *traditional sex roles* more readily than laterborns. According to this hypothesis, firstborn females should score high on tests measuring conventional femininity and firstborn males should score high in conventional masculinity (Edwards et al. 1973).

Child Samples. When kindergarten children were questioned for masculine and feminine game and job preferences, firstborns appeared more strongly sex-typed in job preference (Laosa et al. 1970). This result was not confirmed by another kindergarten sample, where children were studied with the "it" scale (a picture of a sexually neutral child is related to sex-typed objects), a questionnaire, and teachers' ratings for sex-role adoption (Laosa et al. 1972). Sears (1970), following up 40% of his original kindergarten sample at 12 years of age, found no birth order influence on the masculinity scale of the CPI. In a sample of male high school students, no difference by birth rank was found in the masculinity-feminity scale of the MMPI (Farley et al. 1971).

College and University Student Samples. A questionnaire compiled from various personality scales was given to a large sample of male and female subjects. In females femininity was inversely related to sibship size, only children being highest and girls with two sibs lowest. There was, however, no association with birth rank (Gormly 1968). Equally negative results were reported for female students with pertinent scales from the MMPI and the CPI (Landers 1970) and with the CPI scale in a large population of males and females (Marquette 1972).

Studying male students with at least one male sib with the semantic differential, no association of masculinity with birth rank emerged (Nash 1970). When a values inventory was given to male and female students (only children or children having one or two sibs), perception of the own-sex role was independent of birth order and sibship size (Barrett 1975).

Four studies investigated sex role-related traditionalism in females. In a mailed questionnaire (return rate 90%) female students gave their opinion of social roles and personality characteristics of women. Birth rank differences were not significant, though in the majority of questions firstborns proved more traditional (Kammeyer 1966). Altus (1970) investigated sex role satisfaction in female students with one sib. Firstborns reported dissatisfaction less often than laterborns.

A group of college women who had described themselves as career-oriented on a questionnaire were compared with home-oriented subjects. First- and laterborns were equidistributed among both groups (Oliver 1975). A similar result was found in a sample of university females (Edwards et al. 1973) who were questioned on their intention to take up traditional feminine work roles.

Nonstudent Adult Samples. Sex role-related traditionalism was investigated in Israeli women taking a course for homemaking (Weller et al. 1975). Firstborns appeared more traditional than laterborns.

7.6.15.1 Conclusions

Table 38. Birth order and sex role

Author	N	Age	Social class controlled	Sibship size controlled	Highest sex-typing
Game preferences, "it" scale					
Laosa et al. (1970)	96	Kindergarten (males, females)	–	–	Firstborns
Laosa et al. (1972)	96	Kindergarten (males, females)	–	–	–
Masculinity-femininity scales					
Sears (1970)	140	12 years (males, females)	–	+	–
Farley et al. (1971)	288	High school (males)	–	–	–
Gormly (1968)	359	College (males, females)	–	+	–
Landers (1970)	200	College (females)	–	–	–
Marquette (1972)	2,407	College (males, females)	–	–	–
Semantic differential, value inventory					
Nash (1970)	210	College (males)	–	–	–
Barrett (1976)	857	College (males, females)	–	+	–
Measures of traditionalism					
Kammeyer (1966)	209	College (females)	–	–	–
Altus (1970)	118	University (females)	–	–	Firstborns
Oliver (1975)	74	College (females)	–	–	–
Edwards et al. (1973)	272	University (females)	–	–	–
Weller et al. (1975)	138	Adults (females)	–	–	Firstborns

The finding that at kindergarten age firstborns are more strongly sex-typed was not replicated with a second sample and a more thorough method.

Masculinity-feminity scales did not reveal differences accoding to birth rank even in a very large sample.

Stronger sex-typing in females was found in two samples of six in which sex role satisfaction and traditionalism were measured with ad hoc questionnaires; however, sibship size, social class, religious denomination and rural or urban habitation were not controlled, though all of these variables are known to influence attitude toward sex role. There is consequently inadequate evidence for stronger sex-typing in first- than in laterborn women and no evidence at all for differences in sex-typing by birth order in men.

7.6.16 Sex Role Differentiation and Sex of Sib

There are two hypotheses concerning the influence of sex of sib on sex role differentiation. The *imitation hypothesis* states that the presence of a different-sex sib leads to an attenuation of sex role. Girls with brothers, for instance, will appear less feminine than girls with sisters. The *contrast hypothesis*, on the other hand, expects a different-sex sib to enhance sex role in subjects; girls with brothers are supposed to be more strongly feminine than girls with sisters (Leventhal 1970; Sutton-Smith et al. 1970, pp. 18–24).

Sex Role Differentiation and Sib Sex in Sibships of Two

Child Samples. In the Koch sample (1956a) (see p. 93), kinderarten children were rated by their teachers for sissiness and tomboyishness, i.e., for socially disapproved feminine behavior in boys and masculine behavior in girls. Tomboyishness in girls was not related to birth order, sex of sib, or spacing. Results on sissiness in boys were inconclusive.

Koch's data were reanalyzed by Brim (1958). The rated variables were subjected to another rating by four judges for instrumentality (deemed typical of male behavior) and for expressivity (deemed typical of female behavior). Koch's protocols were then evaluated for the number of masculine and feminine traits found to differentiate between her subgroups. This time, the imitation hypothesis was confirmed for both sexes (though levels of significance were not given): girls with brothers were less feminine than girls with sisters. Firstborn boys did not appear strongly influenced by sex of sib; however, younger boys appeared more feminine when the older sib was a girl rather than a boy. Age spacing dod not influence results.

A sample of elementary school children in sibships of two were given a play and game preference scale, the items of which had been rated for masculinity and femininity. In agreement with Koch and Brim, in sibships of two it was found that boys with a brother scored higher on masculinity than boys with a sister, while girls with a sister scored higher on femininity than girls with a brother (Sutton-Smith et al. 1964; Rosenberg et al. 1964b).

Using a sample of middle-class kindergarten children in sibships of two and a control group of only children, Bigner (1972) found with the "it" scale (see p. 171) that males with an older brother had more masculine sex preferences than males with an older sister, and that girls with an older sister were more feminine than girls with an older brother. All results were significant and independent of spacing.

College and University Student Samples. Sample sizes vary between 100 and 250. Scores in the masculinity-femininity scale of the MMPI in male and female students, either single children or in all positions of birth order, sex, and sex of sib in sibships of two, varied with sex of sib in males but not in females. Femininity in males with a sister was significantly higher than in males with a brother (Sutton-Smith et al. 1970). The opposite result was found by Leventhal (1970) when studying male college students with one sib with the femininity scale of the CPI: Men with an older sister tended to be less feminine than men with brothers. In male university freshmen who were given the MMPI by the same author, sex of sibling was not associated with scores on the masculinity-femininity scale. When, however, a population of over 1,000 freshmen with one sib was studied with an interest and activity sheet, males with an older sister were found to be more masculine than men with an older brother, while firstborns were not different by sex of sib. Landers (1970) studied two groups of female college students with one sib with the masculinity-femininity scales of the MMPI and the CPI. There were no consistent and reproducible sibling effects on sex typing. Male university subjects in all positions of birth order and sex of sib were tested with a questionnaire compiled from preexisting personality inventories (Kahn et al. 1972) under the hypothesis that males with an older sister would differ in their sexual attitudes from men in other positions. The result was in the expected direction of higher femininity in these subjects, but not above chance level.

Sex Role Differentiation and Sib Sex in Sibships of Three or More

Child Samples. The Sutton-Smith et al. (1964) result (see above) was not reproducible in sibships of three. One large sample of preschool and one of elementary school children were rated by their teachers on a masculinity-femininity scale (Vroegh 1971). In both samples ratings were independent of the sex composition of the sibship and of the next older sib's sex. Brown (1956) studied kindergarten children for sex preference with the "it" scale (see p. 171). Girls were not influenced in sex preference by sex of sib. In boys, however, having only female sibs tended to lead to less masculine preference. Grotevant (1978) studied a sample of adopted and biologically related adolescents with the scale of sex differences in interest of the Strong Campbell inventory. Boys were not influenced by sex of sibs; in girls, however, having three or more female sibs was associated with less feminine interests.

In a small sample of male high school students (either single children or having only brothers or only sisters) scores on the MMPI masculinity-femininity scales were independent of number and sex of sibs (Farley et al. 1971).

College and University Student Samples. Here sample sizes vary between 300 and 900. In a study on sex-specific working preferences conducted with female subjects (Edwards et al. 1973) there were interactions of position with sex of sibs. The results, however, do not make sense. In an inventory of masculine and feminine values given to a population of male and female freshmen, perception of the own sex role was independent of the sex composition of the sibship (Barrett 1975). A questionnaire on the emancipation of women was given to females (Clowers 1977): Attitudes toward emancipation were independent of the presence of male sibs and of age spacing between subjects and next younger or older brother. Male and female subjects were studied by Lamke et al. (1980) with the Bem sex role inventory. Women with high scores on both masculinity and femininity tended to have more brothers and more older brothers and to be more often laterborn than other women. In males, high scores on both variables were not related to number or sex of sibs.

Sex Discrimination

Schell et al. (1968) used the "it" scale to measure sex discrimination. In a sample of 64 kindergarten children, who had to attribute sex-typed objects to a neutral figure that was presented either as a girl or a boy, children with sibs had higher scores on sex discrimination than only children. Bigner (1972), in the sample described on p. 174, also found with the same method that children of either sex who had an older brother had more masculine preferences than only children.

7.6.16.1 Conclusions (see Table 39)

In studies of children with one sib there is, at kindergarten and elementary school age, some support for the imitation hypothesis: Subjects with one different-sex sib present behavior and interest traits of the other sex. In children in larger sibships and in young adults a consistent influence of sib sex is not found. These findings may be explained by the assumption of a transistory sib sex influence not on sx-typing but mainly on sex discrimination and on interest in the activities of the other sex. The studies of Bigner and of Schell et al. point to this: In both, attribution of sex-typed objects to the "it" figure was higher in children with sibs than in only children. This is a parallel to the studies demonstrating that the presence of an older sib leads to greater discrimination of power relations in younger sibs than in children (Bigner) (see p. 97f.). At a later age, all children have learned to discriminate the sexes, and sib sex loses its former importance. Influence of sib sex perhaps mainly takes place in a cognitive connotation, i.e., a sib helps children to discriminate the sexes at an earlier age. The hypothesis that sex of sib has no general and lasting influence on personality has not been refuted. This, of course, does not exclude the possibility that in *some* families sib sex may have a strong influence on a person's development.

Table 39. Influence of Sex of Sib on Sex-typing

Imitation hypothesis supported	*N*	Contrast hypothesis supported	*N*	Neither hypothesis supported	*N*
Sibship of two					
Children					
Brim (1958)	384 Kindergarten				
Sutton-Smith et al. (1964)	214 Elementary school				
Bigner (1972)	216 Kindergarten				
College and university students					
Sutton-Smith et al. (1970)	253 (supported in males)	Leventhal (1970)	218 males	Leventhal (1970)	624 males
		Leventhal (1970)	1,079 males	Landers (1970)	150 females
				Kahn et al. (1972)	128 males
Sibship of three or more					
Children					
Brown (1956)	146 Kindergarten (males with all sisters)	Grotevant (1978)	425 adolescents (females with 3 or more sisters)	Sutton-Smith et al. (1964 b)	214 Elementary school
				Vroegh (1971)	639 Kindergarten and elementary school
Kindergarten + elementary school					
				Farley et al. (1971)	70 High school
College and university students					
				Edwards et al. (1973)	300 females
				Barrett (1975)	857 males, females
subjects					
				Clowers (1977)	361 females
females					
				Lambke et al. (1980)	454 females

7.6.17 Personality and Sex of Sib

Sutton-Smith et al. (1970, p. 142) have sketched characteristic traits of children in sibships of two by birth order and sex of sib, referring mainly to Schachter's affiliation studies, Koch's research, and MacFarlane's. Berkeley longitudinal study (Schachter 1959; MacFarlane et al. 1954; Koch 1955 a, b). Inconsistencies between these investigations are reconciled by a developmental concept: For example, the younger male sib of an older brother is said to be masculine and fearless at 6 years of age, then to become dependent and submissive until adolescence, and then to return again to independence, low anxiety, and dominance. For each position by sex of sib a similar sketch is given. Sex of sib is supposed to influence a sibs' personality very strongly, a younger male with an older male sib developing "male" personality characteristics, e.g., a preference for entrepreneurial and managerial activities, but a younger male with an older sister developing high anxiety and low self-esteem, which, however, changes at adolescence (because the sister leaves the home) to high self-esteem and low anxiety. As the evidence presented here does not support the hypothesis that sex of sib is generally highly influential in the modeling of a person's sex role and of sex role-related traits, such far-reaching conclusions do not seem warranted. If the concept of development is used so arbitrarily, any hypothesis becomes irrefutable.

7.6.18 Birth Order, Interpersonal Relations, Mate Selection, and Quality of Married Life

7.6.18.1 Selection of Mate by Birth Rank

This variable has been studied upon the assumption that birth order is a pervasive influence on personality and that marriage is more frequent between partners having similar character traits. Accordingly, similar birth rank among marriage partners can be expected.

The following studies were performed with 150–450 subjects. Altus et al. (1970 a) compared the reported birth rank of the parents of American students and concluded that middle children intermarry more often than expected by chance. Ward et al. (1974), studying birth rank in a random sample of faculty members and their wives, found that first- and laterborns tended to marry persons of the same birth rank. However, both studies stressed that, social background variables not being controlled, the results could be understood as following from the intermarriage of persons belonging to the same social class and/or denomination (laterborns being biased for larger sibships). Touhey (1971 a), on the other hand, did not find any association of the birth ranks of husband and wife among passersby in a large American city, nor did Kemper (1966) among businessmen.

7.6.18.2 Toman's Duplication Hypothesis

Toman (1960, 1961, 1962, 1963 a, 1964 a, 1965, 1966, 1968, 1970, 1971 a, b; Toman et al. 1961, 1970, 1973) set up the hypothesis that extrafamilial relations are successful to the degree that they duplicate earlier, long-lasting intrafamilial relations (duplication hypothesis). Birth rank and sex of sibs supposedly determine character to a large extent: An older brother of brothers is supposed to be a leader and a good worker; a youngest sister of brothers is supposed to be feminine, pliant, a good wife, and so on. Duplication is mainly important because it facilitates power relations: older sibs are supposed to direct, younger sibs to conform. The duplication hypothesis implies the two factors of complementarity of birth rank and of sex of sibs. Consequently the marriage of an older brother of sisters to a younger sister of brothers (and vice versa) is expected to be most successful, one of the partners being accustomed to conforming to directions from a person of the other sex and the other to directing a person of the other sex. In middle children the presence of older as well as younger sibs dilutes complementary, as does the presence of sibs of both sexes. No complementarity is present in the case of an oldest brother of brothers marrying an oldest sister of sisters. A poor outcome may similarly be expected when one or both partners are single children, complementarity not being possible. Contrary to the hypothesis discussed in the preceding paragraph, success in marriage would seem to be related not to similarity but to oppositeness of character traits.

Paper-Pencil Tests

Questionnaires on Partner Satisfaction and Problem Solving. By means of a questionnaire Kemper (1966) studied marital satisfaction in business executives in relation to birth rank and sib sex. The duplication hypothesis was not supported. Weller et al. (1974) gave a marital happiness questionnaire to Israeli women taking homemaking courses. He found a significant association of reported satisfaction with birth rank of self and partner, which, however, does not correspond to Toman's hypothesis. Pinsky (1974), on the other hand, studied newly married student couples, dividing them for complementarity according to Toman into a well-matched and poorly matched group. The hypothesis that birth rank would influence power distribution in marriage was not supported by a questionnaire on how domestic problems were solved. A similar negative result was found by Levinger et al. (1965) in married couples. Neither study found differences in need for dominance on the EPPS according to birth rank.

From 500 university students participating in an experimental computer dating program, Mendelson et al. (1974) selected 64 pairs who were divided into four same-sized groups with different degrees of sex and rank complementarity (both rank and sex, either, neither). Within each pair participants were matched for sibship size, religious denomination, occupation of father, race, and attractiveness. Satisfaction reported on a questionnaire and tested for validity by the number of reported dates with the computer-selected partner was significantly related to rank and sex complementarity. This finding was not confirmed by Critelli (1979), who studied volunteer couples from a university who had been dating for some time. Degree of complementarity was defined as by Mendelson et al. (1974). For mate selection the duplication hypothesis was not supported, nor was complementarity of influence on five variables measuring the partners' satisfaction with their relationship.

Questionnaires on Parental Conflict. At one American university a large freshmen population was questioned on parental birth order, dominance of father or mother, and presence or absence of interparental conflict. Dominance was not related to complementarity, while presence of conflict was significantly related to rank complementarity but not to sex complementarity. As, according to Toman, complementarity is mainly important because of dominance/submission relations, the isolated finding for rank does not fit well into his hypotheses (Baxter 1965).

Duplication and Interpersonal Conflict. According to Toman, choice of friends is also governed by duplication. This hypothesis was studied by Scheidt et al. (1974), who found that among female and male pairs of college dormitory roommates interpersonal problems (measured by a dichotomized scale) tended to be more frequent among pairs with conflicting birth rank than among those with nonconflicting rank. The study was replicated with the same result on a second group of subjects (Scheidt et al. 1976). This finding was not confirmed by Schuh et al. (1977) in a prospective study in which 28 pairs of students were matched as roommates on the basis of nonconflicting birth rank, and 31 pairs on the basis of conflicting birth rank. After a month a questionnaire on interpersonal stress did not differentiate the two groups. Birtchnell et al. (1977) compared birth rank, sex, and number of sibs of a comparatively large number of British undergraduates with those of their closest friends. No deviation from chance was found.

Real-Life Situations

Toman tested his duplication hypothesis using a child in psychiatric treatment as an indicator of a disturbed marriage (Toman et al. 1961). Parents of children from a guidance center were compared with parents of college students and with couples in the Boston area (selection unknown). It was found more often in the control groups than in subjects that one of the partners was from the first and the other from the second half of the sibship. There was also a nonsignificant tendency in the controls to have more sibs of the opposite sex than the subjects.

Of course, a child in psychotherapy is no cirterion for an ill-assorted marriage. Subjects and controls are probably from different social backgrounds. That marriage improves in quality with increasing number of different-sex sibs, and not merely with their presence, is an ad hoc introduced hypothesis.

A second attempt at verification (Toman et al. 1973) was based on reports on parents of six samples (total 2,673 subjects) containing high school and college students from various German and Swiss towns, neurotic children from German and Austrian child guidance clinics, juvenile delinquents from three German youth prisons and male and female criminals from three West German penitentiaries. Sixteen positions in the sibship for sex, rank, and sib sex were distinguished. Under the supposition of random intermarriage there are 256 possible combinations for birth rank and sib sex in marriage partners. They were distributed over a 12-point index of complementarity. Choice of partner in the parents of the subjects was found to be independent of complementarity.

Success and failure of marriage was determined by subjects reporting their parents' divorce. A lower frequency of divorce was found among marriages of high complementarity. As the probability of an intermediate complementarity increases with sibship size (presence of different-sex sibs being more probable in large sibships) and as large sibship size may be related to a style of life discouraging divorce (older age, catholic denomination, rural habitation), the high complementarity-low divorce association was examined for 467 marriages where both partners together had four or five sibs. It was found again. The result, however, should not be given much weight. The study is based on an extraordinary combination of populations different in social class, age, religious denomination, and nationality and of course widely different in the possibility their parents had to divorce after an ill-matched marriage.

One finding from this study was a higher divorce rate of single children than of persons with sib. In a longitudinal study of 742 couples, Hall (1965) found that single childrens' marriages ended more frequently in divorce than those of subjects with sibs. Levinger (1965) criticized the concept that only children per se are unfit for marriage and quotes a study proving higher divorce rates in partners from broken homes. That only childrens' homes are more often broken than those of children with sib was shown on p. 26.

Levinger et al. (1965) compared birth order and birth rank in a small sample of couples consulting a family agency with those in parents of elementary pupils. The groups did not differ.

Birtchnell et al. (1977) examined Toman's theory with a British national representative sample contacted by a market research organization. There were 982 subjects reporting a successful and 1,012 subjects reporting an unsuccessful marriage (ending mostly in divorce or separation). Subjects were compared with their partners for 16 positions, according to birth rank and number and sex of sibs. Successful and unsuccessful marriages did not differ in complementarity. Of the subjects, 27% indicated a particular fondness of a different sex sib. Men who were especially fond of an older sister tended to marry, more often than other men, a woman with one younger brother or no sibs. No corresponding choices were found in men who were fond of a younger sister or in women. Apart from this one finding, positions of marriage partners were unrelated.

7.6.18.3 **Conclusions** (Table 40)

Table 40. Birth order and interpersonal relations

Author	*N*	Age	Social class con-trolled	Sibship size con-trolled	Birth rank influence
Intermarriage for birth rank					
Altus et al. (1970 a)	452 couples	Adult	–	–	+ (Middle children)
Ward et al. (1974)	146 couples	Adult	+	–	+ (Middle children)
Touhey (1971 a)	200 couples	Adult	–	–	–
Kemper (1966)	246 couples	Adult	–	–	–
Marital satisfaction and complementarity (Toman)					
Kemper (1966)	246 couples	Adult	–	–	–
Weller et al. (1974)	239 couples	Adult	–	–	–
Pinsky (1974)	40 couples	Student	–	–	–
Levinger et al. (1965)	60 couples	Adult	–	–	–
Mendelson et al. (1974)	64 couples	University	+	+	+
Critelli (1979)	123 couples	University	–	–	–
Baxter (1965)	1,503 couples	Adult	–	–	+ (Rank only)

Table 40. (continued)

Author	N	Age	Social class controlled	Sibship size controlled	Birth rank influence
Choice of friends and complementarity					
Scheidt et al. (1974)	77 pairs	College	–	–	+
Scheidt et al. (1976)	68 pairs	College	–	–	+
Schuh et al. (1977)	61 pairs	College	–	–	–
Birtchnell et al. (1977)	329 pairs	University	–	–	–
Divorce and complementarity					
Toman et al. (1961)	402 couples		–	–	–
Toman et al. (1973)	2,673 couples		–	–	+
Levinger et al. (1965)	60 couples		–	–	–
Birtchnell et al. (1977)	1,994 couples		–	–	–

The hypothesis that people tend to marry persons of similar birth rank has to be rejected as long as there is no investigation controlling for sibship size and social class (Table 40). The duplication hypothesis is rejected. There is no evidence that birth order is of any importance in interpersonal relations, be it between friends, lovers, or married couples.

7.6.19 Birth Order and Sociometric Popularity

In sociometric tests subjects have to choose group members for certain functions, e.g., friend, working partner, and so on. Popularity is related to the number of choices a person receives. Sociometric popularity has become an issue in birth order research because firstborns were considered by some to be less popular because of their allegedly greater dependency (Finneran 1958). Another line of reasoning is based on firstborns having their parents for models and laterborns their sibs, which might lead to laterborns being more interested in peers than firstborns and consequently being more popular (Sutton-Smith et al. 1970, p. 118).

Child Samples. The following studies are based on entire school populations. The elementary grades three to six in two Texan school districts were studied with sociometric tests (Sells et al. 1963). Only and youngest children were highest in popularity, then second children with one or two sibs, and then firstborns. Middle children in large sibships were last. Among the pupils of an elementary school in the rural South there was no association of popularity with birth rank in white and black girls or in white boys. In black boys, however, lastborns were most popular (Baughman et al. 1968). Miller et al. (1976) studied first graders in a California school giving them three questions: with whom they wanted to work, to sit, and to play. With race and sex controlled, there was a small, significant positive correlation of birth rank with popularity as measured by seating and playing preference: Lastborns were most and firstborns least popular. Birth rank explained 1% of the variance in popularity. A second analysis was restricted to sibships of three and four. An explained variance of the same size resulted. Controlling for school grades did not change the association of popularity with birth rank. In a study measuring popularity of an unknown number of elementary school children in spring and autumn of 2 consecutive years and controlling for sex and social class, birth rank was not related to scores (Adams 1967).

Three studies were done with adolescent subjects. A sample of high school males from 30 schools and having one or two sibs was studied by Alexander (1966, 1968). In five of six social classes firstborns had highest popularity scores. In a cross-section of male students from 12 English secondary modern schools (Murray 1971), sibship size and social class being controlled, two measures of popularity (one sociometric) were not associated with birth rank.

College Student Samples. Schachter (1964) sent questionnaires to 833 fraternity and sorority members, asking them with whom they wanted to share their room and their recreation time; 7% of the sample answered. Firstborns were nominated significantly less often than laterborns. On the other hand, when two samples of academy freshmen were rated by their peers for leadership, personality, and compatibility, in one sample firstborns were not different from laterborns, while in the other they were rated higher. In both samples only children proved the most popular subjects (Payne 1971).

Teachers' Ratings of Social Skill in Children. In the Koch (1956b) sample of 5- to 6-year-old children (see p. 93) there were only interactions with spacing and sex of sibs in ratings for attitudes toward peers. The Miller et al. sample (1976) (see p. 181), on the other hand, was rated by the teachers by means of an adjective checklist with nine adjectives referring to social skills: on five laterborns were rated higher than firstborns.

Ratings of Own Popularity. Among sixth graders the degree to which subjects believed to be liked by their peers did not vary with birth rank (Simon et al. 1971).

7.6.19.1 Conclusions (Table 41)

Table 41. Birth order and popularity

Author	*N*	Age	Social class controlled	Sibship size controlled	Highest in popularity
Sociometry					
Sells et al. (1963)	1,003	Third to sixth grades	–	+	Only and youngest children (middle child lowest)
Boughman et al. (1968)	988	Elementary school	–	–	Youngest (interaction sex, race)

Table 41. (continued)

Author	N	Age	Social class controlled	Sibship size controlled	Highest in popularity
Miller et al. (1976)	1,750	First grade (males, females)	–	+	Youngest (firstborns lowest) Explained variance 1%
Adams (1967)	?	Elementary school (males, females)	+	–	–
Alexander (1966, 1968)	1,410	High school (males)	+	+	Firstborns
Murray (1971)	709	High school (males)	+	+	–
Various measures					
Schachter (1964)	833	University (males, females)	–	–	Laterborns
Payne (1971)	574	Academy (males)	–	–	Only children
	449	Academy (males)	–	–	Firstborns, only children
Teachers' ratings					
Koch (1956b)	384	5–6 years (males, females)	+	+	–
Miller et al. (1976)	1,750	First grade	+	+	Laterborns
Perceived popularity					
Simon et al. (1971)	129	Sixth graders	–	–	–

In three of four studies done with elementary school samples youngest children appear most popular. Among older samples the evidence is against a consistent influence of birth rank on popularity. A particular position of the first child does not appear, nor are self-ratings for popularity dependent on birth rank.

7.6.20 Personality and Spacing

Three investigations concern personality veriables in relation to spacing between sibs. Cornoldi et al. (1974) selected from a sample of Padovan senior high school students 32 pairs of firstborns who were matched for age, sex, social class, sibship size, and residence but differed in distance to the secondborn child (less than 34 or more than 38 months). On the EPPS narrowly spaced firstborns were higher on 2 of 15 scales: They tended to report themselves as more succorant and affiliative. The authors interpreted their finding as a consequence of a more intensely felt dethronement in more narrowly spaced firstborns. Hoffman et al. (1979) selected from a freshmen population 191 male and female college students with one sib with a spacing of less than 15 years. When two groups (those spaced less than 36 months and those spaced 36 months or more) were compared on the Eysenck personality inventory and on Rotter's locus of control scale, there were no significant differences in either sex. Dividing the sample at a spacing of 45 months led to more widely spaced males scoring as slightly more responsible on the Rotter scale, while there was no difference in females and on the Eysenck inventory. According to the authors wide spacing leads to less mutual dependency and thus to a more favorable environment for male character development. Hornbostel et al. (1980) studied 120 college students with one sib using the EPPS. Among females those spaced 25 or more months scored higher on need achievement than those with a more narrow spacing. Among males there was no difference with spacing.

Nuttall et al. (1979) studied associations of spacing with personality in a sample of 533 13- to 18-year-old subjects from Boston suburbs (selection unknown), who had either one or four or more sibs. Differences in personality tests appeared only in the large sibships and only when distance between sibs was less than 18 months: Subjects with a distance of less than 18 months to the next older sib were more self-sufficient on a test of academic motivation and more stable and more sober on the Cattell high school personality questionnaire, while subjects with a distance of less than 18 months to the next younger sib appeared more self-sufficient on a dogmatism scale. While there is some agreement between the Italian and the formerly described USA studies in that more independence and need-achievement was found in sibs of large spacing, in this investigation in small sibships no spacing effects were found and in larger ones self-sufficiency and stability were associated with a small distance between sibs. As usual in this field, findings are contradictory.

Zucker et al. (1972) studied smoking and drinking habits in relation to spacing in a sample of male high school students and drop-outs that was stratified for heavy and light drinking. Though narrow spacing is associated with large sibship size, the latter variable was not controlled. There was a significant result only for firstborns: A small gap to the next younger child was associated with more smoking and drinking than a large one. This result may well be spurious and due to higher consumption by firstborns in large sibships, whose atypical situation will be discussed in connexion with psychiatric disorder in children (see p. 230 ff.).

Pfouts (1980) studied the effects of spacing in a highly selected upper-middle class sample of 37 male sib pairs in two-child families, 5- to 15-year-old and stratified for spacing. In the Bene-Anthony family relation test, spacing of less than 2 years was associated with more negative feelings of both sibs toward each other and the father and of the younger sib toward the mother. Thus there is some confirmation of the Bigner (1974a) finding that power relations between sibs are negatively correlated to spacing.

The data on spacing reported here seem to indicate that even according to studies where sibship size is controlled, narrow spacing seems to lead to some interpersonal stress. A part of this effect may be due to the fact that parents of narrowly spaced children could be different in many ways from those having their children at larger intervals.

7.7 Summary of Research on Birth Order and Personality

In the introductory chapter evidence was presented that birth order and sibship size are differentially related to age, social class, denomination, and habitation. At the beginning of this chapter data were given demonstrating that differential sibship size (or rather the variations in social background of which differential sibship size is an indicator) is associated with differences in personality. Accordingly, only studies that take into account background variables at least to some degree will be accepted as evidence for personality differences through birth order (Table 42)

1. Anxiety. There ist no methodologically satisfactory evidence that firstborns are more anxious than laterborns. Their greater propensity to fear in real-life situations is a firstborn-laterborn difference that is usually found when sibship size and social class are not considered. On the other hand, firstborn infants reacting more strongly to being left alone by their mothers fits well with the data on "dethronement."

2. The tendency to associate (dependency, conformity, affiliation, etc.). Evidence of a stronger tendency to associate in firstborns (higher conformity in personality scales, greater conformity of firstborn males of school age in an Asch-type situation) has to be regarded with the same reservation as in "Anxiety". The findings of higher acceptance of traditional values by firstborns and their being rated higher for conformity and dependency are restricted to methodologically insufficient studies. There is one investigation in which sibship size was taken into account where males at elementary-school age were rated as more conforming by their teachers. Exposure to possible bodily harm does not influence firstborns' conformity or affiliation, which is an argument that their supposedly greater fearfulness as well as their conformity may be an artifact of intergroup differences. The studies demonstrating a greater readiness to volunteer in firstborns were done without accounting for sibship size. Generally speaking, clear definitions of constructs such as dependency, conformity, and affiliation are lacking. When measured by similar methods, their respective scores may be correlated, so that little meaning can be attached to them and their association with birth order (Campbell 1959).

3. Need for achievement. Results favoring firstborns are not found when sibship size is taken into account. In self-ratings for academic achievement, birth order usually explains a minimal amount of the variance. There is, however, one exception: in the ratings given by teachers for academic motivation the older of two sibs was rated higher (same sample as quoted above for conformity).

4. Aggression. Evidence of more inhibited aggression in firstborns is lacking (partly because of insufficient operationalization of the concept).

5. Authoritarianism, dominance, dogmatism. There is no evidence of higher scores in firstborns.

6. Values and interests. There is no evidence of their association with birth order. A stronger interest in ideas than people was consistently found in firstborns rather than laterborns. This finding is opposed to the greater pliability of firstborns in the Asch-type situation. Both results appeared without control of background variables.

7. Creativity. Differences favoring firstborns disappear when social class and sibship size are taken into account. Findings of a greater mastery of language in firstborns were obtained when the latter variable was excluded. Greater creativity of firstborns would be opposed to their supposedly higher conformity and adherence to traditional values.

8. Self-esteem. There is no evidence of lower self-esteem in firstborns.

9. *Adjustment*. There is no evidence of lower adjustment in firstborns.

10. *Introversion*. Evidence for firstborns being more introverted is lacking. Two studies in which higher ratings for introversion as assessed by parents and teachers were reported did not consider background variables.

11. *Empathy*. There is no evidence of superior empathy in laterborns.

12. *Responsibility*. One study reported more responsibility in firstborn male students with one sib.

13. *Differences in personality through birth order*. Established personality tests and scales constructed according to theories of birth order do not bring to ligth any consistent differences. *A firstborn personality, however, usually appears when self-selected parents compare the characters of their children.* Firstborns are described as more sensitive, serious, and responsible and as less impulsive, happy, socially active, and outgoing. A consistent picture of personality in other birth ranks does not appear.

14. *Sex-typing*. There is no evidence of stronger sex-typing in firstborns.

15. *Sex-role differentiation and sex of sib*. There is no evidence that sex of sibs has a lasting influence on sex-role differentiation. Children with sibs of the opposite sex may discriminate sex differences earlier than those without sibs or with sibs of the same sex.

16. *Choice of friends or marriage partners*. There is no evidence that birth order and/or sex of sib or sibs influences the choice of friends or marriage partners of the course of friendships and marriage.

17. *Popularity*. Evidence of firstborns being less popular is inconsistent.

What remains of a large body of studies is *the discrepancy between the very tenuous results obtained by tests, experiments, and real-life observations* (where often inter- and intrafamilial differences cannot be separated) *and the unanimity of parenteral ratings*, which establish a definite firstborn personality. This is the more astonishing because whenever studies of *sibs within the same sibship* were carried out, no differences in personality or personality traits associated with birth order were found. Whenever *studies of representative adult samples* were carried out with an unobjectionable method, birth order differences were nil. Whenever it was possible to estimate the *amount of variance* explained by birth order it was negligible.

The Importance of Background Variables

To give more weight to our assertion that most differences between first- and laterborns are artifacts of their being differentially distributed due to age of parents, social class, religious denomination, habitation, and other background variables, a list of attitudes, personality variables, and types of behavior is presented here that has been found to differentiate between persons of different social class.

1. *Educational aspirations* are positively correlated to social class (Jencks 1972, p. 135).

2. Middle-class pupils are rated higher by their teachers for *good behavior* than lower-class pupils (Berelson et al. 1964, p. 441).

3. *Language mastery* is positively correlated to social class (Jencks 1972, p. 78; Lukesch 1976, p. 194).

4. *Volunteering* is positively correlated to social class (Rosnow et al. 1969).

5. *Birth control* and *use of medical care* are positively and frequency of *crimes and delinquency* are negatively correlated to social class (Berelson et al. 1964, pp. 598, 627; Suchman 1965, West et al. 1973).

6. *Political interest* and making a *career in the military service* are positively correlated to social class (Berelson et al. 1964, p. 423).

7. Giving an *opinion* in an interview is positively correlated to social class, as is freedom in discussing *sexual behavior* (Berelson 1964, pp. 486, 302).

8. In general *the middle class may be considered as behaving more conformingly* (Berelson et al. 1964, p. 486).

9. In males, higher *conformity* is correlated with a higher IQ (Maccoby et al. 1975, pp. 131–132). Accordingly, firstborn-laterborn differences in conformity were found more at elementary- and high-school age than at college level, where a selection for IQ and social class has already taken place (see p. 111 ff.). Social-class differences in conforming *behavior* do not exclude lower scores by middle-class than lower-class subjects in written tests investigating conformity, as reported on p. 75.

Previous smaller surveys support our mainly negative conclusions. Warren (1965), Sampson (1965), Clausen (1966), and Adams (1972) rejected other findings as inconclusive but accepted higher conformity in firstborns. De Avila (1971) and Doren (1972) rejected even these results because of a lack of an explanation for the association of socialization through birth order with personality, a lack of conceptual clarity, a lack of generalization with regard to age, a lack of background information, and finally because of methodological insufficiency (particularly regarding Schachter 1959). Peuckert (1974) considered higher conformity in firstborns to be probable, but found no evidence of a greater need for achievement, a greater need to affiliate under stress, or greater anxiety.

Invalid Tests or Overestimation of Environmental Factors?

Birth order does not appear to be a very strong influence in molding personality in a definable way. Adler's far-reaching (and incoherent) hypotheses are not supported by empirical data. This could be a consequence of a want of reliable and valid tests. The fact that experimental or behavioral data sometimes support firstborn-laterborn differences whereas written tests do not (whether the differences found are inter- or intrafamilial is another question) could indicate that birth order does influence personality but that we are unable to define this influence in tests, ratings, and questionnaires. On the other hand, in some of these seemingly unreliable and invalid tests, *sex differences* appear quite consistently (Maccoby et al. 1975; Block 1976).

Differential socialization by birth order, on the other hand, has been well established at least for firstborns in comparison to secondborns and at infancy and preschool age. Firstborns are better cared for in infancy and live through a kind of "dethronement;" their language and toilet training is accelerated and they are treated with less affection than secondborns. These differences in socialization, however, do not seem to leave indelible traces that can be predicted.

Table 42. Data supporting personality differences by birth order, with at least sibship size controlled

Trait	Children and college students			Adults	Sib in the same sibship
	Experiments	Self-ratings, ratings by others	Real-life behavior		
Anxiety	No difference	No difference	First born infants more afraid being left by mother.	No difference	Not investigated
Disposition to associate (affiliation, conformity, etc.)	No difference	Firstborn male school children rated higher by teacher for conformity (Same sample)	No difference	No difference	Not investigated
Need for achievement	No difference	Firstborn school children rated higher by teacher for need for school achievement (Same sample)	Not investigated	No difference	No difference
Aggression	No difference	No difference	Not investigated	Not investigated	Not investigated
Authoritarism, conservatism, dogmatism	No difference	No difference	No difference	Not investigated	Not investigated
Interests and values	Not investigated	No difference	Not investigated	No difference	Not investigated
Creativity	Not investigated	No difference	No difference	No difference	No difference
Self-esteem	No difference	No difference	Not investigated	Not investigated	No difference
Adjustment	Not investigated	No difference	Not investigated	Not investigated	Not investigated
Introversion	Not investigated	No difference	Not investigated	Not investigated	Not investigated
Empathy	No difference	No difference	Not investigated	Not investigated	Not investigated
Responsibility	Not investigated	Firstborn male students higher	Not investigated	Not investigated	Not investigated
Personality in general	Not investigated	No difference	Not investigated	No difference	Ratings by parents ("firstborn personality")
Sex-typing	Not investigated	No difference	Not investigated	No difference	Not investigated
Influence of sex of sib(s) on sex role	Not investigated	Earlier discrimination of the sexes in children with sib of opposite sex	Not investigated	Not investigated	Not investigated
Influence of birth order on marriage, choice of friends	Not investigated	No difference	No difference	No difference	Not investigated

Socialization in infancy and early childhood may be of *lesser importance* in personality development than was believed when psychoanalytic theories were at their apogee and when the heritability of certain personality variables was unknown or denied. Thus, a "dethronement" experience may lead to a personality suffering from proneness to anxiety only under conditions of genetic vulnerability and reinforcement of early childhood experiences in later childhood. In our view, this is why differences in personality through birth order are so elusive and of so little general importance, although birth order still may be an important environmental factor for *some* individuals.

Chapter 8 Birth Order and Mental Illness

8.1 Introductory Remarks

Because of the relative scarcity of diagnosed psychiatric illness in the general population, the large majority of authors study birth order or birth rank of patients within a given diagnosis, using birth order as the dependent variable. The question (often not explicitly formulated) behind this type of research is the following: Are there factors related to the psychological situation of the first- (or second- or later-) born, which are apt to lead to schizophrenia or some other disorder more frequently than in other positions?

Even if the answer for a given diagnosis were affirmative, e.g., if after application of sound methods firstborns were found to be overrepresented among schizophrenics, research would be incomplete as long as the next question remains unanswered: Which are the psychological factors related to being firstborn that promote schizophrenia? Efforts to answer this question are extremely scarce if not nonexistent. An author who has found, with whatever method, firstborns to be overrepresented among schizophrenics, is usually quick to hypothesize that firstborns are under more parental pressure than laterborns or more introverted, and that parental pressure or introversion promotes schizophrenia. Awareness that these ad hoc hypotheses have to be verified is not always present. There is a tendency to jump to conclusions, which is the more inadequate as very often their premise (differential birth order in different psychiatric diseases) may be attacked for various methodological reasons.

8.2 Methodological Pitfalls

Methodological pitfalls were discussed for psychiatric birth order research extensively by Spiegel et al. in 1959, to no avail, and again by Hare et al. (1969, 1970 a) and Schmidt et al. (1977). (Our survey is much indebted to these latter studies.)

Most psychiatric birth order investigations are done in an *institution*, usually an in- or outpatient psychiatric clinic. It is well-known that different institutions attract different clienteles. In- and outpatients differ in mean age, sex distribution, and possibly social class (Petroni et al. 1970), and both groups differ again in these variables from the general population. Since the Hollingshead et al. (1958) fundamental study on social class and mental illness, many others have followed which demonstrate the selectivity of institutions for demographic variables. The relation of these to sibship size and birth order was discussed in Chap. 1.

Another pitfall for birth order studies is the questionable *validity and reliability of psychiatric diagnoses*. Fashions change quickly, and international criteria are not yet everywhere accepted. Consequently the combination of results found at different times and/or different places is a hazardous undertaking. Also questionable is the widespread custom of using old case histories without at least an attempt at rediagnosis.

A third pitfall is hidden in the fact that *many diagnosis are found in groups specific for age, sex, and social class*. Chronic alcoholic inpatients in public institutions are usually of middle age and lower class. The social background of institutionalized female chronic alcoholics may be even more depressed than in males. Female schizophrenic inpatients may have a higher mean age than their male counterparts because chronic paranoid schizophrenia occurs more often in females and is mostly found in older patients. Juvenile delinquents in public institutions, on the other hand, are usually from large lower-class families.

Patient selection for diagnosis offers a further pitfall. The extreme sample shrinking in some studies due to missing data introduces a possible bias. Other biases are the consequence of selecting a sample of first admissions, any admissions, discharges, or patients present at an institution at a key-date. The proportion of chronically ill patients (who differ in age and social class from the patient population in general) varies with each group.

In some psychiatric disorders *broken homes* are more frequent than in others. This will introduce a bias towards only children and small sibships. The proportion of broken homes varies with age, ethnicity, urban or rural extraction, habitation and denomination. Within the same diagnostic group (e.g., alcoholism) older inpatients in a state hospital may come from homes broken by divorce less often than younger patients seen at a university outpatient clinic, but more often from very large families.

A last source of error is *the age of manifestation and the age of being admitted to treatment*. When a sample is very young (e.g., in child psychiatry) it will contain a large proportion of incomplete sibships and accordingly a large number of firstborns. When a sample contains many elderly subjects it will be biased for younger sibs (some of the older sibs being already dead) (see p. 10).

The differential relations of psychiatric diagnosis, institution, and patient selection to demographic variables such as age, sex, social class, urban or rural extraction, and habitation make psychiatric birth order research *absolutely dependent on control groups resembling the samples as closely as possible*. Usually birth order research assumes equidistribution for birth order by sibship size. As we have seen (see p. 6 ff.), this is true only for a demographically stable population. The hypothesis that psychiatric patients are part of a stable population must be verified before equidistribution can be assumed. The "general population" is not a satisfactory control group because of the demographic selectivity of institutions and diagnoses.

8.3 Sibship Size and Mental Illness

8.3.1 Methodological Difficulties

Even the seemingly simple question of whether patients suffering from a given mental disorder are different for sibship size from the general population is full of pitfalls, as described by Gregory (1958c).

1. The Greenwood-Yule correction for sibship size (see p. 3f.) has been introduced into psychiatric birth order research by this author (Gregory 1958). If patients are compared for sibship size with census data (where the number of children per mother is reported), this will lead to patients appearing to have a larger mean sibship size than the general population.

2. Parents of patients and parents in the control group must belong to the same age cohort. If sibship size in patients, as frequently happens, is compared with mean sibship size of the general population according to the last census data, parents of adults are compared to parents in general, many of whom are young and have not yet reached complete family size.

3. Because of the selection of patients treated in institutions according to social variables, it is possible that the patient population contains fewer subjects from the upper and upper-middle class than the general population. As there is a negative correlation between social class and sibship size, this will lead to a spurious larger sibship size in patients.

4. Census data may not record children who have left home or may record children per married woman (including the childless).

All these hidden difficulties in the assessment of sibship size in psychiatric patients tend to *make it appear larger* than sibship size in the general population.

8.3.2 Sibship Size of Psychiatric Patients in General

Birtchnell (1970) used patients entered into a psychiatric case register of the north-eastern region of Scotland, containing all adult cases treated in institutions or in private practice for psychiatric disorder under the National Health Service 1963–1967 (2,861 males, 3,934 females). A control group was created by mailing a questionnaire to a systematic random sample of 4,000 adults registered with general practitioners in the same region. Replies were received from 3,425 of these subjects, i.e., 85.6%. (It will be remembered that the control sample does not consist of patients but *potential* patients and that under the British National Health Service the overwhelming majority of inhabitants are registered with a practitioner: So the Schmidt et al. (1977) criticism that the controls do not represent the general population seems unfounded.) There was a significant relationship between age and sibship size (older controls having more sibs) and between social class and sibship size (smaller sibships being more frequent in the upper-middle and upper class). When patients and controls were compared for sibship size by age there was no difference between the groups. It is of particular interest that the patient sample contained 7.1% only children and the population sample 6.7%. The difference is not significant and makes a particular vulnerability of the only child improbable. The author divided the psychiatric register cases into five diagnostic groups. Diagnoses were equidistributed for social class, but not for age. When patients were compared by diagnosis with controls of the same age distribution, only one diagnostic group was significantly different by sibship size: "Neurosis other than depressive" tended to occur in smaller sibships. The author concludes that sibship size bears no significant relationship to mental illness.

Clum et al. (1970) followed up a group of 11,000 Navy enlistees in their first 4 years of enlistment. During this time 600 subjects were admitted to a psychiatric inpatient service. These men were compared with a control group of 230 randomly selected nonpatients. The groups did not differ in the proportion of only children or in the proportion of small and large sibships.

Vogel (1979) compared all inpatient admissions to a psychiatric university clinic in Berlin between 1968 and 1975. Data on patient's sibship size were compared with German census data by age cohort of parents, and the Greenwood-Yule correction was made. For the whole population and the diagnostic subgroups schizophrenia, affective psychoses, neuroses, and organic disease, smaller sibship size than in the general population was found. Only children were overrepresented among the patients. As the census data exclude illegitimate births and as the patients' distribution by social class may not correspond to the general population, the author draws only the conclusion that patients certainly do not have more sibs than the general population of the same age.

8.3.3 Sibship Size in Schizophrenia

Nonpsychiatric Control Group. Two authors (Wahl 1954, 1956a; Johanson 1958) compared sibships of schizoprenic admissions with children per family in the general population. As the Greenwood-Yule correction was omitted, the sibships of schizophrenics appeared larger. Gregory (1959) made the correction and found patients' sibships to be comparable to the general population of the same age. Goodman (1957) and Smith et al. (1963) used the Greenwood-Yule correction on both groups when comparing schizophrenic admissions with patients of general hospitals. There was no significant difference in sibship size. In the Bleuler (1972) sample, various (not strictly comparable) control groups of somatic patients were used; the author concludes that the sibships of schizophrenics were certainly not larger than the controls'.

The excellent method of Birtchnell (1970) has been discussed (see p. 192). When his subgroup "psychosis other than depressive" (which contains a large proportion of schizophrenics) consisting of 771 patients, was compared with his control sample by age distribution there was no difference in sibship size.

Psychiatric Control Group. In these studies psychiatric control groups were selected from the same institutions and by the same method as schizophrenic patients. In each study care was taken to have a similar mean age. Under these conditions no significant difference between sibship size of schizophrenics and that of other diagnostic groups was found by Burton et al. (1963); Smith et al. (1963); Tsuang (1966); or Hare et al. (1970a).

8.3.4 Sibship Size in Alcoholism

Bakan (1949) published sibship data on two samples of males convicted of "public intoxication" in an American state. Gregory (1960), recalculating the samples, found the larger one contradictory for birth order and sibship data and rejected it. In the second very much smaller sample, Gregory used the Greenwood-Yule correction and found sibship size to correspond to his 1959 sample (see p. 193) and accordingly to the general population of comparable age.

Wahl (1956), in a study repeating the methodological errors of 1954 and 1956 a (see p. 193), found sibship size in institutionalized alcoholics to be significantly larger than in the general population.

Smart (1963 a) compared chronic, institutionalized male alcoholics with the Ontario general population 30 years ago. Though applying the Greenwood-Yule correction, the author found sibships of alcoholics to be considerably larger. Gregory (1965) compared Smart's data with a census sample comparable to the patients for social background and proportion of completed families. The remaining incongruencies (more only children among alcoholics, less sibships of ten and more) were explained by Gregory as possibly being due to different proportions of broken homes and of persons from rural background. Smith (1965) compared Smart's material to his control sample of medical ward patients (Smith et al. 1963) and found the alcoholics' mean sibship size to be somewhat smaller.

Birtchnell (1970) (see p. 192) compared Scottish alcoholics with a sample of the general population by age. In the Pacini et al. (1975) sample, Roman lower-class alcoholics were compared with men of the same age and background found in tax registers. In neither study were there any differences for sibship size.

8.3.5 Sibship Size in Psychoneurosis

In the psychiatric disorders discussed here, reliability and validity of diagnosis are particularly questionable. Samples may differ for social class distribution according to inclusion or noninclusion of personality disorders.

The Norton (1952) random sample of patients attending the psychiatric department of an English general hospital was compared by Gregory (1958) for sibship size with the completed sibships of the nonmanual class in England and Wales. There was no difference. Gregory's own sample of psychoneurotic inpatients (1958) had a lower mean sibship size and a greater proportion of only children than the comparable Ontario population. Broken homes were not equalized in the two samples.

Hau et al. (1966), unaware of methodological pitfalls, found in inpatients of a West German psychosomatic inpatient department larger sibships than in controls from an institution for child psychiatry (Beck et al. 1965; Lempp 1967) and in the general population of the province. Incomplete sibships in the control groups were not excluded and the Greenwood-Yule correction for sibship size was not made. The authors conclude, quite unwarrantedly, that large sibships have a "neurotogenic effect." Comparing patients of a psychosomatic station with census data, Meiners (1975) arrived at the same erroneous result.

Bettray (1970), on the other hand, applied the Greenwood-Yule correction when comparing sibship size of psychoneurotic inpatients with census data at the time when the patients were a mean 6–7 years old, but does not consider the greater frequency of incomplete sibships in the general population. Consequently the mean sibship size in the sample appears much larger than in the general population.

The only deviation found by Birtchnell (1970) (see p. 192) in sibship size for different diagnostic groups in comparison with a control sample of the same age distribution was a tendency for 851 neurotic patients to be members of smaller sibships (two to five) more frequently than the controls. Since in the subjects diagnoses were equidistributed over the social classes this result cannot be a consequence of differential fertility by social class. It is possible that patients who are given the diagnosis of "neurosis" have powers of insight and description which are related to higher IQ and better education within social class. There is a well-known, though small IQ/sibship size correlation (see p. 30). In the Birtchnell sample only children are not overrepresented among neurotics and it is difficult to see why small sibship size should promote neurosis but not personality disorder or alcoholism. In the Hare et al. (1970a) study, on the other hand, there was no difference for sibship size between 1,761 schizophrenics and 7,270 neurotics (see p. 202). Lidberg (1976) found, among Swedish males consulting a specialized institute for sexual dysfunction, more only children than in a census population of the same age. Before concluding that sibship size is in any way related to neurosis, samples that exclude patients who have grown up in broken homes (leading to small sibship size) ought to be studied.

8.3.6 Sibship Size and Personality Disorder

Gregory (1959) found in patients admitted to a Canadian psychiatric hospital smaller sibship size and more only children than in the general population. In the Birtchnell (1970) study of a psychiatric case register this subgroup did not differ from a general population sample with the same age distribution (see p. 192).

8.3.7 Conclusions (Table 43)

All studies reporting larger sibships in patients than controls are methodically inadequate. There is no evidence that psychiatric patients in general or persons suffering from schizophrenia, alcoholism, psychoneurosis, or personality disorder have more sibs on average than adequate control groups. They may even have less. In four samples only children were overrepresented. There was, however, no control for broken homes.

The Hare et al. (1979) finding that in two large series of patients of a London psychiatric clinic parental age at birth was significantly higher than in a comparable segment of the general population gives weight to the hypothesis that sibship size in psychiatric patients may be smaller than average. The difference was significant in all diagnostic subgroups but largest in schizophrenic patients, amounting

Table 43. Sibship size in psychiatric disorders

Author	Controls	N	Larger sibships in patients
Psychiatric case register			
Birtchnell (1970)	Practitioners' registers	6,795	–
Clum et al. (1970	Enlistees	11,000	–
Vogel (1979)	Census (corrected)	2,518	–[a,b]
Schizophrenia			
Wahl (1954, 1956 a)	Census (uncorrected)	392 562	+
Johanson (1958)	Census (uncorrected)	138	+
Gregory (1959)	Census (corrected)	440	–
Goodman (1957)	Somatic patients	352	–
Smith et al. (1963)	Somatic patients, psychiatric patients	283	–
Bleuler (1972)	Somatic patients	208	–
Birtchnell (1970)	Pracitioners' registers	771	–
Hare et al. (1970 a)	Psychiatric patients	1,761	–
Burton et al. (1963)	Psychiatric patients	241	–
Tsuang (1966)	Psychiatric patients	1,620	–
Alcoholism			
Bakan (1949) Gregory (1960)	Census (corrected)	110	–
Wahl (1956)	Census (uncorrected)	109	+
Smart (1963 a) Gregory (1965) Smith (1965)	Census (corrected, somatic patients)	242	–[b] –[a]
Birtchnell (1970)	Practitioners' registers	516	–
Pacini et al. (1975)	Tax registers	260	–
Psychoneurosis			
Norton (1952) Gregory (1958)	Census (corrected)	500	–
Gregory (1958)	Census (corrected)	138	–[a, b]
Hau et al. (1966)	Census (uncorrected)	450	+
Meiners (1975)	Census (uncorrected)	1,016	+
Bettray (1970)	Census (partially corrected)	1,535	+
Birtchnell (1970)	Practitioners' registers	851	–[a]
Hare et al. (1970 a)	Schizophrenic inpatients	7,737	–
Lidberg (1976)	Census (corrected)	235	–[b]
Personality disorder			
Gregory (1959)	Census (corrected)	89	–[a]
Birtchnell (1970)	Practitioners' registers	721	–

[a] Smaller sibship size in sample than controls
[b] More only children in sample than in controls

to 1–2 years in mothers and fathers. In the second series no difference in the *sex ratio* of full sibs between patients and the general population of the same age was found: In each subgroup and for both sexes males were overrepresented (Hare et al. 1980) (see p. 15).

8.4 Birth Order and Mental Illness

8.4.1 Birth Order in Psychiatric Patients in General

The rationale behind the analysis of birth order in psychiatric patients in general is the not particularly well-founded expectation that birth order influences is so penetrating that it will appear in all diagnostic categories.

8.4.1.1 Studies Without Control Groups

Among patients admitted to the psychiatric ward of a general hospital, birth order did not deviate from chance (Gregory 1962). Tsuang (1966) studied birth order in discharges from a large London psychiatric Hospital during 1961–1962. He found no significant deviation from chance expectation for all male and female patients. By applying the Slater index, a tendency appeared for males to be later in birth order than females. The author considers it possible for this tendency to be present in the general population as well, since reproduction could be stopped when a son is born.

A sample of outpatient cases in a New York mental health center (terminated 1947–1972) were studied by Riess et al. (1973). The author's most significant finding was an overrepresentation of firstborns in sibships of two and three and of lastborns in large sibships. Considering that their sampling covers 25 years with corresponding changes in fertility, the result is not surprising (see p. 6 ff.).

8.4.1.2 Studies Using a Control Group

Smith et al. (1963) compared psychiatric admissions into different Canadian hospitals with medical admissions. In these groups birth order and birth rank did not differ.

Breslin (1968) analyzed birth order in psychiatric admissions. Comparing them with "vital statistics," he found an overrepresentation of youngest children among the subjects. Details on the control group are not given, and it may have contained more incomplete sibships.

By far the largest material presented is that of Hare et al. (1969). The authors examined almost 2,000 discharges from a large London Hospital during 1958–1966 and pooled birth order data on all diagnostic groups excluding schizophrenic patients. An excess of first- over lastborns in sibships of two and three and an excess of last- over firstborns in sibships of five and more was found. The sample was divided into cohorts by year of birth (1888–1947), and the two youngest cohorts (born 1938–1942 and 1943–1947) were compared for birth order distribution with the corresponding cohorts in the general population of the Greater London area. The first cohort corresponded very closely to the control group; in the younger one, however, firstborns were overrepresented. The authors consider illegitimacy, larger proportion of patients in higher social class and consequently in smaller sibships, and an increased predisposition of firstborns to mental illness. In 1979 (a) Hare et al. concluded with regard to this sample that the deviation from census data was due to a diagnostic subgroup with an excess of youthfull subjects: personality disorder.

Two studies of mentally ill soldiers used the normal soldier population which they were a part of as a control group. Vogel et al. (1963) compared a small sample of psychiatric patients from a military hospital with healthy soliders. The control group was equated to the subjects by sex, age, education, mean number of sibs, and absence of broken homes. There was no difference in birth order between the two groups. Only children were overrepresented among the patients.

Taintor (1970) compared the birth rank of recruits entering a USA training camp during 15 months with those referred to a psychiatric service during the same period. The psychiatric group contained significantly more only children and significantly fewer firstborns than the control group. There is no information on sibship size, ratios of broken homes, or comparability of subjects and controls for social class.

8.4.1.3 Non-Western Samples

No Control Group. Rao et al. (1964) and Rao (1969), in admissions to three Indian mental hospitals, showed an overrepresentation of firstborns in sibships of four and more. Chakraborty (1969/1970), on the other hand, found equidistribution by birth order for sibship size in a small outpatient institution in Calcutta.

Control Group Present. Sethi et al. (1973) and Abraham et al. (1973) compared Indian psychiatric patients with medical ward patients. Among both patients and controls firstborns were overrepresented. Tsuang (1972) studied 677 discharges (schizophrenia and affective disorder) from a Taiwan mental hospital comparing them with 206 patients with neurological disorder. In the latter group earlier- and laterborns were equally distributed by the Slater index. Among mental patients firstborns were overrepresented. There was no control for age.

Hare et al. (1970 a) related the overrepresentation of firstborns in all sibship sizes to increases in birthrate and marriage frequency. Indian cities attract immigrants who cannot find work in the country and who are, probably, mostly young adults ready to start families. The institutions from which the samples are drawn are mostly situated in cities. In order to do justice to the various studies from developing countries, local demographic data would be necessary.

8.4.1.4 Birth Order and Outcome of Psychiatric Illness

Vogel et al. (1963) in their small and Clum et al. (1970) in their large military sample (see p. 193) found outcome of psychiatric illness, measured by being discharged or remaining in service, to be worse for single children. The prevalence of broken homes was not equalized. Taintor (1970), on the other hand, found that broken homes were strongly overrepresented in recruits who were discharged from service for psychiatric reasons.

Sims (1975) followed up an annual set of 146 neurotic patients treated at Birmingham and traced 97% after 12 years. Outcome was independent of number of sibs and birth rank.

8.4.1.5 Conclusions (Table 44)

Table 44. Birth order of adult psychiatric case loads

Author	Controls	*N*	Result
Gregory (1962)	–	370	No deviation from chance
Tsuang (1966)	–	1,298	No diviation from chance
Riess et al. (1973)	–	2,474	Firstborns in small, laterborns in large sibships
Smith et al. (1963)	Somatic patients	404	No deviation
Breslin (1968)	Census	896	Overrepresentation of youngest sib
Hare et al. (1969)	Census (corrected)	1,966	Overrepresentation of firstborns in one cohort of 2
Vogel et al (1963)	Soldiers	79	–
Taintor (1970)	Recruits	323	Overrepresentation of laterborns
Five non-Western samples			Equidistribution or overrepresentation of firstborns

Results are inconsistent for the Western samples. The consistent equidistribution or overrepresentation of firstborns, on the other hand, among case loads in developing countries can be explained by specific demographic changes in the cities where psychiatric institutions are localized: immigration and increasing birth rate. There is no evidence that any birth order position entails a particular vulnerability for psychiatric disorder in general, or has an influence on outcome.

8.4.2 Birth Order and Schizophrenia

8.4.2.1 Studies Without Control Groups

Sample Size 100–1,000. In a rural Swedish population (demographic stability is mentioned), Böök et al. (1953) studied schizophrenics who were hospitalized some time between 1909 and 1947. They were not deviant from chance expectation of birth order. The same result, also in a Swedish rural population, was obtained by Hallgren et al. (1959).

Goodman (1957) analyzed male and female admissions to a large London hospital. There was no deviation from chance in birth order by sibship size. When birth rank was analyzed, youngest males were overrepresented in comparison with oldest males, which, according to the author, may be a feature of the general population (see p. 196).

Equidistribution by the Slater index was found by Tsuang (1966) in London psychiatric discharges with a diagnosis of schizophrenia. The Gregory (1959) population of consecutive patients admitted to a Canadian hospital contained a subgroup of schizophrenics: They did not differ from chance in birth order for sibship size or for birth rank. Equidistribution of first- and lastborns was also found by Wahl (1954, 1956a) in a sample of consecutive state hospital admissions (very much diminished due to missing information).

A sample of first admissions with schizophrenia into two North Carolina state hospitals dwindled to 40% because of missing data. In the whole sample, sibs from the later half of the sibship were overrepresented and among them women and patients with an unsatisfactory outcome. Unfortunately, age differences between the groups were not considered. Older patients may be overrepresented among women and the chronically ill (Farina et al. 1963).

A similar result was found by Schooler (1964) in male and female admissions to a state hospital. In women, but not in men, there was an overrepresentation of those born among the later half of the sibship. Again, possible age and social class differences by sex were not controlled. Schooler (1972a) quotes an an "eight-hospital collaborative study" which was not accessible to us. In this study 500 schizophrenic admissions in eight eastern USA hospitals were analyzed for birth order, and there was an overrepresentation of firstborns in sibship sizes two to four and of lastborns in larger sibships. There was also an excess of middle- and lastborns among female schizophrenic inpatients at an Israeli hospital (Weller et al. 1978). On the other hand, Solomon et al. (1967), in a young sample of male schizophrenics from five USA mental hospitals where upper-class patients were overrepresented, found that more patients were born in the first than in the second half of their sibship.

An investigation by Wild et al. (1974) is of interest for birth order research in general. In a sample of 490 male schizophrenic inpatients selected from six Boston hospitals there was a birth rank difference between those whose parents lived in Boston in an unbroken marriage and were less than 70 years old, in comparison with those patients whose parents did not fulfill these conditions. Patients in the first group were better educated, more often firstborns, and less often lastborns or only children than those in the second group.

In a German hospital Leonhard (1976) studied chronic and acute patients (method of selection is not given). Both groups were elderly and tended to be born in the later half of their sibships. The author explains his result by decreasing sibship size since the time the patients were born.

Sample Size 1,000 or More. Barry et al. (1967) and Barry (1967) studied all schizophrenic admissions into a Pittsburgh hospital. In men there was an overrepresentation of earlierborns in sibships of two and three and in both sexes an overrepresentation of laterborns in large sibships. Again, possible differences in age distribution were not considered.

A population of consecutive admissions to 11 New York mental hospitals during 1934–1936 and 1954–1956 were investigated by Erlenmeyer-Kimling (1969). Diagnoses were revised by the author. Womens' birth order distribution did not deviate from chance, but in men there was an overrepresentation of earlierborns (Slater index) in small sibships.

Granville-Grossman (1966a, b) studied over 1,000 randomly selected London hospital discharges (1949–1962). Female patients were equidistributed, while in males there was an overrepresentation of lastborns in all sibship sizes. According to Erlenmeyer-Kimling (1969, 1970), however, the result is due to an overrepresentation of lastborns in sibships of five and more.

Studies Combining Research at Different Times and Places. This procedure is methodologically unsound, as already discussed (see p. 191). Accordingly, results of such studies are inconsistent. Hinshelwood (1968, 1970), uniting subjects from six English, Canadian, and USA studies, found an overrepresentation of penultimate children and concluded that there was a psychological disadvantage to this position. Barry et al. (1970) pooled four USA studies and found an overrepresentation of firstborn males, but not females, in small sibships. The authors take this finding for evidence against the importance of demographic change which concerns men and women equally. They do not consider possible age differences between male and female schizophrenic inpatients. On the other hand, Schooler (1972a), pooling seven USA studies (sampled 1930–1964), found an overrepresentation of lastborn women in small as well as in large sibships, a result which the author gives little weight.

Samples from Nonindustrialized Countries. In all the following studies either equidistribution or overrepresentation of firstborns (or, according to method, overrepresentation of earlierborns in all sibship sizes) has been found: Raychaudhuri (1956), Rao et al. (1964), Sundaraj et al. (1966), and Teja (1967) for India; Antrobus et al. (1965) for a Hawaiian-Japanese sample; Rassidiakis et al. (1971) for a Greek sample; Bathaae et al. (1977) for an Iranian sample; Sandler et al. (1978) for the males in a Brasilian sample; and Weller et al. (1978) for Israeli women of Asian or African origin.

8.4.2.2 Studies Using a Control Group

Control Group Consisting of Psychiatric Patients

Sample Size 100–1,000. Smith et al. (1963) compared schizophrenic and nonschizophrenic patients for birth order by sibship size and birth rank and found no significant differences. The same result was found by Burton et al. (1963) comparing schizophrenic state hospital admissions to nonschizophrenic admissions, excluding organic psychoses.

Sample Size Over 1,000. The Hare et al. (1970a, b) extensive investigation concerned all in- and outpatient discharges from a London psychiatric hospital during 1958–1966. A sample of 1,761 schizophrenics was compared with 7,270 neurotic patients for birth rank by sibship size. There was no significant difference. When earlierborns, however, were compared with sibs from the later half of the sibship, there was a tendency toward an excess of laterborn schizophrenics in sibship sizes two to four. Age distribution did not differ between the sample and the control group.

In a second analysis, 1,761 schizophrenics were compared with 18,642 nonschizophrenic discharges by age cohorts. It will be remembered (Hare et al. 1969) (see p. 197f.) that the control group had been compared with the greater London area census data by two age cohorts, and that in the younger cohort firstborns in small sibships were overrepresented among the psychiatric patients. This time the comparison of all schizophrenic discharges with all other discharges was made by nine cohorts comprising all subjects born within 10 years (1888–1917) and then within 5 years (1918–1947). In four of the five cohorts born before 1933 there was overrepresentation of schizophrenic patients in later birth orders at sibship sizes two to four. The difference was larger for males than females.

In 1969, Hare et al. discussed the possibility that in their psychiatric sample (schizophrenics excluded) an increased predisposition of the young adult firstborn for mental illness was appearing. In 1970(a) the authors concluded that in small families laterborn children may be at higher risk for schizophrenia. In 1979(a) Hare et al. came to the result that the excess of laterborns in older cohorts was due to the high mortality rate of schizophrenics and particularly of schizophrenic males: Death risk is higher in the earlierborn members of a sibship and leaves the younger sibs for inclusion in a sample.

Nonpsychiatric Control Group. Wahl (1956a) compared a large series of male schizophrenic admissions to a USA naval hospital with data on 100,000 naval inductees: Sample shrinking due to missing information was considerable. The patients had a larger mean sibship size, a larger proportion of only children, and a smaller proportion of oldest than the inductees. There is no information on the comparability of sample and controls for social class, or the proportion of those coming from broken homes. A sample of schizophrenics and patients from a medical ward were compared by Mentzos et al. (1972). The authors considered it typical for schizophrenics to be only children, but prevalence of broken homes in the samples was not considered. The Birtchnell (1972) psychiatric register study again deserves particular attention (see p. 192) with patients diagnosed "psychosis, non-depressive" compared with an age-adjusted sample of controls from the registers of general practitioners. The majority of these patients were schizophrenic. The sample corresponded to the controls in birth order for sibship size. The Hare et al. (1970a) result was not confirmed.

8.4.2.3 Non-Western Samples (Control Group)

Psychiatric Control Group. There are two studies comparing Indian schizophrenics with neurotics and "other psychoses" (Chakraborty 1969/1970; Prabhu et al.

1973). The samples did not differ from each other or from chance expectation. In a Japanese study (Yamaguchi et al. 1965) 601 schizophrenics and 904 neurotics from a university clinic were compared, and female schizophrenics were overrepresented in the second half of the sibship. This corresponds to other findings (see p. 200f.) and may be a consequence of female schizophrenics being older and of changes in fertility. In another Japanese study of schizophrenic admissions to one hospital, 1,207 patients of either sex were compared with an equally large control group of neurotics. Lastborn males were overrepresented (Kimura et al. 1978). In a sample of 150 schizophrenic patients from six clinics in a Brasilian district birth order did not differ from psychiatric controls in either sex (Bucher et al. 1980).

Nonpsychiatric Control Group. El Islam (1971) compared 179 schizophrenics (unknown selection method) with 200 medical patients in a Cairo hospital. There was no difference between the groups for either sex on the Slater index.

In an Indian medical college, 437 schizophrenic admissions were compared with 227 medical admissions (Abraham et al. 1973). These were older and more often female than the schizophrenics. In both samples and in all sibship sizes firstborns were overrepresented; in the schizophrenic sample, this was significant for females and, in medical patients, for males.

8.4.2.4 Comparison of Sibs in the Same Sibship

Erlenmeyer-Kimling (1968) verified diagnoses of 1,922 schizophrenic admissions between 1934 and 1936 and 1,415 admissions between 1954 and 1956 to a New York state hospital. For 1,610 index cases *all sibs were known*. There were 217 cases where at least one sib had been hospitalized for schizophrenia and where the diagnosis could be verified. The index cases had 264 schizophrenic sibs and 667 other sibs who had reached at least the age of 16 without falling ill. Age at risk was considered and the author concluded that there was little remaining risk, given the age distribution of the sibs. Index cases and affected sibs did not deviate from chance distribution. There was also no tendency to cluster in oldest or youngest positions, or evidence that the severity of the illness (measured by frequency and length of hospitalizations) varied by birth order.

8.4.2.5 Conclusions (Table 45)

The data show no consistent difference in birth rank or birth order whether schizophrenics are compared with the normal distribution, with psychiatric patients, or with nonpsychiatric control groups. The overrepresentation of laterborn males in small sibships found by Hare et al. is not confirmed elsewhere. In the studies with schizophrenic patients where an overrepresentation of only children was found, broken homes were not controlled. Erlenmeyer-Kimling's study on sibs gave no evidence for an influence of birth order on the manifestation of schizophrenia. Thus the hypothesis that schizophrenia occurs independently of birth order is not refuted.

Table 45. Birth order in schizophrenia: sample size 100 or more with no control group (A), with control group (B), and distribution of sibs within the same family (C)

	Author	Country	*N*	Overrepresented
A	Böök (1953)	Sweden	103	–
	Hallgren et al. (1959)	Sweden	214	–
	Goodman (1957)	England	306	Lastborns (males)
	Tsuang (1966)	England	206	–
	Gregory (1959)	Canada	440	–
	Wahl (1954, 1956 a)	USA	309	–
	Farina et al. (1963)	USA	167	Laterborns
	Schooler (1964),	USA	724	Laterborns (females)
	(1972 a)	USA	500	Firstborns, lastborns
	Weller et al. (1978)	Israel	264	Middle- and lastborns (females)
	Solomon et al. (1967)	USA	291	Earlierborns (males)
	Wild et al. (1974)	USA	409	Firstborns (city males)
	Leonhard (1976)	Germany	466	Laterborns
	Barry et al. (1967)	USA	1,009	Earlierborns (males) Laterborns
	Erlenmeyer-Kimling (1969)	USA	1,347	Earlierborns (males)
	Granville-Grossman (1966 a, b)	England	1,252	Lastborns (males)
	Nine non-Western samples			First- and earlierborns

	Author	Population	Country	Control	*N*	Over-represented
B	Smith et al. (1963)	Case load	USA	Psychiatric patients	283	–
	Burton et al. (1963)	Admissions	USA	Psychiatric admissions	241	–
	Hare et al. (1970 a)	Discharges	England	Neurotic discharges	1,761	
				Nonschizophrenic discharges		Laterborns in small sibships (males)
	Wahl (1956 a)	Admissions	USA	Naval inductees	568	Laterborns, only children
	Menzos et al. (1972)	Case load	USA	Somatic patients	400	Only children
	Birtchnell (1972)	Case register	Scotland	Practitioners' registers	666	–
	Seven non-Western samples					Inconsistent results
C	Erlenmeyer-Kimling (1973)	Admissions	USA	Sibs	264	–

8.4.3 Birth Order and Alcoholism

Almost without exception studies have investigated in- and outpatient samples which, according to the institution where they were treated, may have varied for age, social class, duration of illness, and, accordingly, demographic change.

8.4.3.1 Studies Without Control Group

Inpatients: Wahl (1956 b) found no significant difference between the proportion of oldest and youngest sibs in 109 male state hospital admissions. The Navratil (1956, 1959) sample consisted of 600 middle-aged peasants and laborers admitted to an Austrian state hospital. The author found lastborns in sibships of two and those in sibships of five and more to be at highest risk. Vogel-Sprott (1962) recalculated the sample and found a significantly higher proportion of last children only in sibships of two.

Among male admissions to a Toronto specialized clinic, Vogel-Sprott (1962) found an overrepresentation of firstborns in sibships of two. Smart (1963 a) studied male alcoholics, partly discharges from and partly admissions to three Ontario clinics. The sample was equidistributed by birth order for sibship size. Vogel-Sprott (1962), however, found an overrepresentation of firstborns in sibships of two. In a female sample admitted to a Toronto clinic, which was much reduced due to missing data, Smart (1963 b) instead found an overrepresentation of laterborns. Gregory (1965) recalculated the sample and found an overrepresentation of last children in sibships fo four or more. Unfortunately, there is no comparison of the male and female sample for age or other social variables.

A female sample admitted to a Toronto clinic was also studied by De Lint (1964): When women from broken homes were excluded, the sample showed equal proportions of first- and lastborns. In a patient subsample who experienced broken homes before their fifth birthday, lastborns were very significantly overrepresented. According to Blane et al. (1971), Steen (1966) studied hospitalized Norwegian alcohol abusers and found more last- than firstborns.

On the other hand, in male admissions to a Pittsburgh detoxification ward, Blane et al. (1975), found an overrepresentation of firstborns over lastborns which decreased with sibship size. In a Japanese sample of male inpatients, firstborns were overrepresented (Kosugi et al. 1976).

Outpatients. An overrepresentation of last- over firstborns was found in Norwegian alcoholic sailors by Kjølstad (1964), but equidistribution was found in male and female alcoholics in Sydney for the whole sample and for each sex by Koller et al. (1969 a).

The largest sample was investigated by Blane et al. (1971): among mostly middle-aged men, treated in outpatient clinics in two large American cities, lastborns in sibships of four or more were overrepresented. In the female sample ($n=$ 158) there was a tendency for laterborns to be overrepresented.

Bakan's (1949) large sample is widely quoted in birth order research as a proof that youngest children are at an increased risk of alcoholism. The author's subjects are not alcoholics in the usual sense, but 1,493 men arrested for crimes involving misuse of alcohol (mostly public intoxication). In comparison to a state hospital sample, we may expect Bakan's sample to be younger and perhaps more inhomogeneous for social class. The author found an underrepresentation of earlier- and an overrepresentation of laterborns. Gregory (1960) rejected the whole sample because of numerical inconsistencies. Schmidt et al. (1977) recalculated Bakan's sample and did not find the alleged overrepresentation of youngest children but fewer oldest children than expected. In a second independent sample of 110 subjects, however, Bakan (1949) himself found no deviation from chance.

8.4.3.2 Studies Using a Control Group

A sample of New York skid-row alcoholics was compared with alcoholics hospitalized in a rehabilitation camp for elderly skid row men and with nonalcoholic men from a lower-class neighborhood in Brooklyn (Bahr 1971). The groups were randomly selected. There was no significant difference in the proportion of lastborns among skid-row and Brooklyn men, but among the elderly camp inhabitants lastborns were slightly overrepresented. In both alcoholic groups there was a significant overrepresentation of only children in comparison with the normal population of the same age and social class. Broken homes were not taken into consideration.

Birtchnell (1972) compared alcoholics from the psychiatric register of the northeastern region of Scotland with a sample of inhabitants of the same region registered with general practitioners by year of birth. The only significant finding for birth order by sibship size was an overrepresentation of firstborns in sibships of two among the alcoholics. The largest alcoholic sample compared with a normal control group was studied in Minnesota. Over 3,000 alcoholics treated at a private facility were compared for birth rank with subjects from a Michigan population survey. Social class of parents, denomination, and ethnicity did not differ, but age was not controlled. Only children and lastborns in sibships of seven or more were overrepresented among alcoholics of either sex. About one-fifth of each group had lost one or both parents in childhood; unfortunately it was not indicated whether parents missing because of illegitimacy, divorce, and separation were included in this number (Conley 1980).

The following study was done with a psychiatric control group: Schuckit et al. (1977) compared outpatients of 12 USA Navy clinics with outpatients of other diagnoses. The alcoholics were older and more often an oldest or only child. Sibship size was not controlled.

Drinking Behavior. Battegay et al. (1977) studied a large representative sample of 3,870 Swiss recruits. Only and youngest children were more often found to consume large amounts of alcoholic beverages than first- or middleborns. Though there was a social class gradient as well as a gradient for different regions with differential age structure in alcoholic consumption, sibship size, broken homes, social class, urban or rural habitation, and region were not controlled. Consequently any psychodynamic conclusions based on this finding seem premature.

8.4.3.3 Studies Combining Research at Different Times and Places

Blane et al. (1973; Barry et al. 1972, 1977) united 27 samples of male alcoholics studied between 1937 and 1971 in USA, Canada, Australia, and some European countries. The authors calculated the lastborn/firstborn ratio and found lastborns to be overrepresented in 20 of the studies, and significantly so in nine of them. A demographic explanation of these facts is not accepted because in eight samples where birth rank could be studied in detail, only the position of the youngest child was significantly different from chance expectation. As the overrepresentation of youngest children was not found to that extent in female samples, the authors concluded that a dependency conflict in youngest sons is one of the factors leading to alcoholism. The possibility that the overrepresentation of male lastborns could be the consequence of a reduced mean life expectancy in alcoholics males was not considered.

8.4.3.4 Conclusions (Table 46)

Table 46. Birth order in alcoholics: sample size 100 or more with no controls (A) and with control groups (B)

	Author	Country	Sex	N	Overrepresented
	Inpatients				
A	Wahl (1956 b)	USA	Males	109	–
	Navratil (1956, 1959)	Austria	Males	600	Lastborns (sibship of two)
	Vogel-Sprott (1962)	Canada	Males	100	Firstborns (sibship of two)
	Smart (1963 a), Vogel-Sprott (1962)	Canada	Males	242	Firstborns (sibship of two)
	Smart (1963 b), Gregory (1965)	Canada	Females	254	Lastborns (sibship of four or more)
	De Lint (1964)	Canada	Females	276	Lastborns in broken homes
	Steen (1966)	Norway	Males	500	Lastborns (in comparison to firstborns)
	Blane et al. (1975)	USA	Males	410	Firstborns
	Kosugi et al. (1976)	Japan	Males	295	Firstborns (in comparison to lastborns)
	Outpatients				
	Kjolstad (1964)	Norway	Males	114	Lastborns (in comparison to firstborns)
	Koller et al. (1969 a)	Australia	Males, females	210	–
	Blane et al. (1971)	USA	Males, females	623	Lastborns (sibship size of four or more, males only)
	Bakan (1949)	USA	Males	1,493	Laterborns (in comparison to firstborns)
	Bakan (1949)	USA	Males	110	–

	Author	Country	Sex	Controls	N	Overrepresented
B	Bahr (1971)	USA	Males	Brooklyn	402	Lastborns (in an elderly subsample)
	Birtchnell (1972)	Scotland	Males, females	Practitioners' register	432	Firstborns (in sibship size two)
	Conley (1980)	USA	Males, females	General population	2,454	Lastborns in sibships of seven or more; only children
	Schuckit (1977)	USA	Males, females	Outpatients	160	Firstborns and only children

Of 14 studies without controls, two found firstborns with one sib to be overrepresented, and another firstborns mainly from small sibships; in addition a Japanese study found firstborns to be overrepresented in comparison with lastborns. In opposition to these four investigations, six showed greater risk among later- and lastborns: Two found more last- than firstborns among alcoholics, two found lastborns to be overrepresented only in sibships of four or more, one found lastborns with one sib in greater number than expected, and one found that firstborns were underrepresented in comparison with laterborns. The last four samples did not deviate from expected numbers.

Of the four studies with a control group only Birtchnell's compared alcoholics with a sample of the normal population by age, finding overrepresentation of firstborns with one sib among the former. This finding was isolated and, according to the author, made no sense. Lastborns were overrepresented in an elderly subsample of New York alcoholics and lastborns – only in very large sibships – in a Minnesota sample. When, on the other hand, alcoholics from the American Navy were compared with other outpatients with the same military background, firstborns were found in greater number than expected (perhaps because of lack of control for sibship size).

The picture concerning *alcoholics* is, to say the least, inconsistent. *Alcohol consumption* among young Swiss men seems to be highest in youngest and only children – but there is not the slightest control of background variables. Generally in samples where elderly or rural or lower-class alcoholics are overrepresented younger and youngest sibs in large sibships may prevail, but in younger or urban samples, where broken homes are frequent, only and oldest children. In the investigations discussed here no consistent relationship between birth order and alcoholism emerges.

8.4.4 Birth Order and Smoking Behavior

Among 804 male and female college students, Forbes (1970) found the highest proportion of smokers in lastborns and the lowest in firstborns; middle children were intermediate, and only children smoked least of all. No association of smoking with sex or sibship size was found. Srole et al. (1973) correlated birth rank and smoking behavior in the population of midtown Manhattan. The percentage of subjects describing themselves as nonsmokers was lowest in only children, increased over youngest to middle children, and was highest in oldest sibs. Passersby in a shopping center (all 25 years old or more) were interviewed by Simon (1973) (253 males, 385 females). Lastborns were more likely to smoke than first- and middleborns.

These results seem to point to youngest children as least and to oldest as most resistant to smoking behavior, while results for only children vary. Srole et al. (1973) did establish a social class gradient for smoking, and there are sex and age differences in smoking (Staecker et al. 1973, pp. 9–11), yet no study controlled for these variables. Since among lastborns, older, less educated, and lower-class subjects may be overrepresented, the conclusion is obvious that there is insufficient evidence for a relationship of birth rank with smoking behavior.

8.4.5 Birth Order and Use of Drugs

Studies Without Control Samples. In a large sample representative of all Swiss recruits between 1972 and 1973, Battegay et al. (1977) (see p. 206) found that only and youngest sons were overrepresented among drug users. Separate data for the two groups were not published and social class and prevalence of broken homes were not taken account of, though social class differences in the use of drugs had been established.

Linder et al. (1972a, b, 1975/1976) studied 1,530 students from fourth grade to college from the San Francisco area. They found that only children more often used tranquilizers than first-, middle-, or lastborns. The prevalence of broken homes was not controlled.

Studies Using Control Samples. Rosenberg (1969) constructed three groups of male and female inpatients below 30 years of age (50 neurotics, 50 alcoholics, 50 drug addicts). Using the Slater index the author found drug addicts as well as alcoholics to be early in birth order, while neurotics were equidistributed.

A sample of 95 male inpatients (randomly chosen from the inpatient population at a Texan research center) were studied by Linarducci (1972). Their birth order was compared with national statistics of birth order in 1969. There was no difference between the subjects and the general population. As the author does not report making allowance for incomplete sibships in the general population or for comparing sibs with children per mother, this could signify that his sample contains a large proportion of small sibships. Subjects from broken homes were not excluded. In a sample of 198 hospitalized heroin addicts only children were strongly overrepresented in comparison with census data (Lerner et al. 1975). In this case the presence of incomplete sibships in the general population tends to reduce the difference between subjects and controls. Simon et al. (1974) gave a questionnaire on marijuana use to 199 female undergraduates; 29 described themselves as regular users and 147 as nonusers. Birth rank was not different for users and nonusers.

Conclusions

There is some direct and indirect evidence that among drug users there may be an overrepresentation of small sibships and only children. In no study, however, has the prevalence of broken homes been controlled. A consistent influence of birth order on drug addiction has not been demonstrated. No large scale study has as yet met the requirement of a control group comparable for age and social class.

8.4.6 Birth Order and Depression

The term "depression" is particularly vague. In an outpatient clinic most "depressives" may be younger subjects with depressive reactions or neurotic depressions, while in a state hospital catering mostly for chronic patients, "depressives" may be elderly. In a university inpatient clinic the proportion of acute, severe manic-depressive psychoses may be larger than in the other facilities mentioned. To some degree the delineation between different forms of depression is optional and very much influenced by trends and traditions. It is difficult to imagine a consistent correlation of birth order with a diagnosis that covers such a variety of behavior.

Samples Without Control Groups

In the Gregory (1959) material of 1,000 admissions to a Canadian psychiatric hospital there were 70 manic-depressive psychoses. Their birth order did not deviate from chance. The London psychiatric hospital discharges studied by Tsuang (1966) contained affective disorders and depressive reactions, and both groups were equidistributed according to the Slater index (see p. 197). A Swedish sample of patients with involutional melancholia did not deviate from chance distribution by birth order (Stenstedt 1959). Granville-Grossman (1968) recalculated the birth order distribution with the Slater method and found in the male subsample an overrepresentation of subjects born late in their sibships, which is not surprising given that the sample was elderly and that males have a shorter mean life expectancy. In another Swedish sample of hospitalized manic-depressive and unipolar depressive patients, birth order in both samples was distributed according to chance expectations. The two samples were not different from each other (Perris 1966).

Samples with Control Groups

Munro (1966) compared consecutive admissions for primary depressive illness in the Edinburgh area with general hospital patients matched for age, sex, social class, residence, and religion. Samples did not differ by mean sibship size, birth order, and birth rank. In a subgroup of 49 moderate depressives, more subjects were from middle and penultimate rank than the controls.

Birtchnell (1972), among his Scottish psychiatric register cases (see p. 192f.), studied 2,305 "depressed" patients. When they were compared with a control sample on the basis of year of birth there was only one significant difference: In sibships of seven there was an underrepresentation of first- and an overrepresentation of second- and seventhborns.

Two non-Western samples are presented by El Islam (1971) and Tsuang (1972): In the first study done in Cairo manic-depressives and neurotic depressives were compared with medical controls, and depressives were overrepresented in intermediate positions on the Slater index. In Tsuang's Taiwan sample discharged patients with affective disorders did not differ by the Slater index from discharged schizophrenics. Subjects in the first half of their sibships were overrepresented in both groups.

8.4.6.1 Suicide Attempts and Suicides

Persons who attempt and persons who commit suicide are demographically different. Among attempters, young people, particularly young women, are overrepresented but among suicides older persons, particularly men. One may thus expect studies relating birth order to suicide attempts to find an overrepresentation of earlierborns and those relating birth order to suicides, one of laterborns.

Attempts. Suicide attempts in children were studied in hospitalized samples by Lawler et al. (1963), Rosenberg et al. (1966), Haldane et al. (1967), and Cantor (1972). As expected in these young subjects, firstborns were overrepresented.

A sample of 42 enlisted men, treated at a military medical center for a suicidal gesture, were compared with 20 other psychiatric patients in the same center and with 30 well-adjusted soldiers. All subjects were in their early twenties. There was no difference in sibship size or birth rank between the groups (Tucker et al. 1966).

Koller et al. (1969 b) used a random sample of short-term prisoners and all long-term prisoners in an Australian institution. Among them were 53 subjects with a history of attempted suicide. Each subject was individually matched to five other prisoners comparable for age, social class, and marital status. In the attempter sample, youngest children were overrepresented.

Suicides. Forty-one public school suicides (Jan-Tausch 1963) in New Jersey contained, as was to be expected in this young sample, a very large proportion of firstborns.

There are two studies using large samples and controls. A series of 492 currently reported New York suicides were investigated by Kallman (1949): the proportion of only children among them was no different from the proportion in completed New York families. Paffenbarger et al. (1966) obtained university records of 225 students who later died by suicide. For each subject there were two controls from the same school and the same case-taking year. There was no difference between subjects and controls for the first- to laterborns ratio, but in the suicide sample broken homes were overrepresented.

8.4.6.2 Conclusions (Table 47)

All studies on *depressions*, whether controlled or not, show a birth order distribution consistent with a diagnosis that becomes more frequent with increasing age. Accordingly, of the two studies that control for age (Munro 1966 and Birtchnell 1972), one found more middle children only in a subgroup of moderate depression, while the other produced an unexplainable result of higher susceptibility in second- and lastborns with six sibs. The only sample where earlierborns were overrepresented was from a developing country. Consequently there is at present no reason to reject the hypothesis that depressions of all kinds occur independent of birth order.

Table 47. Birth order in depressives: sample size 100 or more with no control group (A) and with control group (B)

	Author	Country	N	Overrepresented
A	Tsuang (1966)	England	240	–
			280 DR[a]	–
	Stenstedt (1959)	Sweden	303	Laterborns
	Perris (1966)	Sweden	138	–
			139	–

	Author	Country	Controls	N	Overrepresented
B	Munroe (1966)	Scotland	Somatic Patients	153	Laterborns (in subgroup of 49 subjects)
	Birtchnell (1972)	Scotland	General practioners' register	2,305	Laterborns in sibships of 7
	El Islam (1971)	Egypt	Somatic patients	50	middle children
				203 DR[a]	
	Tsuang (1972)	Taiwan	Schizophrenics	102	Earlierborns

[a] DR, depressive reactions. The other samples consist of endogenous depressives. Birtchnell (1972) does not differentiate between depressions

Results for *suicide attempts* are inconsistent. In school samples firstborns are overrepresented, but in one well-controlled samples of prisoners, lastborns.

Studies on *suicide* point to an influence of broken homes, but not of birth order. In a survey of birth order and suicidal behavior, Lester (1966, 1970) also reports inconsistency between various studies. The hypothesis that suicidal behavior is related to birth order cannot be accepted on the basis of the reported investigations.

8.4.7 Birth Order and Psychoneurosis

Psychoneurosis, like depression, is a diagnosis which varies a great deal at different times and places. Possibly this diagnosis is preferentially given to subjects with some capacity for introspection and verbalization and with a higher IQ and more schooling than to patients in other diagnostic groups. The diagnosis of personality disorder, on the other hand, may be reserved for younger, predominantly male patients with little education and a lower-class background.

8.4.7.1 Studies Without Control Groups

Case Loads. A population of 1,535 patients who had been treated for psychoreactive illness in a West German university hospital (Bettray 1970) was reduced due to missing information and exclusion of broken homes to 217 female and 199 male patients. Birth order by sibship size was not different from chance distribution. When symptoms (not diagnoses) were related to birth rank, there were some significant results among 44 comparisons. Sex, however, seemed of much greater weight than birth rank; the results have no rationale and, because of sample reduction, are not representative.

Among 7,270 neurotic discharges from a London psychiatric hospital between 1958 and 1966 (see p. 202), firstborns in small, and lastborns in large sibships were overrepresented (Hare et al. 1970 a), as was to be expected because of demographic change (Hare et al. 1969; Price et al. 1969). There was equidistribution between earlier and later halves of sibships and equidistribution between first- and lastborns.

Hysteria. The following samples were ordered according to the time when the subjects were in treatment. Stephens et al. (1962) discussed 50 patients discharged from a USA psychiatric clinic between 1912 and 1920 and the same number of patients discharged between 1945 and 1960. The first sample contained 13% youngest children, whereas the latter contained 37%. Ljungberg (1957) revised diagnoses of hysterical patients treated in three Stockholm clinics between 1931 and 1945: There was no overrepresentation of youngest children. Ziegler et al. (1960) analyzed birth order by sibship size of patients admitted to Johns Hopkins Hospital during the 1950 s and found youngest children to be overrepresented in comparison to firstborns. There seems to be a trend for older samples to bequidistributed and for more recent ones to contain more youngest children. Unfortunately there is no information on social class. The findings fit the hypotheses that the diagnosis of hysteria is often given to female patients from large lower-class sibships, which are becoming less frequent, or that increasingly elderly patients with multiple unsubstantiated somatic complaints are included in this group.

Non-Western Samples of Psychoneurotics. No deviation from chance was found in a large Indian outpatient sample with the Greenwood-Yule method (Chakraborty 1969/1970) or in a Cairo outpatient sample with the Slater index (El Islam 1971). On the other hand, Yamaguchi (1964) found an overrepresentation of firstborns among 904 psychoneurotics seen at a Japanese university clinic.

8.4.7.2 Studies Using Control Groups

Sample Size Less than 100. In a West German clinic, Hau (1962) compared 50 patients with compensation neurosis with an unselected control group of 50 neurotic inpatients without these tendencies. The sample was 10 years older on average and more subjects came from very large sibships. Not surprisingly, middle children were overrepresented in comparison with the control group. The author explains compensation neurosis by the rivalry elicited in middle children from large sibships.

The Kayton et al. (1967) study of outpatients suffering from compulsive neurosis has been widely quoted. They compared 40 subjects (30 men, 19 women) with outpatient controls matched for intactness of family, nationality, race, and sex (but not for social class or sibship size). Among the group of male patients firstborns and only children were very strongly overrepresented in comparison to the control group. Unfortunately, there are no answers to the questions of whether parents of male compulsive neurotics tend to have particularly small families and of whether the result is an artifact of sibship size.

In a private psychiatric hospital 32 discharged patients diagnosed as having hysterical personality were compared with the next discharge comparable for age and sex. Sibship size and birth order did not differ (Slavney et al. 1974). The same result was found when a Canadian sample of 31 patients with hysterical neurosis was compared with matched controls with depressive neurosis (Roy 1979).

In the Taintor (1970) sample (see p. 198) 88 neurotic recruits were compared with those with personality disorders. In the former group firstborns were overrepresented. There was no control of sibship size.

Sample Size of 100–1,000. A sample of students diagnosed as psychoneurotics in an ambulatory students' service (Ingham 1949/1950) were compared with controls selcted for age, sex, and study year from the same university. Mean sibship size, proportion of single children, and mean number of older and younger sibs did not differ in subjects and controls. Norton (1952) compared 500 randomly selected patients with the diagnoses of psychoneurosis, mild depression, and personality disorder who attended the psychiatric department of an English general hospital with 500 medical inpatients from the same hospital. The controls were matched for age, sex, and social class. There was no difference by birth rank (oldest-middle-intermediate) between the groups.

When, in Birtchnell's (1972) (see p. 192) case register sample, 708 neurotic patients were compared with controls from practitioners' registers comparable for age distribution, lastborns were overrepresented in sibships of two and tendencially underrepresented in sibships of three; in larger sibship sizes there was equidistribution. As has been shown (see p. 206), this is contrary to the findings of the same author for alcoholics. It is difficult to find a rationale for this result.

In patients with neurotic disorders found among London psychiatric hospital discharges birth order did not differ from birth order in pathological and immature personalities (Tsuang 1966, see p. 215).

A large series of male and female obsessional neurotics treated at a London psychiatric hospital were compared with controls from a general hospital. Sibship size in the former group was smaller. When the obsessional patients were compared with controls by pairs matched for age, sex, sibship size, and social class, firstborns were overrepresented among males (Snowdon 1979).

8.4.7.3 Non-Western Samples (Control Group)

A sample of 205 patients with neurosis and personality disorder who were admitted to the psychiatric department of an Indian College hospital were compared with 227 medical patients in the same hospital. In the neurotic group but not in the medical group oldest children were overrepresented. With the Slater index, both groups tended toward an overrepresentation of sibs in the first half of the sibship. The age distribution in both groups was the same (Abraham et al. 1973).

In their Indian sample (see p. 198), Sethi et al. (1973) compared 319 psychoneurotics with 1,000 medical patients. In both groups there was (by the Greenwood-Yule method) an overrepresentation of oldest children.

8.4.7.4 **Conclusions** (Table 48)

Again the findings are inconsistent. In the studies without controls the extremely large London sample reflects demographic change in the general population.

Table 48. Birth order in psychoneurosis, sample size 100 or more: no control, group (A), with control group (B), and non-Western samples (C)

	Author	Country	N	Overrepresented
A	Bettray (1970)	West Germany	416	–
	Hare et al. (1970 a)	England	7,270	Firstborns in small, last-borns in large sibships
	Stephens et al. (1962) (hysteria)	USA	100	Youngest (increasing rate over time)
	Ljungberg (1957) (hysteria)	Sweden	380	–
	Ziegler et al. (1960) (hysteria)	USA	100	Youngest

	Author	Country	Control	N	Overrepresented
B	Ingham (1949/50)	USA	Students	138	–
	Norton (1952)	England	Somatic patients	500	–
	Birtchnell (1972)	Scotland	Practitioners' registers	708	Lastborns in sibship size two
	Tsuang (1966)	England	Personality disorders	309	–
	Snowdon (1970)	England	Somatic patients	156	Firstborns (males) ($P \leqq 0.05$)
C	Five non-Western samples (with and without controls)				Equidistribution or first-borns overrepresented

The suggestion that hysterial patients are youngest children is not confirmed in adequately controlled though small samples. Birtchnell's finding of a particular risk in the younger sib of two is not confirmed by any other controlled study. There are two studies, one of them with a relatively large number of subjects, which found a relationship between birth order and neurosis by the method of well-matched pairs: *Among male obsessional neurotics firstborns may be overrepresented.* For psychoneurosis in general or for hysteria there is as yet no evidence for an association with birth order.

8.4.8 Birth Order and Personality Disorder

The findings of Tsuang (1966) and Taintor (1970) were previously mentioned (see p. 214). Birtchnell (1972) found no difference in birth order for 589 patients with personality disorder when they were compared with a population sample on the basis of the age distribution. There are as yet no studies where differences from control samples are found when sibship size and social class are held constant.

8.4.9 Birth Order and Psychosomatic Illness

Hypertonia

Paffenbarger et al. (1968) reviewed medical records of students of the University of Pennsylvania between 1931 and 1940. In 1962 the authors sent a questionnaire to the subjects who could be traced and 80% answered. Of the respondents 659 declared that they suffered from medically diagnosed hypertension. The reliability of the statement was controlled by the investigation of a random sample and found to be sufficient. When hypertonic and normotonic respondents were compared for prevalence of first- versus laterborns there were significantly more firstborns among the hypertonics. Unfortunately, sibship size and proportion of broken homes in subjects and controls were not taken into account.

Myocardial Infarction

There are two studies comparing patients with controls. Oscherwitz et al. (1968) compared 100 male and female patients with controls with a different illness matched for age, sex, and race. Mean birth order in patients was higher. Szaklo et al. (1976) compared 100 female patients with females hospitalized under other diagnoses. Two levels of social class were represented to the same degree. The patients were more often laterborns from large sibships (besides being more often smokers, having married earlier, and being less often Protestant). As there is a social class gradient for smoking and infarction, differential social background not covered by two social levels may be more important for this birth order difference than an ill-defined "stress" of being laterborn.

Duodenal Ulcers

Ruesch et al. (1948), in a sample of 68 male patients, found an overrepresentation of youngest verses eldest sons. Groups of 50 male patients with doudenal ulcers, 50 with gastric ulcers, 50 dyspeptics, and 50 male patients with other lengthy somatic illnesses were carefully matched for age by Hamilton (1950). There was no difference in birth rank between the groups. The same result was obtained by Kellock (1951), who matched a large sample of male patients with duodenal ulcers for age to male patients with other diseases treated at the same hospital. The groups did not differ for social class. There were also no significant differences in sibship size, birth order, and spacing to the next older or next younger sib.

Chronic Rheumatoid Arthritis and Chronic Back Pain

An overrepresentation of youngest sibs and a high proportion of large sibships was found by Stecker (1957) in patients with rheumatoid arthritis and by Gentry et al. (1974) in those with chronic back pain. Ziesat (1978) expected to find in patients with chronic back pain positive significant correlations between birth order, number of siblings and scores on the hypochondriasis and hysteria scales of the MMPI. This was not confirmed. A predominance of laterborn and last children is to be expected in patients suffering from diseases that mostly befall elderly subjects.

Patient Populations of Psychosomatic Wards

Ikemi (1974) found an overrepresentation of oldest children among patients in a Japanese psychosomatic station. Hau et al. (1966) tried to find statistically significant correlations between birth rank of 450 psychosomatic patients and type of disturbance. The few significant results in many comparisons were explained post hoc and in the vaguest terms, e.g., male oldest sibs suffer from psychosomatic diseases of the heart because they are under stress; female oldest sibs, however, suffer from anxiety and depression because they are not under stress and therefore feel unwanted and insecure. Meiners (1975) on the other hand, found no relationship between type of disturbance and birth rank in 1,016 patients with psychosomatic illness.

Psychosomatic Complaints in a Student Population

In 1974 a questionnaire concerning the 5-year incidence of psychosomatic complaints was given to all students at Edinburgh University (Sheldrake et al. 1976) and 75% answered. Among almost 5,000 males, only children reported the greatest number of affections and firstborns the smallest; laterborns were intermediate. Among more than 3,000 females, differences between first- and laterborns and only children were small. While none of 30 comparisons between women of different birth rank is significant, there are four significant comparisons between men. Only children suffered more often than firstborns (but not than laterborns) from nervous tension, high blood pressure, eczema, and hay fever and more often than secondborns from asthma. The general picture is one of a disadvantage for male only children, which may be related to a possible overrepresentation of broken homes among them. Unfortunately this variable was not ascertained. In a random sample drawn from three annual sets of psychology students, Schwab et al. (1978) found no difference in the frequency of reported psychosomatic symptoms by birth rank among males and significantly fewer symptoms in first- than laterborns among females.

8.4.9.1 Conclusions (Table 49)

In uncontrolled studies diseases found mostly among older patients occur more often in laterborns than would be expected by chance. In controlled studies, we find an overrepresentation of firstborns with hypertonia and of laterborns with myocardial infarction. As hypertonia heightens the risk of infarction, this difference, if taken at face value, leads to the assumption of a "firstborn stress" leading to hypertonia and a "laterborn stress" leading to infarction. The tendency of psychosomatic patients to be of later birth rank could be the consequence of their being from larger sibships and/or older than controls. Typically, in the two studies that matched subjects and controls for *age* no birth order differences were found.

Table 49. Birth order and psychosomatic Illness

Author	Illness	Controls	*N*	Overrepresented
Paffenbarger et al. (1968)	Hypertonia	Normotonic students	659	Firstborns
Oscherwitz et al. (1968)	Myocardial infarction	Somatic patients	100	Higher birth orders
Szaklo et al. (1976)	Myocardial infarction	Somatic patients	100	Laterborns in large sibships
Ruesch et al. (1948)	Ulcers	–	68	Youngest (vs firstborns)
Hamilton (1950)	Ulcers	Somatic patients	150	–
Kellock (1951)	Ulcers	Somatic patients	250	–
Stecker (1957)	Chronic rheumatoid arthritis	–	?	Lastborn (vs firstborns)
Gentry et al. (1974)	Back pain	–	56	Laterborns
Hau et al. (1966)	Psychosomatic case load	–	450	Spurious correlation of rank to illness
Meiners (1975)	Psychosomatic case load	–	1,016	–
Ikemi (1974)	Psychosomatic case load	–	157	Firstborns
Sheldrake et al. (1976)	Psychosomatic complaints in students	–	8,022	Only children (males)
Schwab et al. (1978)	Psychosomatic complaints in students	–	308	Laterborns > firstborns (females)

8.4.10 Birth Order and Homosexuality

8.4.10.1 Homosexuality in Males

Slater's birth order index (1962) was introduced into research in relation to a large sample of homosexual males admitted to a London psychiatric hospital between 1949 and 1960. The sample was compared with epileptics admitted to the same hospital during the same period. The latter did not deviate from chance expectation, while the homosexuals were of later birth order. Slater's sample was reanalyzed by Russel-Davis (1962), who found an overrepresentation of last sons in sibships of five and more.

Hare et al. (1979 b) found that the deviation from chance was reduced when the few homosexuals with nine or more sibs were discarded from the sample.

When a later series of male homosexuals discharged from a London psychiatric hospital was compared with a sample of the general population of approximately the same age the two Slater indexes did not differ (Hare et al. 1979 b).

A volunteer sample of male homosexuals was compared by Siegelman (1973) with a random sample of university students. Both groups were similar for age, education, maternal education, and percentage in psychotherapy. Among many comparisons concerning birth order, spacing, and sex of sibs, only a few were significant (e.g., heterosexuals more often having younger sisters, homosexuals more often having two or more sisters, etc.). As these findings make no sense, the author dismisses any birth order influence on male homosexuality.

Zuger (1974) compared 43 boys with persistent effeminate behavior with boys in a psychiatric outpatient clinic with the "usual disorders." There was no significant difference in the proportion of firstborns and secondborns in subjects and controls.

Schubert et al. (1976) studied homosexual outpatients in a psychiatric clinic. Lastborns in sibships of three and firstborns in sibships of four were overrepresented in comparison to the normal distribution. A control group of college freshmen was used only for a comparison of distance to and sex of next sibs. Homosexuals more often had younger sisters than either freshmen or the patient population from which they were taken. For sib spacing there were no consistent findings.

8.4.10.2 Female Homosexuality

Slater (1962) also calculated his index for a small group of female homosexuals. They deviated from epileptics in being late in birth order, similar to the male homosexuals. The finding was not confirmed by Hare et al. (1979b), who found the same Slater index among 117 female homosexuals discharged from a London psychiatric clinic (see p. 218) as among a comparable sample of the general population.

In a further study a questionnaire concerning birth order was mailed to members of a female homosexual organization. Members of a married women's organization were used as controls, being in a similar age range to the subjects. The groups were comparable for social class as well as for sibship size. Birth rank (eldest-second-youngest-middle child) did not differ in sample and controls (Kenyon 1968).

Siegelman (1973) (see p. 219) did a similar study comparing lesbians with female university students. There was no difference in birth order, sibship size, sib spacing, or sib sex between the samples.

Gundlach et al. (1967; Gundlach 1972, 1977) used a sample of lesbians and a nondescript control group matched (as a group) for age, education, and community size. There was a tendency toward overrepresentation of only children and firstborns (forming one category) among lesbians. Broken homes, however, were not excluded and sibship size was not controlled. This control group was used by Perkins (1978) for comparison with another homosexual group (surveyed in Dallas). The author concluded that when only children who had experienced incestuous relations were removed from the sample their overrepresentation among lesbians disappeared.

8.4.10.3 Conclusions (Table 50)

The data show that as yet there is no evidence that homosexuality is influenced by birth order. A finding that male homosexuals have younger sisters more often than controls is opposed by a contrary result.

Table 50. Birth order and homosexuality

Author	N	Sex	Control group	Overrepresented
Slater (1962)	389	Males	Epileptics	Laterborns
Hare et al. (1979b)	623	Males	General population	–
Siegelman (1973)	150	Males	University students	–
Zuger (1974) ('effeminate' boys)	43	Males	Outpatients	–
Schubert et al. (1976)	86	Males	–	Lastborns, firstborns
Slater (1962)	32	Females	Epileptics	Laterborns
Hare et al. (1979b)	117	Females	General population	–
Kenyon (1968)	123	Females	Women's organization	–
Siegelman (1973)	99	Females	University students	–
Gundlach (1967, 1972, 1977)	225	Females	Present, nondescript	Only children and firstborn
Perkins (1979)	212	Females	Present, nondescript	–

8.4.11 Birth Order in Criminals

In the German Democratic Republic the birth order of 439 sexual offenders who had been given a psychiatric examination was compared with normal distribution by Fehlow (1973): 38% were firstborns, and a third of these single children. Age, demographic change, and prevalence of broken homes were not considered.

In all male offenders entering a state correctional system it was found that being a firstborn was connected with a lower risk of recidivism (Horton 1977) and that having older sisters explained 1% of the variance in the number of incarcerations (Horton et al. 1979). Both studies are inconclusive as the probability of former convictions increases with age, as does the probability of being a laterborn in a large sibship.

Mukerjee et al. (1961) found equal proportions of first- and lastborns among Indian criminals. The authors were surprised to find middle children overrepresented, and concluded that middle children are most exposed to abuse and hence to later crime. Middle children's bias for larger sibship size was not taken into account.

There is no evidence that birth order has any influence on the development of criminal behavior. Existing studies are methodologically inadequate.

8.4.12 Mental Illness in Sibships of Two and Three

White (1969) and Walker et al. (1973) selected, from all patients referred to a psychological service, white Anglo-Saxons from unbroken families in sibships of one or two (mean age 25 years, age range 13–61). All subjects were diagnosed as having a "functional mental disorder." There were 614 subjects with one sib and 245 only children. In the whole sample firstborns were overrepresented. When social class and sex were held constant, the overrepresentation of firstborns could be traced to upper-middle class males. When age was held constant as well, firstborns were overrepresented among females of 30–39 years. The sample includes all diagnoses except organic psychoses and mental deficiency. Given the low mean age and the large age range it also probably contains subjects from incomplete sibships. It is impossible to find a rationale for the findings. Overrepresentation of members of the highest social class in firstborns confirms our earlier hypothesis (see p. 10f.) that in samples not specified for social class, firstborns will be predominantly middle class.

The study of Grosz (1968) was limited to sibship size three. A sample of consecutive discharges from a London psychiatric hospital who were diagnosed as having depressive reaction and had two living sibs was compared with schizophrenic discharges and discharges with anxiety reactions. While the other groups were equidistributed for birth rank, in depressives the oldest and the middle children were overrepresented and the youngest was underrepresented. James (1969) offers an explanation: At middle age and later it is less probable for a youngest sib to have two living sibs than for middle and oldest sibs, which will lead to exclusion of youngest children and to a birth order difference between subjects and controls if the depressives are older than their controls.

In the Birtchnell (1971 b) northeastern Scottish register sample (see p. 192) there were 865 subjects from sibships of two and 995 from sibships of three who had complete sibship data (98% of the sample). The subjects were compared with controls registered with general practitioners. There were 469 controls in sibships of two and 514 in sibships of three. The samples were comparable for age and sex. In sibships of two and in sibships of three, patients and controls did not differ by birth order. When the patients were subdivided for diagnoses and sex there was no difference by birth order for depressives, psychosis other than depressive (mostly schizophrenia), and "other diagnoses." There was, however, a slight but significant overrepresentation of secondborns with one sib among neurotic women. In sibships of three, thirdborn neurotic women were slightly underrepresented. Female firstborn patients more often had a younger brother than their controls. This result was found in psychotics and depressives but not in neurotics, where it would be most expected.

Conclusions (Table 51)

Table 51. Risk of psychiatric illness by birth order in small sibships

Author	Sibship size	Diagnosis	*N*	Overrepresented
White (1969) Walker et al. (1973)	One, two	Functional mental disorder	859	Firstborn women (ages 30–39 years)
Grosz (1968)	Three	Schizophrenia	267	Equidistribution
		Anxiety neurosis		Equidistribution
		Depression		First- and secondborns
Birtchnell (1971 b)	Two	Psychosis other than depressive (schizophrenia)	1,860	No difference to controls
		Depression		No difference to controls
		Neurosis		Secondborn women

No result has been replicated in another author's investigations. Though it may be supposed that small sibships are more suitable for the detection of psychological differences by birth order (sib positions being more clearly demarcated in sibships of two than between for instance middle children in sibships of seven), there is no evidence for any consistent birth order influence on neurosis, depression, or schizophrenia in small sibships.

8.4.13 Birth Order and Problem Behavior in Children

8.4.13.1 Introductory Remarks

In birth order research on children *incomplete sibships* may lead to spurious results. In any sample containing young children there will be an overrepresentation of firstborns in small sibships (see p. 9 f.).

Children showing problem behavior often live in *broken homes*. Broken homes lead to small family size and to an overrepresentation of firstborns and only children.

Other spurious results stem from a possible differential use of child psychiatric institutions by *social class*. Rutter (1976, p. 213) reported that in a psychiatric crisis, lower-class women tend to contact social, but not medical agencies. Roach et al. (1958) demonstrated a strong white and middle-class bias in an outpatient clinic population. The same overrepresentation of the middle class was found by Shepherd et al. (1973) when comparing children treated at a clinic with a control group. It has to be remembered that there is evidence that postwar fertility changes were class-specific (see p. 10 f.), the upper-middle class tending to increase fertility. Social class may have yet another effect on incidence or prevalence of children's psychiatric disorder: Rutter et al. (1970, p. 160) compared teachers' and parents' answers to a questionnaire on psychiatric disorder in 10- to 11-year-old children and found parents of large sibships underestimating their children's deviancy in comparison to teachers. Similarly Shepherd et al. (1971) analyzed a number of symptoms are reported by parents in a representative sample of English schoolchildren and found that the percentage of children without symptoms decreased up to sibship size six and then increased again. When Lessing et al. (1967) compared staff ratings and parental ratings for 99 10- to 12-year-old outpatients, they found mothers of firstborns enumerating more symptoms than staff. We may formulate the tentative hypothesis that parents' awareness of symptoms may decline with social class and may be lower in large families.

A last source of spurious results appears in the fact that child-psychiatric institutions are a relatively new branch of psychiatry and tend to cluster in *urban regions*. In the postwar period many suburbs developed with a young population having a high marriage and birth rate, more education and possibly more modern attitudes that may lead to more frequent use of child-psychiatric facilitites than by older parents.

Incomplete sibships, broken homes, selection of middle-class children, selection of children of younger parents, and child-psychiatric institutions being situated in urban or suburban regions are all factors which will result in an overrepresentation of firstborns among child-psychiatric case loads.

8.4.13.2 Sibship Size in Child Psychiatry

Psychiatric Case Loads

Traditionally both being a single child and a member of a large sibship are considered pathogenic in child psychiatry. Only rarely has the proportion of children in broken homes been studied among single children treated for psychiatric disturbance (Ko et al. 1865). When it has been studied, it amounted to 50%–60% (Schindler 1974; Beck et al. 1965; Hau et al. 1966). Ellis et al. (1951) found broken homes to be very significantly overrepresented in single children and in sibships of seven and more. It is evident that the impact of sibship size on psychiatric disorder in children ought to be studied after the exclusion of broken homes.

The pitfalls leading to an overestimation of sibship size in adult psychiatric patients have been described (see p. 192ff.). Sibs have to be compared with sibs (and not with children per family) of the same age, the same social class, and, if possible, the same locus of habitation. Artifacts because of larger proportions of incomplete sibships in census data will be smaller in child than in adult psychiatry, because the sample will also contain incomplete sibships.

Comparisons with census data led to the expected underrepresentation of only children and overrepresentation of large sibships in child psychiatric case loads studied by Descombey et al. (1953), Roach et al. (1958), and Chombart de Lauwe (1959). Tuckman et al. (1967b) compared a sample of children treated in Philadelphia outpatient clinics during 1955 with the general population in 1962. There was no significant difference by sibship size, though there is no evidence that the pitfalls already mentioned were avoided. This suggests a smaller mean sibship size in the subjects than in the general population.

Beck et al. (1965) compared the child psychiatric outpatients treated in Tübingen between 1959 and 1965 with the child population of the corresponding German province, making the necessary corrections. There was still an underrepresentation of only children (due to a lesser proportion of incomplete families) and an overrepresentation of sibships of five and more.

One study (Casadebaig et al. 1976) compared the patients of a child guidance clinic in a district of Paris with school children from the same district. Among the patients, children in homes broken by separation and divorce were overrepresented. There was no difference in sibship size within six social classes.

Psychiatric Field Studies

In field studies it is possible to compare children with and without disorders for sibship size, all having the same chance of entering the study. A structured interview with a stratified random selection of 1,000 Australian mothers on the prevalence of emotional disorder in their children (Cullen et al. 1968) showed disorder to be highest in only children and significantly lower (but constant) in all other sibship sizes. As children from broken homes were not reported to be more often disturbed than children from unbroken homes and as social class and age of the children were not controlled, at least a part of the difference might be due to younger mothers of incomplete families reporting more emotional disorder.

Holding constant two social classes, Rutter et al. (1970) studied all 10- to 11-year-old school children in the Isle of Wight and found, among intellectual retardates and children with reading difficulties, significantly more members of large sibships than among controls. The number of symptoms indicative of antisocial disorder on a questionnaire given to parents increased with sibship size, though parents of large sibships tended to underestimate their childrens' symptoms in comparison to teachers' ratings (see p. 222). However, in this case social class was not controlled and differences tended to disappear when childrens' IQ was held constant. In an investigation of 10-year-old school children in an Inner London area, Rutter et al. (1975), employing the same method, found that a higher proportion of children with psychiatric disorder came from large sibships than was the case among normal controls. Social class was again not accounted for, but the sample may be assumed to have been homogeneous.

Shepherd et al. (1971) studied a representative sample of all 5- to 15-year-old school children in an English county ($N=6{,}453$). Behavioral disorder was assessed by a questionnaire given to parents. The percentage of children with high scores increased up to sibships of six and was lowest in only children. There was no control for social class. In the Davie et al. (1972) national sample of 15,468 7-year-old children, teachers' ratings for adjustment at school were dependent on sibship size: Children from large sibships were less well adjusted, sex and social class being controlled. Sibship size explained as much variance as sex and somewhat less than social class. The overall explained variance, however, was only 6%. The same sample was again studied at 11 and 16 years of age. Changes in behavior ratings at school were related to sibship size: Very significantly more children with at least three sibs remained deviant or became so during the interval from 7 to 16 (Ghodsian et al. 1980).

The Belmont (1977) finding for psychiatric diagnoses in 19-year-old Dutch inductees is contrary to the results of the above-mentioned field studies. In the non-manual social class, risk of being given a psychiatric diagnosis decreased in last- but not firstborns with increasing sibship size. In the manual social class, risk decreased for both with increasing sibship size. Unfortunately this large and valuable material has not been adequately studied (see p. 39).

Symptoms Varying with Sibship Size

Dechêne (1967) and Sankar et al. (1976) found, in child psychiatric case loads, that quality of symptoms changed with sibship size. Enuresis, pilfering, quarrelsomeness, and untidiness were more frequent in children with many sibs, and stuttering, being overweight, and compulsiveness in those with few sibs. This fits well with Tuckman et al.'s (1967) finding that frequency of school problems and antisocial behavior increases with sibship size while anxiety and neurotic symptoms decrease (see p. 223).

8.4.13.3 Conclusions (Table 52)

Comparison of outpatient case loads with census data leads to spurious overrepresentation of large sibships and underrepresentation of only children

Table 52. Sibship size and child-psychiatric disorders

Author	Control group	Social class controlled	Larger sibships and fewer only children among patients
Descombey et al. (1953)	Census	–	+
Roach et al (1958)	Census	–	+
Chombart de Lauwe (1959)	Census	–	+
Tuckman et al. (1967 b)	Census	–	No difference
Beck et al. (1965)	Census (corrected)	–	+
Casadebaig et al. (1976)	School children (same district)	+	No difference
Field studies	Control for		Highest symptom frequency
Cullen et al. (1968)	–		Only children
Rutter et al. (1970)	–		Large sibships
Rutter et al. (1975)	–		Large sibships
Shepherd et al. (1971)	–		Sibships of six
Davie et al. (1972), Ghodsian et al. (1980)	Social class		Large sibships
Belmont (1977)	Social class		Small sibships

only children in case loads if the necessary corrections (see p. 223) are not made. One study, comparing a case load with children of the same age and district within six social classes, found no overrepresentation of large sibships among the case load. The majority of field studies, on the other hand, give evidence that the rate of disturbed children increases with sibship size and that antisocial symptoms become more frequent. There is an association between psychiatric disorder and having many sibs.

It might, however, be expected that by equalizing samples and controls to a higher degree, sibship per se would cease to appear as a pathogenic influence. In their prospective study of delinquent boys, West et al. (1973) found that becoming a delinquent was related to large sibship size. When, however, living in a crowded home was taken into account, this was no longer the case (see p. 233). Small sibships and particularly being an only child are associated with broken homes while large sibships are associated with social disadvantage. It may not be sibship size in itself but these relationships that are relevant to psychological development.

It is impressive that thus the association of large sibship size with negative parent-child relations and personality traits is confirmed by psychiatric data (s. p. 75 ff.).

8.4.13.4 Birth Order and Behavior Disorders in Children and Adolescents Seen at Institutions

Birth Order as Dependent Variable

In- and Outpatient Samples (no Controls). Comparing case loads with the normal distribution, an overrepresentation of firstborns with one or two sibs was found by Chombart de Lauwe (1959) in a series of French mental health clinics. Firstborns were overrepresented in an outpatient clinic at Sao Paulo (Katzenstein (1957), in inpatients at Epsom (Annesley 1961), among children with behavior disorders in the middle West (Cushna et al. 1964; Wolf et al. 1965), among outpatients in Munich (Dechêne 1967) and Philadelphia (Tuckman et al. 1967 a), and in Israeli and Japanese case loads (Peskin et al. 1974; Ikemi et al. 1974). Lahey et al. (1980) studied children with one sib referred to a southern Clinic and found male firstborns to be overrepresented.

Inpatient and Outpatient Samples (Controls). The following studies compare case loads with national census data on children born approximately in the same years as the patients, i.e., with a population having a different distribution of social class and habitation. Reasons have already been enumerated (see p. 222) why an overrepresentation of firstborns is to be expected among case loads when such a procedure is adopted. This was the case in the samples of Phillips (1956) and Shrader et al. (1967). Mauco et al. (1951) studied outpatients from the Paris region and found both an overrepresentation of only children and of firstborns. Nissen (1971) found among a West-Berlin sample of inpatients in comparison with national census data an overrepresentation of only children but not of firstborns. In his sample half of the children came from broken homes. A large rate of these, both in postwar Berlin and postwar Paris, may have influenced the Mauco and the Nissen finding.

Only one study using an appropriate control group has come to our notice: in the French sample of Casadebaig et al. (1976) (see p. 223), which was compared with children of the same age and same school district, neither an overrepresentation of only nor of oldest children was found.

Conclusions

Table 53. Birth order and behavior disorders in childhood

Case loads

Author	Overrepresented
Comparison to normal distribution	
Chombart de Lauwe (1959)	Firstborns in small sibships
Katzenstein (1957)	Firstborns
Annesley (1961)	Firstborns
Cushna et al (1964); Wolf et al. (1965)	Firstborns
Dechêne (1967)	Firstborns
Tuckman et al. (1967 d)	Firstborns
Peskin et al. (1974)	Firstborns
Ikemi et al. (1974)	Firstborns
Lahey et al. (1980)	Firstborn males (sibship size 2)

Author	Control	Overrepresented
Comparison to control group		
Mauco (1951)	Census	Only children, firstborns
Philipps (1956)	Census	Firstborns
Shrader et al. (1967)	Census	Firstborns
Nissen (1971)	Census	Only children
Casadebaig et al. (1976)	School children (same district)	–

All studies that compare case loads with the normal distribution find the overrepresentation of firstborns which is to be expected in younger urban populations. Of four studies that used census data for control, two showed firstborns to be treated in greater numbers than expected, one found an overrepresentation of firstborns and only children, and one – investigating children of postwar West Berlin – merely found overrepresentation of the latter group. Neither deviation appeared in the only study with adequate controls.

If care is not taken to compare caseloads and census data for age, the general population will contain more infants and very young children who do not yet have any sibs. Caseloads that do not have fewer only children than the census population probably have more than would be found in a control population of the same age. This need not signify a particular vulnerability of the only child, as children from broken homes will accumulate at psychiatric institutions (see p. 222).

Birth Order as the Independent Variable

The following studies concern the hypothesis that there are differences in kind or severity of symptoms by birth order.

There are two studies comparing children of different birth rank for number of symptoms. Investigating 599 children treated at a New Jersey child guidance clinic, Shrader et al. (1967) found, in a checklist filled out by parents, that firstborns had a larger mean number of problems than lastborns though not a different problem pattern.

Staff ratings for number of symptoms and two symptom checklists given to mothers were compared by Lessing et al. (1967) for a sample of 10- to 12-year-old boys and girls admitted to an American Institute of Juvenile Research. Firstborns had more symptoms than laterborns on one of the list, but not on staff ratings. The authors found that children of middle-class mothers were overrepresented among firstborns and concluded that the heightened incidence of psychopathological disorder was due to their mothers' greater awareness.

In five studies psychiatric case loads were compared by birth rank for *kind* of symptoms. Haeberle (1958) found that among children frequenting a therapeutic nursery, firstborns more often had regressive and compulsive tendencies while laterborns were characterized by tantrums and low frustration tolerance (ratings by nursery teachers). Among 1,800 children with one or two sibs treated at an Illinois institute, firstborns more often had feeding problems and lastborns more often had problems with toilet training (Harris 1961). That between-group differences can be present even in a sample were sibship size is controlled is evident in the following investigation: Tuckman et al. (1967b) studied referral symptoms in over 1,000 outpatients in a Philadelphia child psychiatric clinic in sibships of two and three. The oldest child was more often referred for anxiety, aggression, and interpersonal problems and the youngest for mental retardation. In a similar study from Jowa, Cushna et al. (1964) reported more behavior disorders and aggression in firstborns and more congenital disorder and withdrawing in lastborns. As the social gradient for retardation is well-known, the findings are indicative of differences in background between oldest and youngest children.

Beck et al. (1965) found anxiety states most frequent in only children and behavior disorder most frequent in middle children.

Dechêne (1967) related symptoms found in case histories at a psychosomatic clinic in Munich to birth rank (including those symptoms that were not observed, but merely reported by parents). There were some significant findings leading to a completely incoherent picture. A sample of children and adolescents from six child guidance centers in a region of West Germany was rated by psychologists for severity of all present symptoms. The main symptom was then associated to one of five forms of neurosis (the reliability and validity of this method are not discussed). Oldest children tended to have schizoid traits, middle children obsession, and youngest children depression. Age, social class, and sibship size were not controlled (Langenmayr 1975 a, b).

Conclusions (Table 54)

The finding that more symptoms are reported for first- than laterborns by parents is in agreement with the finding (see p. 167 f.) that parents describe their firstborn children as more troubled and introverted than laterborns. It is, however, contrary to the finding that there is no evidence for differential adjustment by birth order in normal samples (see p. 157 ff.).

Differences in kind of symptoms (firstborns being inclined toward anxiety, compulsion, and schizoid traits, youngest children toward temper tantrums and school retardation) could be considered as evidence for greater socialization and introversion in firstborns. In none of these studies, however, have between-group variables been controlled, though there is evidence that first- and later- or lastborn children have different backgrounds.

Table 54. Birth order, number and kind of symptoms in child-psychiatric samples

Author	Symptoms reported by	*N*	Highest number of symptoms
Shrader et al. (1967)	Parents	599	Firstborns
Lessing et al. (1967)	Parents	99	Firstborns
Author		***N***	**Kind of symptoms in first vs. later- or lastborns**
Haeberle (1958)		67	Regression, compulsion vs. impulsivity
Harris (1961)		1,800	Feeding vs. toilet problems
Tuckman et al. (1967 b)		1,297	Anxiety, aggression vs. mental retardation
Cushna et al. (1964)		1,255	Behavior disorder vs. congenital disorder
Dechêne (1967)		416	Incoherent results
Langenmayr (1975 a, b)		163	Schizoid traits (oldest) vs. obsession (middle) vs. depression (last)
Beck et al. (1965)		56	Anxiety (onlies) vs. behavior disorders (middle children)

8.4.13.5 Birth Order and Field Studies of Psychiatric Disorder

The unsatisfactory results in studies of populations seen in in- or outpatient institutions can be explained by selective use of these institutions by parents of different social class, cohort, and education. This objection to the validity of results concerning birth order does not hold against field studies, where a representative sample of the population is investigated and self-selection is largely excluded.

Birth Order as Dependent Variable

Studies Using No Control Group. Belmont (1977) has published results on the psychiatric investigation of 400,000 Dutch inductees born between 1944 and 1947. The risk of receiving a psychiatric diagnosis was studied, controlling for two social classes and for sibship size. Only children were at greatest risk in both social classes. Within each sibship size lastborns were at greater risk than firstborns. Middle children's risk was not reported. As will be seen, the investigation contradicts other field studies performed with better methods though on a much smaller scale (see p. 230).

Teachers' referral of school children for treatment of emotional disorder was studied in the whole school population of over 8,000 children (first to tenth grades) in an Arkansas town by Kanter (1971). Only children were overrepresented (prevalence of broken homes was not controlled); otherwise all birth ranks were referred with the same frequency.

Studies Using a Control Group. In an unpublished London thesis Mitchell (1965) compared 677 English school children who were rated as deviant by their mothers with well-matched controls. Among the subjects youngest children were underrepresented.

In the Rutter et al. (1970) survey of all 10-year-old children on the Isle of Wight, parents and teachers were given questionnaires and the children screened by this method as having symptoms were interviewed by psychiatrists. Among over 2,000 children, 42 neurotic and 63 antisocial children were found. In comparison to a randomly chosen control group, neurotics were more often oldest children, while antisocial children did not differ from controls. Antisocials, however, tended to have more sibs than neurotic children. On the other hand, no difference in social class between neurotic and antisocial children was found.

Birth Order as the Independent Variable

A sample of 1,000 Australian mothers, selected for size of locality and representing over 3,000 children, were questioned in structured interviews on behavior disorders in their children. Prevalence fell from the first to the sixth child (only children and firstborns included in one category). Data on age and prevalence for birth order within sibship size were not given (Cullen et al. 1966) though a decline in awareness of symptoms by lower class parents of large families is possible (see p. 222).

In the Jonsson (1967) study of Swedish juvenile delinquents, a random sample of 7- to 16-year-old Stockholm school boys is mentioned. They underwent a thorough child-psychiatric examination (including interview with parents and teachers and use of medical records). Oldest and youngest boys did not differ for number or kind of symptoms.

All 5- and 6-year-old children living on the Danish island of Samso, as well as a random sample of children residing at Aarhus, were studied by Kastrup (1976). High symptom loads were found in only children and in those from broken homes. Symptom loads varied with birth rank insofar as youngest children were particularly low on psychiatric disorder. The method of assessment is not described in the English summary.

In the Shepherd et al. (1971) sample (see p. 231) the relationship of birth order to the number of symptoms reported by parents on a questionnaire was analyzed. Number of symptoms was higher in oldest and middle than in youngest children. When sibship size was controlled, oldest children with four or more sibs had the largest ratio of high scores. When age and sex were controlled, oldest girls less than 11 years of age in large sibships appeared particularly disadvantaged.

Frederking (1975) studied a random sample of Mannheim fourth graders by sending a questionnaire to parents. Only children and children from broken homes were reported to have more symptoms than children in other situations. In sibships of two and three birth order was not associated with number or kind of symptoms.

In the large Newcastle Survey of Child Development, the number of older sibs ascertained at birth was unrelated to teachers' reports of abnormal behavior at age 10 years with sex, birthweight, social class, and care of child being controlled (Neligan et al. 1967). Ghodsian et al. (1980) related changes in behavior ratings by mothers and teachers concerning the children in the British National Child Development Study to birth order. The subjects were born in 1958 and followed up at 7, 11, and 16 years of age (see p. 17). Firstborns were underrepresented among the children who became deviant at home during this interval, and fourth- and laterborns were very strongly underrepresented among those who were rated as nondeviant at school each time. Thus a pronounced disadvantage of laterborn children with many sibs appears.

Gallagher et al. (1977), in samples of firstgraders from 2 consecutive years in a New York area, found no consistent difference by birth order in teachers' reports of adjustment problems when sex, school, location, social class, and sibship size were controlled.

Conclusions (Table 55)

Of 12 field studies, three found first- and middleborns to be at greatest risk of psychiatric disorder. Four studies failed to show an association of risk with birth order; two found firstborns to be most disturbed, one laterborns with at least three sibs, one lastborns, and one only children. There is no evidence thas psychiatric risk clusters in any birth position.

Some studies point to a particular resistance of youngest children. In order to understand how this favorable position of the youngest child may be accounted for, the only study that gives a birth order distribution by sibship size of 682 disturbed children has to be considered more thoroughly.

Table 55. Birth order and psychiatric symptoms in children: field studies

Author	N	Source of information	Overrepresented among the disturbed
Birth order as dependent variable			
Belmont (1977)	400,000	Army psychiatrists	Only children, lastborns
Mitchell (1965)	677	Mothers	Middle- and firstborns (controls)
Kanter (1971)	8,017	Teachers	Only children
Rutter et al. (1970)	105	Parents, teachers	Firstborns (neurotics) (controls)

Author	N	Source of information	Behavior disorder found most often in
Birth order as independent variable			
Cullen et al. (1966)	1,000	Mothers	Firstborns (only children included)
Jonsson (1967)	222	Psychiatrists, parents, teachers	–
Kastrup (1976)	175	Not given	Middle- and firstborns
Shepherd et al. (1971)	6,463	Parents	Middle- and firstborns
Frederking (1975)	419	Parents	–
Neligan et al. (1976)	3,443–4,651	Teachers	–
Ghodsian et al. (1980)	1,251	Teachers, mothers	Fourth- and laterborns
Gallagher et al. (1977)	697	Teachers	–

Shepherd et al. found, among their representative sample of school children in an English county, 682 subjects with behavioral symptoms. They were distributed as follows:

	Sibship size		
	Two	Three to four	Five or more
Firstborns	12%	13%	27%
Middle children		13%	13%
Lastborns	7%	9%	7%

If this distribution is compared with the distribution of all Scottish 11-year-old children in 1947 (see p. 9), in both samples firstborns in small families are overrepresented, as is to be expected with young subjects. Instead, however, of an overrepresentation of lastborns in large sibships (due to decrease of sibship size and incomplete families), in the disturbed sample first and middle children are overrepresented in intermediate and large sibships.

This is exactly what is found when samples of juvenile delinquents are compared with well-matched control groups (see p. 233 f.). The delinquents are members of large families that are started at a time when among controls larger sibships are mainly represented by later- and lastborns. In distributions of disturbed children, lastborns in large sibships are underrepresented for the same reason, which makes these subjects intellectually superior to first- and middleborns with many sibs (see

p. 37). Parents of last children in large sibships are older and belong to a cohort in which having a large family was not exceptional. The overrepresentation of first and middle children among those with behavioral disorder may signify that children in large families founded by young parents have a social and biological background leading to greater risk.

The two investigations finding firstborns to be at greatest risk should also be briefly discussed. In the Rutter et al. sample (see p. 229) there was no control for broken homes, though they may have resulted in smaller sibship size and a higher rate of firstborns among neurotics. Prevalence of broken homes may be of large weight when the number of disturbed children is so small. In the Cullen et al. study only children were not differentiated from firstborns and age was not controlled. There was a stepwise decrease in prevalence of disorder from the first to the sixth child, which is suggestive of interfamilial differences.

Even if these results were, despite our hypothesis that they are derived from demographic change, considered sufficient evidence for lastborn children being at lower or firstborn children being at greater risk of psychiatric disorder, the data on adjustment (see p. 158f.) ought to be remembered. There, if anything, greater adjustment in firstborns was found and considered a spurious finding because of their bias for smaller sibship size. Neither would firstborns' supposedly greater susceptibility to psychiatric disorder agree with what was reported previously concerning psychiatric illness in adults. There, no support for differential vulnerability by birth rank was found. Since at least *some* connection between behavioral disorders in childhood and adult psychiatric disorder is established (Robins 1966), this disagreement either favors our hypothesis that the results discussed here are due to confounding interfamilial with intrafamilial differences or are due to the fact that birth order influences on personality disappear at adult age.

8.4.13.6 Birth Order and Minimal Brain Dysfunction

Jayasekara et al. (1978) studied a random selection of 48 6- to 14-year-old boys at a center for dyslexia treatment. Rate of firstborns did not deviate from census data. Teachers in three counties of Florida rated 5- to 12-year-old elementary school children. On this basis 43 hyperactives were found and compared with a random sample of normal children. There was no birth order but a highly significant sex difference (Campbell 1979). Thus there is at present no evidence for an association of birth order with minimal brain dysfunction, just as none was found for an association of birth order with handedness (see p. 18f.).

8.4.13.7 Psychosomatic Disease in Childhood

Among a representative sample of Aberdeen school children 121 asthmatic children were found. In comparison to the whole sample, secondborns were overrepresented. There was no information on sibship size (Dawson et al. 1969).

Tolstrup (1953) investigated 40 obese children who were found partially by a Danish medical school board and partially in hospitals. These were compared to a sample of nonobese children, found through the same school board and matched for sex and age.

Social class, housing conditions, mean sibship size, and psychogenic symptoms entered into school board case histories were similar in both groups. Among the obese sample, only children were significantly overrepresented. This was also seen when comparing a sample of 230 obese children in Düsseldorf with children treated for infections at the same hospital. In the obese sample, broken homes were overrepresented (Bolte et al. 1969).

Conclusions. There are as yet no well-controlled and representative studies in sufficient number to allow any statements on a relationship between psychosomatic disease in childhood and birth order. It is, however, plausible that only children are most at risk of obesity, if it is remembered that they are not affected by social class differentials in height and age at menarche (see p. 19ff.), both of which are connected with nutrition.

8.4.13.8 Birth Order and Delinquency

Sibship Size and Delinquency

In their unsurpassed investigation of 500 male juvenile delinquents who were matched individually for age, sex, IQ, race, and neighborhood to 500 controls, Glueck et al. (1950) found a larger mean sibship size in delinquents. Rhodes (see Carr-Saunders et al. 1942) matched almost 2,000 English delinquent boys to non-delinquents at the same schools. Sibship size was larger for delinquents. Cowie et al. (1968) compared a sample of English delinquent girls with Rhodes' control subjects and obtained the same result. In a prospective London study male delinquents were compared with their schoolmates in six primary schools. Delinquents' sibship size was significantly larger (West et al. 1973).

In three studies British delinquents were compared with representative samples of school children of the same age without controlling for social class (Berg et al. 1967; Douglas et al. 1968; Rutter et al. 1970). As lower-class origin of delinquents has been well-documented (Douglas et al. 1968; Rutter et al. 1976; West et al. 1973) and as there is a negative correlation between sibship size and social class (see p. 30) the results invariable showed larger sibship size in delinquents.

In other studies control groups are less adequate (Koller 1971; Biles 1971; Schindler 1974): Mean sibship size in delinquents appears extremely large when compared with census data (reporting children per mother and including young incomplete families).

Delinquents' origin from larger sibships than controls in the same social class is well-established. Beyond that, it was repeatedly found that the *rate* of delinquency or maladjustment scores increases with sibship size (Ferguson 1952; Cowie et al. 1968; West et al. 1973; Murrell 1974).

Birth Order and Delinquency

Studies Without Controls. In 165 delinquents among 1,314 14-year-old male school leavers in Glasgow, Ferguson et al. (1952) found equidistribution for birth order.

This was also the case in the Barry et al. (1969) small study of adolescent delinquents. In the Cowie et al. (1968) sample of consecutive female admissions to an approved school in London, earlierborns were overrepresented according to the Slater index.

In a small random sample of Australian training school girls, Koller et al. (1971) found an overrepresentation of first- and middleborns and an underrepresentation of lastborns. Among a very large series of children who had appeared in 1966 in an Australian court, Biles (1971) found middleborns to be at greatest risk, followed by firstborns. Lastborns were underrepresented in comparison to first children.

Studies with Control Groups. A sample of 502 delinquents was compared by birth rank with boys in one grammar and four secondary schools in Nottingham. Middle children and those from broken homes were overrepresented among the delinquents (Lees et al. 1954).

Berg et al. (1967) compared birth order of about 800 Scottish approved schoolboys with birth order in 11-year-old Scottish schoolboys (sample of the National Educational Survey). The control sample deviated significantly from the normal distribution in favor of firstborns in small sibships of two and three. The delinquent sample deviated significantly from both the normal distribution and the control sample: Delinquents were overrepresented in early birth orders in sibships of four to ten.

West et al. (1973) compared delinquents from six London primary schools by birth order with their schoolmates. Among delinquents, middle children were overrepresented.

Studies Using an Individually Matched Control Group. Fifty children treated for delinquency and 50 children treated for neurosis at an English child guidance clinic were matched by Bennett (1960) for age, sex, and IQ. As the clinic was in a rural area and free of charge, the author assumes the samples were socially homogeneous. The proportions of firstborns, lastborns, and only children were equal: Both groups contained about 50% firstborns.

The individually matched Glueck et al. (1950) sample has been mentioned already on p. 233. Among the delinquents middle children were overrepresented.

All inmates of a Swedish youth prison paroled in 1951 were matched for age, sex, and place of birth with a control group (Johanson 1968). Sibship size was not significantly different, though offenders tended to come from larger sibships. Among single-child delinquents, broken homes were significantly more frequent than among single children in the control group. Birth order in both groups was random.

Truancy. Tennent (1970) compared birth order of a small sample of truants from a London remand home to that of property offenders of the same age. Among the former youngest children were overrepresented. This result is in accordance with the Berg et al. (1972) study: The authors compared school-phobic male adolescents of an English inpatient unit with admissions having other diagnoses and with a random sample of secondary schoolboys. In opposition to both control groups, by the

Slater index the subjects tended to come more often from the second half of their sibships. Baker et al. (1978), on the other hand, found that over 50% of 99 cases of school phobics treated at an English child guidance clinic were firstborns. A control group was not used.

Conclusions

That delinquents have a larger mean sibship size than comparable controls is a well-established fact (see p. 233) and is the reason why middle children are overrepresented among them. In Table 56 the same favorable position of the youngest child appears as for the association between psychiatric symptoms in general and birth order (see p. 230ff. and Table 55). The overrepresentation of first- and middleborns is due to the families of delinquents not sharing the reduction of fertility to the same degree as the normal population. This most clearly emerges from the Berg et al. (1967) comparison of a population of delinquents to a national educational survey.

Data on school phobia and truancy are preliminary and inconsistent.

Ultimately, all deviations from appropriate controls can be understood as consequences of variations in sibship size. As the correlation of juvenile delinquency

Table 56. Birth order in juvenile delinquents, sample size 100 or more: no control group (A), with unmatched controls (B), and with individually matched controls (C)

	Author	Country	N	Overrepresented
A	Ferguson et al. (1952)	Scotland	165	–
	Cowle et al. (1968)	England	368	Earlierborns
	Barry et al. (1969)	USA	97	–
	Koller et al. (1971)	Australia	121	First- and middleborns
	Biles (1971)	Australia	3,692	First- and middleborns
	Truants			
	Baker et al. (1978)	England	99	Firstborns

	Author	Country	Controls	N	Overrepresented
B	Bennett (1960)	England	Neurotics	100	–
	Lee et al. (1954)	England	Grammar and secondary school	206	Middle children
	Berg et al. (1967)	Scotland	Survey	799	Earlierborns in large sibships
	West et al. (1973)	England	Schoolmates	84	Middle children
	Truants				
	Berg et al. (1972)	England	Secondary school	100	Laterborns
C	Glueck et al. (1950)	USA	Neighborhood	500	Middle children
	Johanson (1968)	Sweden	Neighborhood	128	–

to alcoholism and crime in adults is well-known (Robins 1966), birth order in juvenile delinquents may be compared with the results found in these groups (see pp. 207f., 220). In the few investigations with criminals, firstborns and middle children were overrepresented, since criminals are mostly young men. Among alcoholics, on the other hand, in some samples youngest children predominate. It would be extremely difficult to explain the latter result by psychodynamic theories, as youngest children and children in small sibships seem at a particularly low risk of juvenile delinquency.

8.4.13.9 Autistic Children, Schizophrenia in Children, and Birth Order

Ando et al. (1975) compared 119 autistic children, 292 children with cerebral palsy, and 146 children with Down's syndrome (all in the same Japanese hospital; mean age 4.5 years) with healthy kindergarten children from the same area. Autistic children were not different from the control group by birth rank. Among the two other patient groups there were significantly more single children and lastborns.

Lowe (1966) analyzed admissions to the only existing child-psychiatric inpatient clinic in the state of Indiana. Among 65 autistic children, 34 chronic schizophrenic children, and 146 generally disturbed children firstborns were represented in the same proportions.

8.4.14 Mental Deficiency in Children and Adults

Mental deficiency is a syndrome that may be caused by genetic variation, pre- or postnatal illness, birth trauma, or disorders related to the mother's age or the number of previous pregnancies. The syndrome is differentially associated with social class: Moderate deficiency is negatively correlated with social class, while the higher grades are equidistributed over class.

As early as 1931 Brugger found in a Swiss sample that feeble-minded subjects tended to be born in the second half of their sibships. The same result was found by Böök et al. (1953) and Hallgreen et al. (1959) in low-grade mental defectives from a Swedish rural area and by Saunders (1977) in a review of 28 studies on moderately subnormal children. An overrepresentation of lastborns was found by Gregory (1959) in hospital admissions for mental deficiency in Canada and by Davies (1963) in severely retarded children. Among birth trauma-deficient subjects, Malzberg (1950a, b) found an overrepresentation of firstborns, but in cases of deficiency due to congenital spastic paralysis an overrepresentation of fifthborns. According to Sternlicht et al. (1975) and Biswas (1975), firstborns were overrepresented among retarded children and adults.

The accumulation of these results does not seem helpful, when there is no differentiation of causes or comparison with a control group equalized for sibship size and social class and when the investigations do not serve to examine well-defined hypotheses.

8.4.15 Birth Order in Epileptics

Malzberg (1973) studied 3,906 admissions to the only public institution for epileptics in New York state. For both idiopathic and symptomatic epilepsy, he found small sibship sizes and overrepresentation in early ranks. The sample partially consisted of children from possibly incomplete sibships. Sethi et al. (1973), on the other hand, found no difference for birth rank between a small sample of Indian epileptics and medical controls, and Slater (1962) found epileptics discharged from Maudsley Hospital (London) to be equidistributed for birth order. There is no mention of children in these samples.

8.5 Birth Order and Psychiatric Illness: Conclusions

The findings emerging from the survey presented here are as follows: In one well-controlled study neurosis was related to small sibships; in two others obsessional neurosis to being an oldest male. Obesity may be related to being a single child. There is a large body of evidence proving that juvenile delinquents have larger sibships than controls. Psychiatric disorder in children may be associated with the background large sibships stand for at a time of decreasing fertility.

The scarcity of results arising from a large number of investigations is disappointing. Earlier (see p. 6ff.) the associations of birth order and sibship size with age, social class, and parental cohort were discussed. They are particularly important in the study of psychiatric illness, as differential diagnosis and differential modality of treatment are related to patients of different age and social background. Additionally, broken homes may introduce a bias toward small sibships and overrepresentation of firstborns.

Studies comparing birth order in psychiatric patients with a chance distribution usually find an overrepresentation of firstborns in younger middle-class city dwellers and an overrepresentation of later- and lastborns in older lower-class patients. This is particularly evident in studies on schizophrenia: Males tend to be first- and females laterborns. Rather than explain this by "laterborn stress" increasing risk in females and "firstborn stress" increasing it in males, the well-known difference in mean age between male and female schizophrenics should be considered.

The studies using control groups, on the other hand, are scarce and often contradictory or sample-specific. There is evidence, based on one well-controlled study, that among alcoholics firstborns in sibships of two may be overrepresented. There is evidence, also based on one well-controlled study, that among criminals lastborns are prone to attempt suicide (while among attempters of school age, firstborns are overrepresented). Confirmation of both findings by other controlled studies is missing.

There is a large body of evidence that, among case loads of child-psychiatric outpatient clinics, firstborns are overrepresented. However, one study in with these young patients were compared with a well-chosen control group supported the hypothesis that the overrepresentation of firstborns is due to the demographic characteristics of the particular segment of the population they derive from, rather than to higher risk of psychiatric illness in firstborns.

One might expect field studies of psychiatric disorder or disturbing behavior in children to disclose the real connection with birth order. In fact the results are divergent, probably due to their varying methodological levels. The overrepresentation of first and middle children among the disturbed, found several times, may be explained by large and incomplete sibships rather than by a particular resistance of the youngest child.

The hypothesis that psychiatric illness is unrelated to birth order has yet to be refuted. As in research on IQ, achievement and personality, sibship size seems to be a far more important variable than birth order, since small sibship size may be related to neurosis and large sibship size is evidently related to juvenile delinquency. It is probable, however, that small sibship size does not promote neurosis because of unceasing parental attention, but because broken homes are overrepresented among small sibships. it is also probable that large sibship does not promote juvenile delinquency because of diluted parental attention, but because parents who have more children than they can financially and psychologically afford have biological and cultural characteristics leading to a heightened risk of delinquency. This interpretation of the influence of sibship size is supported by the evidence regarding IQ as well as personality: that sibship size explains only very small amounts of the variance when other background variables are controlled.

Chapter 9 Summary and General Conclusions

In Chap. 1, the methodological fallacies of research on the correlaton of birth order and sibship size to intelligence and other personality variables are enumerated. In segments of the population undergoing differential demographic change the distribution of birth order can be expected to deviate from normality. Because of class-specific changes in postwar fertility and postwar educational and occupational upgrading, among firstborns middle-class subjects will be overrepresented and vice versa.

In Chap. 2, the question of whether there are biological differences by birth order that may cause differences in personality variables or intelligence is examined. Research on prematurity, birth weigth, stillbirth, and death in infancy provides evidence for social class differences between subjects of different birth order and those born by mothers of different ages. There are no indications, on the other hand, that IQ in the normal range is influenced by biological influences during pregnancy, and none that in normal populations birth order influences the risk of minimal brain dysfunction.

In Chap. 3, data on twins and only children are discussed. Having no sibs or a sib with spacing zero, they may be said to occupy the extremes of birth position. For the slightly slower intellectual development of twins, the contact with a sib of the same age seems to be of less importance than their often substantially subnormal birth weight. Findings regarding only children, on the other hand, are inconsistent both for personality and IQ. Studies were only children are compared with children with sibs matched for background variables (particularly for the prevalence of broken homes) do not provide evidence of an "only child personality." Research both in twins and only children implies that presence for absence of sibs may be of less importance for intelligence and personality than is generally believed.

In Chap. 4, the correlation of birth order and sibship size to IQ is discussed. Large sibships and narrow spacing between sibs may be related to lower IQ not because of reduced contact with adults, but because both are connected with social and biological variables in parents that are not conducive to high IQ in children. This finding is an agreement with the twin results mentioned above. Birth order differentials in IQ approach zero with increasing control of background variables and when sibs from the same family are compared. These results correspond well to the generally accepted findings on the heritability of IQ.

In Chap. 5, school achievement is discussed according to measures of school grades, achievement tests, and educational attainment. The study of achievement in relation to family size comes to a conclusion similar to that drawn in connection with IQ: Large sibship size may be an indicator of an environment impeding high achievement rather than a direct inhibitor. Achievement differences by birth order approach zero with control of background variables or the use of adequate control groups. This is confirmed by several studies of sibs. There is no evidence that firstborns are overachievers (as they ought to be if they are equal to laterborns in IQ but higher in school achievement).

In Chap. 6, birth order differences in occupational status are examined. They are found in studies lacking control groups, but do not appear when satisfactory methods are used or in studies of sibs within the same family.

In Chap. 7, the correlation of birth order and sibship size to personality variables is studied. When social class is controlled, increasing sibship size is associated with unfavorable socialization influences, such as parent's lack of interest in school, punitiveness, and unsatisfactory parent-child relations. Though the association is very weak, it is contrary to the hypothesis that *large sibships are an advantage for socialization*. There is also *a consistent tendency for socialization to be less favorable in the lower class*. Personality variables are extremely tenuously correlated to sibship size when social class is controlled. As far as personality variables are concerned, there is a tendency for *less confidence, activity, and self-esteem to be associated with lower social class.*

Personality variables by birth order must be based on *differential socialization*. Firstborns are better cared for and enjoy more linguistic stimulation in infancy than laterborns, but at preschool age they tend to be treated with slightly more criticism and slightly less affection. There is, however, no evidence that this somewhat harsher socialization outlast preschool age, and differences are only small. *"Dethronement"* is present in the sense that the birth of a younger sib considerably disturbs the firstborn's relation to his/her mother and frequently leads to behavior disorders during the first months. There are very preliminary and incomplete data showing that dethronement does not necessarily leave a lasting impression.

As far as *parent-child relations* are concerned, there is some evidence that *firstborns describe themselves as more strongly identified with parents and readier to accept their authority*.

How far does the *presence of sibs* influence socialization? There is evidence that the presence of older sibs makes children aware of power interactions and that there is more antagonism between adjacent pairs than between jump pairs. There is, however, as yet no evidence that *what is learned by interactions with sibs is transferred to interactions outside the family*.

How far does a special relationship to parents and how far do relations to sibs affect personality? The evidence for differences in personality by birth order is separately summarized for experiments, paper-pencil tests, and observations of real-life behavior. Results are very often inconclusive because of *failure to control background variables*, which leads to mistaking interfamilial differences for differences between sibs. By this insufficient method contradictory results are obtained: Firstborns appear more anxious, but at the same time more verbally creative and no less well-adjusted or lower in self-esteem than laterborns. They appear more conforming, but at the same time higher on need for achievement, creativity, and task-orientation. They appear more introverted, but at the same time no less popular and more highly rated for leadership than laterborns.

If little weight is given to objectionable methods, it will be possible to explain all these characteristics by "dethronement", i.e., by the temporary "cooling off" of relations to the mother in early childhood, which would then supposedly have a lasting influence on personality. If this explanation were true, however, greater anxiety and conformity would appear in paper-pencil tests as well, as many pertinent tests consistently reveal sex differences.

In research where, on the other hand, at least sibship size is controlled, evidence for birth order differences becomes extremely tenuous: This discussion will not be taken up again (see p. 184ff.). The main finding is that, in accordance with firstborns' special relationship to parents, the latter describe them in a special way: i.e., as more introverted, neurotic, and striving than their younger sibs. This leads to the conclusion, if the finding were to be confirmed by studies with unselected samples of parents, that firstborns behave in a special way toward their parents. There would then be no "firstborn personality" in the sense of specific traits, but *a situation-specific firstborn behavior*, which is not necessarily, transferred to persons outside the family. Incidentally, such a result supports those trends in modern psychology that depart from the description of "traits" in favor of descriptions of situation-specific behavior.

Inconsistent evidence is not missing evidence. With better methods such as comparing sibs of the same sex and at the same age (data might be found in the archives of career counselors), more consistent findings may appear. Results as they stand, and particularly the fact that there are no data on adults that are not easily explained by well-known social class differences, make it possible to predict that *if any consistent personality differences between sibs are found with better methods, they will represent only a small part of the variance.*

In Chap. 8, studies of birth order, sibship size, and mental illness are considered. It was found that among younger patients firstborns are overrepresented and among older patients laterborns, as expected because demographic change. The only findings emerging from an enormous amount of often ill-conducted research are that juvenile delinquency is related to large sibships, that neurotics may come from small ones, that obsessional neurosis may be more frequent in firstborn males, and that obese children may more often be only children than controls.

The scarcity of findings, again not comparable to the large and frequent sex and social class differences in mental illness, confirm our view that, even with better research methods resulting birth order differences in personality will be slight. If birth order strongly influenced personality, some repercussion at least on "psychogenic" illness might be expected.

Our survey demonstrated that

1. Evidence of differential parental behavior toward children of different birth order is weak.

2. Birth order differences between nonrelated subjects tend to disappear with increasing control of social background variables.

3. Birth order differences disappear when sibs of the same family are compared.

4. Studies on birth order influences on the adult personality are rare and negative.

Our survey thus allows the conclusion that *birth order influences on personality and IQ have been widely overrated*. This result is in agreement with modern research on the *heritability of certain personality variables*. If temperamental characteristics are based on polygenic inheritance, each child in a sibship will interact in a novel way with the environment and, from the first day on, will mold it and be molded by it in a highly individualistic way. Each sib in a sibship will react differently to parents and sibs. The idea that birth order indelibly imprints personality in a predictable way starts from the assumption that a newborn child is a "tabula rasa."

All this does not signify that being an oldest, middle, or youngest child may not be of the greatest importance for the personality of *some* individuals. It seems however, that the times where sweeping generalizations in "dynamic" or "depth" psychology and psychiatry were possible are over.

The influences of the "schizophrenogenic mother" on schizophrenia, toilet training on "anality," and being an oldest or youngest child on personality have not been confirmed by controlled experience. *It seems increasingly important to consider the interaction of each individual person with his or her individual environment*. Psychodynamic psychology and psychiatry will not become more simple by getting rid of unwarranted theories, but perhaps more rewarding. We hope that the present survey of birth order research contributes to this development.

Part II Analysis of Empirical Data

Chapter 10 Examination of Hypotheses Concerning Birth Order and Sibship Size by Multivariate Analysis of a Representative Young Adult Population

10.1 Introduction and Purpose of this Study

Siblings growing up in the same family differ considerably in physical appearance, personality, intelligence, school achievement, and other characteristics. It is a basic human need to explain these differences. If the general assumption is true that mainly environmental conditions influence human development, birth order should be of paramount importance. Being one of the few clearly defined environmental factors, it is open to scientific investigation.

There seems to exist a common-sense "knowledge" that being born as a single, eldest, or youngest child determines to a large extent the development of personality. While discussing with friends and psychologists the problem whether birth rank is an important factor in human development, we were amazed at how many contradictory opinions about the importance of birth order were expressed. Birth order is supposed to explain school performance, character traits such as introversion and extraversion, dominance, and submission, but also major and minor emotional disorders, mental illness, and addiction.

As genes are randomly transferred from parents to child, consistent differences in personality related to birth rank cannot be explained by genetic differences. Therefore, the evidence that birth order influences human characteristics would establish an environmental factor of high general validity. But if birth order does not influence human development to a considerable extent, we have to conclude that at least one marked environmental characteristic is unimportant. This may lead to the examination of other hypotheses about the influence of environmental variables that are less well-defined, and encourage a more critical view of current theories on human development mainly based on environmental factors.

The aim of this study is to evaluate a possible influence of two well-defined environmental factors, birth order and sibship size, on school achievement, some personality dimensions (extraversion, neuroticism, and others), and consumption habits (tobacco, alcohol, cannabis, hypnotics, minor tranquilizers, and analgesics). Special emphasis is placed on the analysis of interfering social variables, so as to minimize spurious correlations, more accurately estimate the relative weight of birth order and sibship size, and thus avoid false conclusions.

10.2 Methodology

10.2.1 Samples

In 1971 the Research Department of the Psychiatric University Clinic, Zurich, carried out a study on the epidemiology of tobacco, alcohol, and drug consumption among a representative sample of 6,315 19-year-old male and 1,381 20-year-old female inhabitants of the canton Zurich. This district is situated in northeastern Switzerland and contains 1.1 million German-speaking inhabitants. More than half of them live in the two major cities of the region, the others residing in rural and subalpine areas. Besides a questionnaire on alcohol, tobacco, and drug consumption, a personality test (Freiburger Personality Inventory, FPI) including a lie scale was given, and information on several social variables, birth order and sibship size was gathered.

The *male sample* was examined at the compulsory military draft (but independently of the military examination) in groups of ten. The subjects were carefully informed of the purpose of this study. Medical secrecy was guaranteed and confirmed by a personal letter signed by the project manager. Fewer than 1% refused to participate. Half of the questionnaires were anonymous and the other half had to be signed. The results of the two groups of questionnaires were not significantly different. Some methodological aspects of the project were published in earlier papers (Angst et al. 1973 a, b; Ruppen et al. 1973). Reliability and consistency of the answers were high.

The majority of the *female sample* was collected at several schools offering a compulsory house-keeping course. The rest were questioned at other schools. The questionnaires were answered in the classrooms. Among the female group, persons with higher education are overrepresented.

Due to missing data, a high lie score in the personality questionnaire, and/or signs of inconsistency in a number of slightly modified questions, 1.5% of the subjects had to be dropped.

10.2.2 Assessment of Sibship Size and Birth Order

The subjects had to indicate the number of their sibs. For the analysis three distinct groups were formed: single children, sibships of two, and sibships of three or more children. Table 57 shows the male and female samples broken down by birth order within sibship size. Despite the difference in size of the samples, the proportions of the subgroups are the same for both sexes.

10.2.3 Statistics

In this study birth order and sibship size are treated as independent variables. In analyzing their relationship with personality traits, school achievement, or alcohol and drug consumption, bivariate and multivariate strategies were used to find out the influence of other independent variables, such as number of inhabitants in

Table 57. Distribution of the sample by birth rank

Birth order (sibship size)	Males		Females	
	N	Percent	*N*	Percent
Single child	588	9.5	110	8.0
Firstborn (two)	932	15.0	231	17.0
Secondborn (two)	836	13.4	188	13.8
Firstborn (three or more)	1,144	18.4	253	18.6
Middle (three or more)	1,718	27.6	360	26.4
Youngest (three or more)	1,002	16.1	220	16.2
Total	6,220	100.0	1,362	100.0

place of residence, marital status of parents, and fathers' occupational status. The size of the female sample did not allow all analyses that were carried out with the male sample.

The statistical analyses are based on the program libraries SPSS (Statistical Package for Social Sciences) (Nie 1975) and OSIRIS (Andrews et al. 1975). Findings at a significance level of 5% or less are accepted. Data showing particularly strong associations are boxed. They are usually in agreement for males and females.

10.3 Birth Order and School Achievement

In the foregoing review of literature the following hypotheses were found to be important and have been reexamined by means of our representative samples (see pp. 52f., 29, 40, 86):

1. There is a negative correlation between sibship size and school achievement.
2. Firstborns show better school achievement than laterborns.
3. Youngest children achieve less than their elder sibs.
4. School achievement is inversely related to birth order within sibship size.
5. School achievement of single children is lower than that of firstborns.
6. Single children show lower school achievement than children with sibs.

School achievement is measured by *educational attainment* (see p. 50).

10.3.1 Classification of School Types and Distribution of School Achievement

In Switzerland, school attendance starts at the age of 6–7 years and is compulsory for 9 years. In the canton Zurich all normally intelligent children attend the same type of school for the first 6 years (primary school). Afterwards, there is a subdivision: Students continue primary school or enter secondary school, higher secondary school, or various types of grammar schools. For subnormal children, special schooling opportunities are offered.

Table 58. Distribution of the sample by School achievement

	Males		Females	
	N	Percent	*N*	Percent
1. Special school for subnormal children	144	2.4	2	0.2
2. Primary school	732	12.0	45	3.5
3. Lower secondary school	2,041	33.4	292	22.7
4. Higher secondary school	2,017	33.0	548	42.6
5. Grammar school	307	5.0	172	13.4
6. Grammar school with university entrance examination	870	14.2	226	17.6
Total	6,111	100.0	1,285	100.0

School achievement was assessed by the school types attended at the ages of 19 and 20 years respectively. This led to the following classification (Table 58):

1. Special school for subnormal children
2. Primary school (9 years)
3. Lower secondary school
4. Higher secondary school
5. Grammar school
6. Grammar school with university entrance examination. As already mentioned in Sect. 10.2.1, higher school levels are overrepresented among the female sample.

10.3.2 Birth Order and School Achievement: Bivariate Analysis

School Achievement of Single Children and Firstborns. Single children attain the same school achievement as firstborns (Table 59). This refutes the hypothesis that single children achieve less than children with younger sibs.

School Achievement in Sibships of Two. In both sexes there is no significant difference in school achievement between the older and the younger child in sibships of two (Table 59 a).

School Achievement in Sibships of Three and More. Among sibships of three and more children we compared the oldest with the middle and the youngest child. Table 59 b shows that among the male sample school achievement is not equally distributed among the three groups. At the highest school level the oldest sibs show a better performance than the middle or youngest child. In the female sample there is a nonsignificant trend in the same direction. Later it will be examined whether this finding is due to birth order or to intervening social variables.

10.3.3 Sibship Size and School Achievement: Bivariate Analysis

Sibship size correlates negatively with school achievement (Tables 60 and 61). In the female group, where higher school levels are overrepresented, the negative cor-

Table 59. School achievement in single child versus first of two children versus first of three or more children

	Males						Females					
	Single[a, c, e]		First of two		First of three or more		Single[b, d, f]		First of two		First of three or more	
	N	Percent	*N*	Percent	*N*	Percent	*N*	Percent	*N*	Percent	*N*	Percent
1. Special school for subnormal children	13	2.3	21	2.3	27	2.4						
2. Primary school (9 years)	54	9.4	78	8.7	122	11.0	4	3.7	7	3.2	5	2.2
3. Lower secondary school	167	29.2	283	31.4	358	32.3	22	20.2	41	19.0	43	18.5
4. Higher secondary school	196	34.3	297	33.0	386	34.8	49	45.0	95	44.0	107	46.1
5. Grammar school	49	8.6	58	6.4	51	4.6	13	11.9	36	16.7	32	13.8
6. Grammar school with university entrance	93	16.3	163	18.1	164	14.8	21	19.3	37	17.1	45	19.4
Total	572	100.0	900	100.0	1,108	100.0	109	100.0	216	100.0	232	100.0

[a] χ^2 17.8695,
[c] P NS (0.06),
[e] Contingency coefficient 0.08,
[b] 2.6065
[d] NS.
[f] 0.07

Table 59a. School achievement by birth order in sibships of two

	Males				Females			
	Older		Younger[a, c, e]		Older		Younger[b, c, e]	
	N	Percent	*N*	Percent	*N*	Percent	*N*	Percent
1. Special school for subnormal children	21	2.3	14	1.7	7	3.2	3	1.8
2. Primary school (9 years)	78	8.7	60	7.4				
3. Lower secondary school	283	31.4	254	31.3	41	19.0	35	21.0
4. Higher secondary school	297	33.0	306	37.7	95	44.0	73	43.7
5. Grammar school	58	6.4	34	4.2	36	16.7	23	13.8
6. Grammar school with University entrance	163	18.1	144	17.7	37	17.1	33	19.8
Total	900	100.0	812	100.0	216	100.0	167	100.0

[a] χ^2 8.3838,
[b] 1.8082
[c] *P* NS
[e] Contingency coefficient 0.07

relation is less marked than among males. The contingency coefficients are in the order of magnitude of the data reported on p. 30).

The negative correlation betwenn family size and school achievement may be due to interfering variables (e.g., social status), which are associated with sibship size.

10.3.4 Other Social Factors and School Achievement

The present analysis takes into account the influence of social variables other than birth order and sibship size on school achievement. In a first step school achievement was cross-tabulated with various social data (Table 62). The definitions of the variables are given in the Appendix (see p. 285). It is possible to distinguish two sets of variables: The first set contains those relating to the sociocultural environment of the subject (size of place of residence, denomination, marital status of parents, father's income and occupational status). These variables will be called *structural*. The second set relates to the personal history and situation of the subject (habitation during childhood and adolescence, educational style of parents during the last 3 years, present relations with parents). These variables will be called *individual*.

The main influence on school achievement is exerted by two related structural variables: father's income and occupational status. Other correlations are considerably lower. Higher school achievement is positively correlated with number of inhabitants in place of residence, with parents being married, and with stating no religious denomination. Among the individual variables, this is true for having lived with both parents, for reporting a friendly educational style of, and for persisting relations with parents.

Table 59b. School achievement by birth order in sibships of three or more

	Males						Females					
	Oldest [a, c, e]		Middle		Youngest		Oldest [b, d, f]		Middle		Youngest	
	N	Percent	*N*	Percent	*N*	Percent	*N*	Percent	*N*	Percent	*N*	Percent
1. Special school for subnormal children	27	2.4	38	2.3	27	2.8	5	2.2	18	5.3	8	3.9
2. Primary school (9 years)	122	11.0	259	15.4	135	13.9						
3. Lower secundary school	358	32.3	600	35.8	355	36.7	43	18.5	88	25.8	61	29.9
4. Higher secondary school	386	34.8	504	30.1	310	32.0	107	46.1	133	39.0	81	39.7
5. Grammar school	51	4.6	79	4.7	33	3.4	32	13.8	48	14.1	19	9.3
6. Grammar school with university entrance	164	14.8	197	11.7	108	11.2	45	19.4	54	15.8	35	17.2
Total	1,108	100.0	1,677	100.0	968	100.0	232	100.0	341	100.0	207	100.0

[a] χ^2 27.8863,
[c] $P \leqq 0.002$,
[e] Contingency coefficient 0.09,
[b] 14.7929
[d] NS (0.07)
[f] 0.14

Table 60. School achievement and sibship size: male sample

	Sibship size											
	Single child[a, b, c]	Percent	Two	Percent	Three	Percent	Four	Percent	Five	Percent	Six or more	Percent
1. Special school for subnormal children	12	2.1	36	2.1	36	2.2	23	2.2	15	2.6	22	4.3
2. Primary school (9 years)	51	9.0	145	8.4	165	9.9	122	11.9	112	19.2	130	25.3
3. Lower secondary school	170	29.0	541	31.2	572	34.3	374	36.3	203	34.8	177	34.5
4. Higher secondary school	193	34.0	609	35.2	566	33.9	335	32.6	180	30.9	129	25.1
5. Grammar school	49	8.6	93	5.4	83	5.0	46	4.5	21	3.6	15	2.9
6. Grammar school with university entrance	93	16.4	308	17.8	248	14.9	129	12.5	52	8.9	40	7.8
Total	568		1,732		1,670		1,029		583		513	

[a] χ^2 231.3882
[b] $P \leqq 0.0001$
[c] Contingency coefficient 0.19

Table 61. School achievement and sibship size: female sample

	Sibship size											
	Single child[a, b, c]	Percent	Two	Percent	Three	Percent	Four	Percent	Five	Percent	Six or more	Percent
1. + 2. Special school for subnormal children, primary school	3	2.8	10	2.6	6	1.7	17	7.1	4	3.9	7	7.8
3. Lower secondary school	20	18.9	79	20.3	80	22.7	59	24.6	28	27.2	25	27.8
4. Higher secondary school	49	46.2	172	44.1	163	46.3	83	34.6	40	38.8	39	43.3
5. Grammar school	13	12.3	59	15.1	38	10.8	35	14.6	16	15.5	10	11.1
6. Grammar school with university entrance	21	19.8	70	17.9	65	18.5	46	19.2	15	14.6	9	10.0
Total	106		390		352		240		103		90	

[a] χ^2 34.6474
[b] $P = 0.03$
[c] Contingency coefficient 0.16

Table 62. School achievement and social data: bivariate analysis

	Males		Females	
	Contingency coefficient	*P*	Contingency coefficient	*P*
Number of inhabitants in place of residence	0.17	0.00	0.17	0.001
Denomination	0.10	0.00	0.16	0.0012
Marital status of parents	0.09	0.00	0.10	0.015
Occupational status of father	0.36	0.00	0.37	0.00
Income of father	0.36	0.00	0.39	0.00
Habitation during childhood	0.09	0.00	0.11	0.004
Habitation during adolescence	0.11	0.00	0.11	0.006
Educational style of father	0.14	0.000	0.11	0.66 (NS)
Educational style of mother	0.12	0.00	0.11	0.54 (NS)
Relationship with parents	0.10	0.00	0.14	0.005

The hypothesis brought forward (see p. 11 f.) that subjects with different school achievement are differentially distributed by residence, is confirmed. As the canton Zurich is under one educational system, larger differences in achievement by residence can be expected in less homogeneous contexts.

10.3.5 Birth Order, Social Factors, and School Achievement: Multiple Classification Analysis

Social Factors

On the strength of the results obtained by the bivariate analysis, eight social variables were selected for a multivariate classification analysis. As a further variable either sibship size or birth order was introduced. As the correlations of the eight variables with achievement do not change when variables representing various aspects of birth order and sibship size are added, the results will be represented by the multivariate analysis of the single child's school achievement as opposed to that of subjects with sibs (Table 63).

The explained variance in school achievement is 0.17 for males and 0.13 for females. Again, the highest contribution to school achievement is made by a structural variable, i.e., occupational status of father (beta 0.33 for both sexes). All other factors contribute considerably less (beta 0.05–0.12), though in a significant way. The results of males and females are in good agreement.

Structural variables seem to have more weight with females and individual variables with males. Female Catholics have lower school achievement, while among males and females those stating no denomination achieve better. Among males, on the other hand, individual variables come in second and third place. The direction of the correlation is the same as with the bivariate analysis. Achievement is posi-

Table 63. School achievement of single children: multivariate classification analysis

	Males [a, b]	
	Beta	*P*
1. Occupational status of father	0.33	0.01
2. Educational style of mother	0.12	0.01
3. Relations with parents	0.10	0.01
4. Number of inhabitants in place of residence	0.09	0.01
5. Habitation during chidhood and adolescence	0.08	0.01
6. Denomination	0.06	0.01
7. Educational style of father	0.05	0.01
8. Single child	0.05	0.01
9. Marital status of parents	0.02	NS

	Females [c, d]	
	Beta	*P*
1. Occupational status of father	0.33	0.01
2. Denomination	0.11	0.01
3. Relations with parents	0.08	0.05
4. Educational style of father	0.08	NS (0.10)
5. Number of inhabitants in place of residence	0.08	NS (0.10)
6. Habitation during childhood and adolescence	0.08	0.01
7. Educational style of mother	0.05	NS
8. Single child	0.02	NS
9. Marital status of parents	0.008	NS

[a] Multiple R^2 0.17
[b] $P \leq 0.01$
[c] Multiple R^2 0.13
[d] $P \leq 0.01$

Table 64. Effect of occupational status of father on school achievement: Adjusted means

		School achievement	
		Males	Females
Occupational status of father:	High	2.98	3.35
	Middle	2.63	2.97
	Low	2.20	2.64

tively correlated to an unbroken home and to both a friendly and an authoritarian style of education, and negatively to detachment from parents at 19 years of age.

Table 64 presents adjusted means for achievement by occupational status of father for each sex. Females' higher level of achievement is due to selection bias (see p. 246).

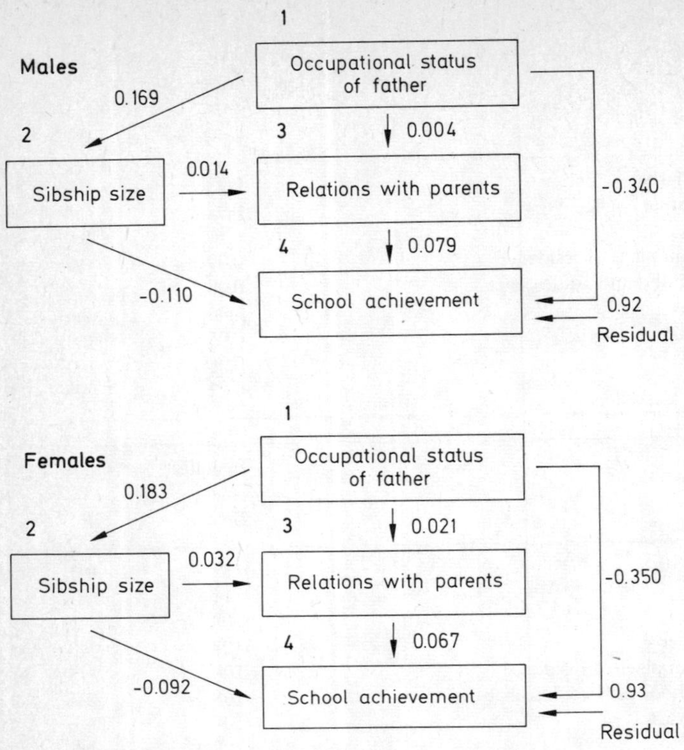

Fig. 4. School achievement: path analysis

Birth Order

Single Children versus Children with Sibs. The only significant result was found among males, where single children show a slightly better school achievement than children with sibs. The difference is not significant among females. Male single children have an adjusted mean of school achievement of 2.75 and all others of 2.58.

Sibships of Two. The older and the younger sibs do not differ significantly in school achievement (adjusted means, 2.74 versus 2.71 for males and 3.09 versus 3.13 for females, respectively).

Sibships of Three or More. Oldest, middle, and youngest children do not differ significantly in school achievement. The oldest male has an average achievement of 2.57 and the middle and the youngest of 2.50: Among females the corresponding values are 3.7, 2.97, and 2.90. Thus the findings of the bivariate analysis are not confirmed.

10.3.6 Social Factors, Sibship Size, and School Achievement: Multiple Classification Analysis

In this section sibship size is introduced. The results are given in Table 65. They are similar to the analysis presented in Table 63. The explained variance of school

Table 65. School achievement and sibship size: multivariate classification analysis

	Males[a, b]	
	Beta	P
1. Occupational status of father	0.32	0.01
2. Educational style of mother	0.11	0.01
3. Relations with parents	0.10	0.01
4. Sibship size	0.095	0.01
5. Habitation during childhood and adolescence	0.08	0.01
6. Number of inhibitants in place of residence	0.08	0.01
7. Educational style of father	0.05	0.01
8. Denomination	0.05	0.01
9. Marital status of parents	0.02	NS

	Females[c, d]	
	Beta	P
1. Occupational status of father	0.33	0.01
2. Denomination	0.11	0.01
3. Relations with parents	0.08	0.05
4. Educational style of father	0.08	NS (0.10)
5. Number of inhabitants in place of residence	0.08	0.01
6. Habitation during childhood and adolescence	0.08	0.01
7. Educational style of mother	0.05	NS
8. Sibship size	0.04	NS
9. Marital status of parents	0.006	NS

[a] Multiple R^2 0.18
[b] $P \leqq 0.01$
[c] Multiple R^2 0.13
[d] $P \leqq 0.01$

achievement among males is 0.18 and among females, 0.13. When other background variables are controlled, school achievement is still correlated to sibship size. The association is, however, weak and reaches significance only in the male sample (beta 0.095, $P < 0.01$). Further analysis shows that the correlation is negative.

10.3.7 Path Analysis (Fig. 4)

Based on the results of Sect. 10.3.5, a path analysis was carried out for the male and female samples, including the factors that were found associated with school achievement in the preceding analysis. Therefore, birth order had to be dropped. The results of this analysis are in agreement with the results of the multivariate classification analysis. The model assumes school achievement to be directly dependent on father's occupational status and on sibship size, possibly also on the reported relationship with parents. Both solutions fit with a remaining residual path of 0.93. By far the strongest positive correlation was found with father's occupational status. A second important connection was found between lower-status occupation of father and larger sibship size. The latter variable was again negatively correlated with school achievement. The path coefficients demonstrate that the subject's evaluation of his relations with parents is of minor importance.

10.3.8 Discussion

With control of a number of structural and individual variables the following conclusions are reached with reference to the hypotheses brougth forward in Sect. 10:

1. Sibship size is negatively, though very slightly, correlated to school achievement among males.
2. The hypothesis that firstborns achieve better than laterborns is not confirmed.
3. Youngest children do not achieve less than their older sibs.
4. School achievement is not negatively correlated to birth order within sibship size.
5. Single children do not achieve less than firstborns.
6. Single male children are slightly superior to male subjects with sibs.

Earlier (see p. 31, 52) it was supposed that the achievement-sibship size correlation would prove spurious when background variables were controlled to a higher degree than is customary in birth order research. On the basis of the results presented here we must, however, conclude *that sibship size has a very slight influence of its own.* Fewer familial resources of attention, supervision, and money may mediate the effect. More resources, on the other hand, may cause single children's slightly higher achievement.

It was supposed (see p. 58, 11f.) that a broken home would have a negative, and living in a large town or city a positive influence on school achievement. Both hypotheses have been confirmed, though the amount of variance explained by them is low.

On the other hand, the Zajonc (1976) "confluence theory" and "teaching hypothesis" are not confirmed (see p. 39f.). There is no significant stepwise decrease of school achievement by birth order. Single children are even at an advantage and youngest children do not have a significantly lower achievement.

The multiple classification analysis explains only a small amount of the variance in school achievement. Nonetheless, the weight of the structural and individual variables makes sense: Female achievement appears more strongly influenced by environmental structure and male achievement by personal history. This is in line with the well-established greater adaptability of women to social demands and men's greater vulnerability to social stress.

10.4 Birth Order and Personality

The following hypotheses taken from the previous review of literature have been examined (see pp. 82ff., 85ff., 25f.).

1. Sibship size has an impact on personality.
2. Firstborns are more nervous than laterborns.
3. Firstborns are less aggressive than laterborns.

4. Firstborns are more depressive than laterborns.
5. Firstborns are less sociable than laterborns.
6. Firstborns are more dominant than laterborns.
7. Firstborns are more inhibited than laterborns.
8. Firstborns are less open than laterborns.
9. Firstborns are less extraverted than laterborns.
10. Firstborns are more neurotic than laterborns.
11. Single children differ unfavorably from firstborns by being more nervous, less sociable, less extraverted, more neurotic.
12. Youngest children differ unfavorably from other sibs.

10.4.1 Assessment

Aspects of personality were assessed with the FPI (Freiburger personality inventory) developed by Fahrenberg et al. (1973). The questionnaire consists of 212 items measuring primary (1–9) and secondary factors (10–12) of personality:

Primary factors

1. Nervousness
2. Aggressiveness
3. Depression
4. Excitability
5. Sociability
6. Calmness
7. Dominance
8. Inhibition
9. Openness

Secondary factors

10. Extraversion
11. Neuroticism (emotional lability)
12. Masculinity

The FPI was applied for measuring personality aspects in correlation with the consumption of tobacco, alcohol, and drugs. These results were published in 1973 by Müller-Oswald et al.

10.4.2 Birth Order and Personality: Oneway Analysis of Variance

Personality of Single Children. Single children were compared with firstborns because the latter have been only children at least for some time in their lives. The results are given in Table 66. Only children of either sex score higher on sociability and extraversion than the first of two or of three or more sibs. Among males single children score lower on the inhibition and openess dimensions. Single children, on the other hand, do not score higher on neuroticism or any of its components (nervousness, aggressiveness, depression, excitability). These findings are not in agreement with psychological folklore, which believes single children to be less sociable, less extraverted and more neurotic than children with sibs.

Personality in Sibships of Two. The older is not consistently different from the younger child in any aspect of personality measured by the FPI. There is only one trend that is valid for both sexes: Dimension 2 (aggressiveness) is slightly elevated among younger sibs ($P<0.10$). Considering the large size of the samples, this finding is insignificant.

Personality in Sibships of Three or More. The 12 FPI personality dimensions were included in an analysis of variance comparing the oldest, middle, and youngest child. Only in one dimension, masculinity, did differences consistently appear in

Table 66. FPI values in single child versus first of two children versus first of three or more children: oneway analysis of variance

FPI	100 × ETA² (%)	Males			100 × ETA² (%)	Females		
		One	Two	Three		One	Two	Three
		Mean values				Mean values		
Nervousness	0.07	10.0	9.7	9.6	0.5	12.1	12.7	11.7
Aggressiveness	0.05	9.2	9.1	9.3	0.8	8.4	7.5	8.0
Depression	0.07	12.1	12.5	12.5	0.2	13.6	14.2	14.0
Excitability	0.2	8.3	7.7	8.1	0.8	10.1	9.6	9.0
Sociability	0.8[a]	17.1	16.3	15.7	1.4[a]	16.8	14.9	15.4
Calmness	0.3	11.5	11.4	11.5	0.5	9.2	9.3	9.9
Dominance	0.1	7.6	7.4	7.7	0.2	6.3	6.6	6.3
Inhibition	0.7[a]	7.5	8.1	8.5	1.0	9.9	11.1	10.7
Openness	0.5[a]	9.7	9.8	10.1	0.1	9.7	9.5	9.6
Extraversion	0.6[a]	13.9	13.2	12.9	1.1[a]	12.7	11.3	11.8
Neuroticism	0.00	10.8	10.9	10.9	0.5	12.9	13.2	12.3
Masculinity	0.05	15.1	15.0	15.2	0.7	11.0	10.6	11.3

[a] $P \leqq 0.05$

Table 67. Sibships with three or more children: masculinity scale; oneway analysis of variance

	100 × ETA² (%)	Oldest ($\bar{X}$)	Middle ($\bar{X}$)	Youngest ($\bar{X}$)
Males	0.2	15.2	15.1	14.8
Females	1.4	11.3	10.7	10.2

both samples. Masculinity is lowest for both sexes in the youngest sib. The explained variance (eta²) is, however, very small (Table 67). In all other aspects birth rank is not related to personality dimensions.

10.4.3 Birth Order, Extraversion, and Neuroticism

Tables 68 and 69 reproduce the mean values of the two personality dimensions extraversion and neuroticism for all birth positions. Single children score higher on extraversion than children with sibs, while the latter do not differ from each other. Neuroticism is not related to birth order. Firstborns, laterborns, and single children appear in no way different from each other or from other birth ranks on this dimension.

10.4.4 Sibship Size and Personality

If the finding that single children are more extraverted and sociable than others is correct, we may expect sibship size to correlate with personality. This is confirmed

Table 68. Birth order and extraversion: oneway analysis of variance

	Males[a]			Females[b]		
	N	$\bar{X}$	S	*N*	$\bar{X}$	S
Single child	569	13,84	4.53	106	12.78	4.42
Firstborn of two	897	13,24	4.67	229	11.34	4.66
Secondborn of two	799	13.49	4.53	186	12.17	4.72
Oldest of three or more	1,108	12.95	4.59	249	11.85	4.79
Middle of three or more	1,669	13.13	4.42	354	11.10	4.46
Youngest of three or more	983	13.08	4.43	212	11.97	4.43
Total	6,025	13.22	4.52	1,336	11.70	4.60

[a] $P < 0.002$, $100 \times ETA^2 = 0.3\%$
[b] NS $100 \times ETA^2 = 1.2\%$

Table 69. Birth order and neuroticism: oneway analysis of variance

	Males[a]			Females[b]		
	N	$\bar{X}$	SD	*N*	$\bar{X}$	S
Single child	569	10.79	5.46	106	12.84	5.29
Firstborn of two	897	10.87	5.28	229	13.16	5.08
Secondborn of two	799	11.24	5.47	186	13.01	5.22
Oldest of three or more	1,108	10.87	5.47	249	12.35	5.43
Middle of three or more	1,669	10.77	5.05	354	12.87	5.26
Youngest of three ore more	983	11.05	5.29	212	12.51	5.04
Total	6,025	10.92	5.30	1,336	12.78	5.22

[a] NS $ETA^2 = 0\%$
[b] NS $ETA^2 = 0.3\%$

by the results of the analysis in Table 70. Extraversion and sociability decrease and inhibition increases with sibship size. Neuroticism or other aspects of emotional lability (nervousness, aggressiveness, depression), however, are not related to sibship size. The variance explained by sibship size is very low (consistently less than 1%). Living with no, one or several sibs has only a minimal impact on personality.

10.4.5 Personality (Extraversion and Neuroticism) and Other Social Variables

The previous analysis of social factors influencing school achievement shows clearly that other structural and individual factors are of more weight than birth order. In our present analysis the same factors will again be included. We may expect neuroticism to be negatively correlated to occupational status of father (as an indicator for social class), but extraversion to be positively correlated to it (Eysenck et al. 1969). School achievement may have a similar connection to neuroticism and extraversion. Having grown up in a broken home, reported educational style of and relations with parents can be supposed to influence neuroticism.

Table 70. Sibship size (one, two, three or more) and personality: oneway analysis of variance

FPI	100 × ETA² (%)	Males: One	Males: Two	Males: Three or more	100 × ETA² (%)	Females: One	Females: Two	Females: Three or more
		Mean values				Mean values		
Nervousness	0.01	6.4	6.2	6.1	0.1	12.1	12.8	12.3
Aggressiveness	0.00	9.2	9.3	9.3	0.2	8.4	7.7	7.9
Depression	0.06	12.1	12.7	12.6	0.06	13.4	14.0	14.0
Excitability	0.05	8.3	7.9	7.9	0.8[a]	10.1	9.5	8.8
Sociability	0.3[a]	17.1	16.4	16.1	0.6[a]	16.8	15.4	15.2
Calmness	0.1[a]	11.5	12.3	11.6	0.1	9.2	9.4	9.6
Dominance	0.1[a]	7.6	7.4	7.6	0.3	6.3	6.4	6.0
Inhibition	0.4[a]	7.5	8.1	8.4	0.6[a]	9.8	10.8	11.1
Openness	0.6	9.7	9.9	9.9	0.09	9.7	9.5	9.6
Extraversion	0.3[a]	13.9	13.4	13.1	0.4	12.7	11.7	11.6
Neuroticism	0.03	10.8	11.1	10.9	0.2	12.9	13.1	12.6
Masculinity	0.02	15.1	15.0	15.1	0.1	11.0	10.6	10.7

[a] $P \leqq 0.05$

Table 71. Social data and personality: oneway analysis of variance

	Extraversion: Males	Extraversion: Females	Neuroticism: Males	Neuroticism: Females
	100 × ETA² (%)		100 × ETA² (%)	
Number of inhabitants in place of residence	0.3			
Denomination			0.2	
School achievement	0.3[a]	0.8[a]	0.2	
Marital status of parents			0.6	0.3
Occupational status of father	0.4			
Income of father	1.0[a]	0.9[a]	0.2	
Habitation during childhood			0.5[a]	0.8[a]
Habitation during adolescence			0.5[a]	0.4[a]
Educational style of father			2.0[a]	3.0[a]
Educational style of mother	0.07		2.0[a]	2.0[a]
Relationship with parents	0.4		5.0[a]	3.0[a]
Psychiatric treatment	0.08		2.0[a]	1.0[a]

[a] $P \leqq 0.05$. The framed numbers are significant for both sexes

The correlations between several social variables, extraversion, and neuroticism are described in Table 71. Only significant results are given (by means of the explained variance eta², based on a oneway analysis of variance). *Extraversion and neuroticism correlate with a completely different set of social data:* Extraversion is influenced by structural, and neuroticism by individual factors.

Extraversion. Extraversion is positively associated with father's income, and in males with father's occupational status. Extraversion has a curvilinear relationship to school achievement. High and low achievers are more introverted than those in an intermediate position. Each of variables however, explains only a very small amount of the variance in extraversion.

Neuroticism. In contrast to extraversion, neuroticism is dependent on subjects' evaluation of the relationship with their parents during the last few years. This variable explains 5% of the variance in neuroticism among males and 3% among females. This is also true, though to a lower degree, for the evaluation of parents' educationl style. All these social factors reflect a recent aspect of life or a present view of the relationship with parents. Indicators of a broken home (habitation during childhood and adolescence, marital status of parents) also correlate with neuroticism, but explain less than 1% of the variance.

Two structural factors are not significantly correlated with personality measures: number of inhabitants in place of residence and denomination.

Additional information on all 12 dimensions of the FPI is given in *Tables 72 and 72 a*, which present the variance (eta^2) explained by structural and individual factors. The findings are in agreement with the previous data on extraversion and neuroticism. For instance, father's income, which correlates positively with extraversion, also correlates with higher sociability and lower inhibition. Higher sociability and lower inhibition, on the other hand, correlate with higher occupational status of father. A positive correlation of extraversion with fathers' occupation is, however, only present in males (Table 72). Neuroticism is independent of both indicators of social class.

Factors indicating a broken home (marital status of parents, lodging in adolescence) and factors indicating disturbed relations with parents (educational style of

Table 72. Structural factors and personality (extraversion): oneway analysis of variance

FPI	Number of inhabitants in place of residence 100 × ETA^2(%)		Occupational status of father 100 × ETA^2(%)		Income of father 100 × ETA^2(%)		School achievement 100 × ETA^2(%)	
	Males	Females	Males	Females	Males	Females	Males	Females
Nervousness	0.6			1.0	1.4		1.8[a]	0.2[a]
Aggressiveness								0.2
Depression			0.2			0.2	0.8	
Excitability			0.4					0.9
Sociability			0.6[a]	0.7[a]	1.2[a]	1.2[a]	1.3[a]	0.7[a]
Calmness	0.2[a]	0.7[a]	0.2			0.2	2.1[a]	3.0[a]
Dominance	0.5		1.0			0.3	3.3[a]	0.4[a]
Inhibition	0.3[a]	0.7[a]	0.6[a]	1.0[a]	1.5[a]	1.5[a]		0.4
Openness		0.1	0.1					1.7
Extraversion	0.3		0.4		0.9[a]	1.0[a]	0.9[a]	0.8[a]
Neuroticism						0.2		0.3
Masculinity	0.3		0.2		1.3			1.5

[a] $P \leq 0.05$

Table 72a. Individual factors and personality: (neuroticism) oneway analysis of variance

FPI	Marital status of parents 100 × ETA²(%)		Habitation during adolescence 100 × ETA²(%)		Educational style of father 100 × ETA²(%)		Educational style of mother 100 × ETA²(%)		Relationship with parents 100 × ETA²(%)	
	Males	Females	Males	Females	Males	Females	Males	Females	Males	Females
Nervousness	1.0[a]	0.7[a]	0.4[a]	0.9[a]	2.8[a]	2.4[a]	1.9[a]	2.0[a]	1.6[a]	3.4[a]
Aggressiveness	0.3[a]	0.4[a]	0.4[a]	0.3[a]	1.7[a]	1.4[a]	1.3[a]	1.0[a]	2.5[a]	2.6[a]
Depression	0.7[a]	0.3[a]		0.6	3.6[a]	2.6[a]	2.9[a]	2.5[a]	4.4[a]	5.5[a]
Excitability	0.5[a]	0.3[a]	0.4[a]	0.4[a]		1.0		0.9		1.4
Sociability				0.1	1.1[a]	0.4[a]		0.5	1.4[a]	1.5[a]
Calmness						0.5		0.5	0.7[a]	1.2[a]
Dominance				0.2	0.8[a]	0.6[a]		0.5		0.4
Inhibition						0.3		0.6		1.5
Openness					0.8	0.6	1.4[a]	1.2[a]	2.6[a]	2.0[a]
Extraversion										
Neuroticism	0.6[a]	0.3[a]	0.4[a]	0.5[a]	2.7[a]	2.2[a]	2.3[a]	2.4[a]	3.1[a]	4.7[a]
Masculinity	0.1			0.2	1.2[a]	0.7[a]	0.8[a]	0.8[a]	0.7[a]	2.4[a]

[a] $P \leqq 0.05$

and relationship with parents) are not only related to a higher neuroticism score, but also to primary dimensions of neuroticism, such as nervousness, aggressiveness, depression, and excitability (Table 72a). On the other hand, these factors do not influence extraversion. The dependency of two supposedly orthogonal factors of personality on two sets of social data is an argument for the validity of the FPI.

10.4.6 Birth Order and Personality: Multiple Classification Analysis

A multiple classification analysis of variance was carried out introducing nine social factors as independent variables together with variables for various aspects of birth order and sibship size.

Extraversion. As an example, the results of the multivariate classification analysis are given in detail in Table 73 taking into account the status of single children versus all others. The overall multiple R^2 is only 0.02 ($P \leqq 0.01$), which means that extraversion is more or less independent of all variables analyzed. A very low con-

Table 73. Extraversion: social factors and single child status (multivariate classification analysis)

	Males[a, b]	
	beta	*P*
1. School acievement	0.07	0.01
2. Occupational status of father	0.07	0.01
3. Relationship with parents	0.06	0.01
4. Single child versus others	0.05	0.05
5. Denomination	0.04	0.05
6. Number of inhabitants of place of residence	0.04	0.10
7. Educational style of father	0.04	NS
8. Habitation during childhood and adolescence	0.02	0.10
9. Educational style of mother	0.02	NS
10. Marital status of parents	0.01	NS
	Females[c, d]	
	beta	*P*
1. Relations with parents	0.10	0.05
2. School achievement	0.09	0.05
3. Occupational status of father	0.09	0.05
4. Single child versus others	0.08	0.05
5. Educational style of father	0.07	NS
6. Denomination	0.07	NS
7. Number of inhabitants of place of residence	0.06	NS
8. Habitation during childhood and adolescence	0.04	NS
9. Educational style of mother	0.04	NS
10. Marital status of parents	0.02	NS

[a] Multiple R^2 0.02
[b] *P* 0.01
[c] Multiple R^2 0.02
[d] *P* 0.01

Table 74. Neuroticism: social factors and single child status (multivariate classification analysis)

	Males[a, b]	
	beta	P
1. Relations with parents	0.17	0.01
2. Educational style of mother	0.10	0.01
3. Educational style of father	0.08	0.01
4. School achievement	0.05	0.01
5. Habitation during childhood and adolescence	0.04	0.01
6. Single child versus others	0.02	0.10
7. Marital status of parents	0.02	NS
8. Denomication	0.02	NS
9. Occupational status of father	0.02	NS
10. Number of inhabitants of place of residence	0.01	NS
	Females[c, d]	
	beta	P
1. Relations with parents	0.15	0.01
2. Educational style of father	0.10	0.05
3. Educational style of mother	0.09	0.05
4. Number of inhabitants of place of residence	0.08	NS
5. School achievement	0.07	NS
6. Habitation during childhood and adolescence	0.07	0.05
7. Denomination	0.05	NS
8. Occupational status of father	0.04	NS
9. Single child versus others	0.03	NS
10. Marital status of parents	0.02	NS

[a] Multiple R^2 0.07
[b] $P \leqq 0.01$
[c] Multiple R^2 0.05
[d] $P \leqq 0.01$

tribution to a higher extraversion score is given by higher school achievement, higher occupational status of father, and a more positive evaluation of the relationship with parents.

Among both groups, males and females, single children are more extraverted than subjects with sibs. The adjusted mean for males is 13.93 for single children and 13.19 for other children; the corresponding figures for females are 12.94 and 11.59.

Birth order (first and last child in sibships of two, first, middle, and last children in sibships of three and more) and sibship size were not associated with extraversion.

Neuroticism. The same procedure was used to analyze the correlation of social factors, birth order, and sibship size with neuroticism. Table 74 gives, as an example, some of the results. The ten independent variables listed in Table 74 contribute only 6.6% of the variance ($P < 0.01$), which is disappointingly low. At the top the subjects' evaluation of their relationship with and the educational style of parents are listed with the highest beta. Subjects with higher neuroticism scores describe their parents as more rejecting. The association with school achievement is curvilinear, showing a high neuroticism score among those with high and those with very low school achievement. As expected, subjects who did not live with their parents in childhood and adolescence have a higher neuroticism score.

Introducing birth order and sibship size as one of the independent variables did not lead to any significant results. The figures in Table 74 show an insignificant trend ($P<0.10$) for single children to have a lower neuroticism score than subjects with sibs. Birth order in sibships of two or three and more is not related to neuroticism. Eldest and youngest children do not differ from each other or from middleborns. Neuroticism is also not influenced by sibship size.

10.4.7 Discussion

The results of the *bivariate analysis* of personality variables by sibship size and birth order do not point to a strong influence of the latter. In contrast to expectations, single children of both sexes differ from children with sibs by higher scores on sociability and extraversion. Youngest children in large sibships score slightly lower on masculinity. There is no evidence that single children or firstborns or youngest children are more neurotic than subjects in other positions. None of the stated hypotheses (see p. 258) are confirmed: There is no firstborn and no single child personality. It is of particular interest that no differences pointing to higher conformity or affiliation in firstborn males were found (e.g., lower aggressiveness, lower dominance, lower masculinity, higher sociability) (see p. 113 ff.).

Also the influence of sibship size is slight. Children in large sibships score lower on extraversion and appear more inhibited. Large sibships do not seem to produce more extraverted or sociable personalities.

In the *multivariate analyses* there still appears a slightly higher score of single children on extraversion. Otherwise, *birth order and sibship size have no impact on personality* when the structural variables of sociocultural environment and the individual variables of personal history are controlled.

In opposition to these negative or very tenuous results, extraversion was found to be mainly dependent on structural, and neuroticism mainly on idividual factors. Though the explained variance is low, these associations make sense. They indicate that our negative findings for the dependence of personality on birth order and sibship size are probably not due to deficiencies in the measuring instrument.

10.5 Birth Order and the Consumption of Cigarettes, Alcohol, and Drugs

As discussed in the previous review of literature, youngest children are considered at highest risk of both consumption and addiction (see p. 207 ff.). On the following pages, the hypothesis will be tested that youngest children are more often consumers of tobacco, alcohol, and drugs than subjects in other birth positions.

10.5.1 Assessment of Consumption

We questioned our subjects on presence and quantity of their consumption of cigarettes, analgesics, hypnotics, minor tranquilizers, and hypnotics in combination with tranquilizers. As mentioned in Sect. 10.2.1, no differences in consumption rates were found between subjects remaining anonymous and others. Accordingly, the answers can be considered reliable.

For reasons of simplicity, in the present analysis quantitative aspects of consumption are neglected and the percentage of subjects is used who reported current smoking of cigarettes or having ever used cannabis or licit drugs. The amount of alcohol consumption is measured by the percentage of subjects who reported having ever experienced drunkennes. In an earlier investigation, this fact was significantly correlated with daily alcohol consumption in grams (Sieber et al. 1977).

Table 75 shows the frequency of consumption found by this dichotomizing method among males and females. More males consume cigarettes, alcohol, and cannabis, more females analgesics (mostly in connection with painful menstruation), hypnotics, minor tranquilizers, and both.

10.5.2 Birth Order and Consumption: Bivariate Analysis

Table 76 reports the results for males and females. As the female sample is smaller and the consumer's percentages lower than for males, the frequency of significant results in females will be reduced.

Among both sexes, in sibships of two the youngest child more frequently consumes cannabis and tobacco. In larger sibships the same is true for alcohol and analgesics among males, while cannabis consumption is equally frequent among first-

Table 75. Percentage of consumers

	Males	Females
Cannabis	23,3	13,5
Alcohol	40,8	21,1
Cigarettes	52,8	41,1
Analgesics	29,8	70,2
Hypnotics	7,2	17,5
Minor tranquilizers	4,0	7,2
Hypnotics and minor tranquilizers	9,8	20,8

Table 76. Birth order and percentage of consumers

	Single %	Older of two %	Younger of two %	Oldest of three or more %	Middle of three or more %	Youngest of three or more %	*P*	Contingency coefficient
Males								
Cannabis	25.3	26.5	27.8	22.6	19.0	22.9	0.0001	0.07
Alcohol	40.5	37.8	39.1	40.1	40.0	47.0	0.001	0.06
Tobacco	53.2	49.6	55.5	49.5	52.4	56.4	0.0001	0.08
Analgesics	30.2	28.6	32.7	29.3	27.0	33.2	0.01	0.05
Tranquilizers, hypnotics	13.6	9.9	10.9	8.1	8.6	10.6	0.01	0.05
Females								
Cannabis	18.2	11.7	16.0	11.9	13.1	13.6	NS	
Alcohol	26.4	16.9	25.5	17.4	21.4	23.2	NS	
Tobacco	35.5	34.6	45.2	38.7	42.5	46.4	NS	
Analgesics	70.5	74.1	72.4	68.0	67.4	71.4	NS	
Tranquilizers, hypnotics	24.7	24.9	24.6	16.9	18.2	20.5	NS	

and lastborn males and higher than among middleborns. Among females, youngest children have the highest rate of consumers for all substances, but the differences are not significant.

Single male children consume significantly more tranquilizers and hypnotics than subjects of other birth positions. They are not, however, more often consumers of tobacco, alcohol analgesics, or cannabis than oldest children in large and small sibships. Single female children consume more cannabis and alcohol than subjects of other birth ranks. The differences are not significant.

10.5.3 Sibship Size and Consumption: Bivariate Analysis

The results are presented on Table 77. There is no coherent correlation between sibship size and consumers' rate. Cigarette consumption is independent of sibship size. Alcohol consumption tends to increase with sibship size among males. For cannabis and the consumption of licit drugs there is a consistent tendency in males for higher consumption in small sibships.

10.5.4 Other Social Factors and Consumption

On the basis of the bivariate analysis the hypothesis that *youngest children* are most often consumers of tobacco, alcohol, cannabis, and licit drugs is *confirmed.* In the previous survey of literature, however, similar results have been questioned with the argument that interfering social variables were not taken into account (see pp. 208, 209). One of them is *social class*, the importance of which for birth order research has been extensively discussed (see p. 10 f.) in relation to class-specific changes in postwar fertility. The other variable is childhood in a *broken home*, the

Table 77. Sibship size (one to six or more) and percentage of consumers

	One (%)	Two (%)	Three (%)	Four (%)	Five (%)	Six or more (%)	*P*	Contingency coefficient
Males								
Cigarettes	53.4	52.6	52.4	52.1	51.5	56.6		
Alcohol	40.4	38.5	42.1	38.4	45.3	44.6	0.008	0.05
Cannabis	25.7	27.3	23.2	19.8	19.2	19.1	0.001	0.08
Tranquilizers, hypnotics	13.6	10.3	10.4	7.7	8.3	7.7	0.002	0.06
Analgesics	30.1	30.6	31.7	29.1	26.3	25.8	0.05	0.04
Females								
Cigarettes	35.5	39.7	40.3	45.9	45.5	38.0	NS	
Alcohol	26.4	20.9	20.2	20.6	20.9	20.7	NS	
Cannabis	18.2	13.6	11.5	13.6	16.4	10.9	NS	
Tranquilizers, hypnotics	24.7	24.6	19.2	18.2	19.2	14.3	NS	
Analgesics	70.5	73.6	66.3	72.9	71.3	61.5	NS	

impact of which on research on the single child is also discussed (see p. 25f.). The hypotheses that subjects of different birth order differ in social class and in the rate of broken homes are tested on our representative material.

10.5.4.1 Birth Order and Occupational Status of Father

By occupation of father our subjects were divided into three classes. Among males of large sibships (three or more children) there was a *highly significant difference in social class between first- and lastborns* in that the latter came more frequently from lower-class families ($P \leqq 0.0001$). No such difference was found among subjects from small sibships and among females (who are, as we have repeatedly pointed out, biased for higher school achievement). The difference in social class between first- and lastborn males in large sibships was found in an area without large cities or extreme class differences, and with a high percentage of immigrants in lower-class occupations whose children are not liable for military duty. It is not improbable that, in a more heterogeneous social context (e.g., USA or England), a difference in social class by birth order may be even more prominent.

10.5.4.2 Birth Order and Broken Homes

Single and youngest children have more frequently grown up in broken homes than subjects in other birth positions. This is shown in Table 78, which gives the current marital status of parents. The rate of subjects whose home is broken by divorce is highest among single children, while the death rate of parents is highest among single children and youngest children in large sibships (thus confirming that the latter's parents are not only on average of lower class but also older than parents of subjects in orther birth ranks). Among males, only 71% of single children have grown up in unbroken families, and only four-fifths of the youngest with more than one sib. While not always reaching significance the same trend is found in the female sample.

The fact that single and youngest children have grown up more frequently in broken homes may be related to their higher consumption of tobacco, alcohol, and drugs. This hypothesis can be tested by breaking down the sample by marital status of the parents (Table 79).

When single, youngest, and other children from unbroken and broken homes are compared it is evident that among males the latter's percentage of consumers is higher for all substances apart from alcohol. In females there is no such consistent trend. Differences in consumption by birth order for subjects in unbroken homes are substantially reduced; a slight difference in favor of a higher consumption in the youngest child, however, remains.

In Table 80 the analysis takes into account the type of broken home. Epidemiological studies have shown that parental divorce has more impact on childrens' mental health than death of a parent (Rutter et al. 1976, p. 204). Subjects from intact families are compared with those from families broken by divorce or separation and with those who have lost one or both parents by death. We put forward the hypothesis that more psychological stress in reaction to a home broken by par-

Table 78. Birth order and marital status of parents

	Married		Separated/-divorced		Dead (one or both parents)	
	N	Percent	*N*	Percent	*N*	Percent
Males[a]						
Single	414	71.0	102	17.5	67	11.5
Older of two	800	86.3	79	8.5	48	5.2
Younger of two	692	83.5	76	9.2	61	7.4
Oldest of three or more	1,000	87.7	95	8.3	45	3.9
Middle of three or more	1,491	87.0	121	7.1	102	6.0
Youngest of three or more	804	80.7	79	7.9	113	11.3
Females[b]						
Single	86	78.2	17	15.5	7	6.4
Older of two	206	89.2	10	4.3	15	6.5
Younger of two	151	80.3	19	10.1	18	9.6
Oldest of three or more	221	87.4	24	9.5	8	3.2
Middle of three or more	321	89.2	22	6.1	17	4.7
Youngest of three or more	184	83.6	10	4.5	26	11.8

[a] *P* 0.001 [b] *P* 0.001

Table 79. Broken homes and percentage of consumers

	Single children: Parents			Youngest children: Parents			Other children: Parents		
Males	Mar-ried	Divorced, separated, dead		Mar-ried	Divorced, separated, dead		Mar-ried	Divorced, separated, dead	
N	414	170	*P*	1,496	329	*P*	3,308	499	*P*
	%	%		%	%		%	%	
Cigarettes	50.0	60.6	0.02	53.5	67.5	0.00	49.0	63.7	0.00
Alcohol	37.9	47.6	0.04	42.8	47.1	NS	39.1	42.1	NS
Cannabis	22.5	32.4	0.02	23.7	31.6	0.00	21.0	28.1	0.00
Tranquilizers, hypnotics	11.2	19.3	0.01	10.0	14.7	0.02	8.3	11.8	0.02
Analgesics	29.0	33.1	NS	32.0	37.6	NS	27.6	31.9	NS
Females									
N	86	24	*P*	335	73	*P*	751	98	*P*
	%	%		%	%		%	%	
Cigarettes	32.6	45.8	NS	45.7	46.6	NS	37.7	51.0	0.02
Alcohol	25.6	29.2	NS	25.1	20.5	NS	16.5	38.8	0.00
Cannabis	18.6	16.7	NS	14.9	13.7	NS	11.1	21.4	0.00
Tranquilizers, hypnotics	25.3	22.7	NS	20.7	29.4	NS	18.8	25.8	NS
Analgesics	72.8	62.5	NS	73.3	65.3	NS	68.7	74.5	NS

Table 80. Type of broken home and percentage of consumers

	Single children: Parents				Youngest children: Parents				Other children: Parents			
Males	Married	Divorced	Dead	*P*	Married	Divorced	Dead	*P*	Married	Divorced	Dead	*P*
N	414	103	67		1,496	155	174		3,308	301	198	
	%	%	%		%	%	%		%	%	%	
Cigarettes	50.0	61.2	59.7	NS	53.5	70.3	64.9	0.00	49.0	68.8	56.1	0.00
Alcohol	37.9	45.6	50.7	NS	42.8	47.1	47.1	NS	39.1	42.9	40.9	NS
Cannabis	22.5	35.0	28.4	0.02	23.7	38.7	25.3	0.00	21.0	32.9	20.7	0.00
Tranquilizers, hypnotics	11.2	15.8	24.6	0.01	10.8	18.7	11.0	0.00	8.3	13.5	9.2	0.00
Analgesics	29.0	29.7	38.5	NS	32.0	38.7	36.6	NS	27.6	32.8	30.6	NS
Females												
N	86	17	7		335	29	44		751	57	41	
	%	%	%		%	%	%		%	%	%	
Cigarettes	32.6	52.9	28.6	NS	45.7	51.7	43.2	NS	37.7	54.4	48.8	0.03
Alcohol	25.6	29.4	28.6	NS	25.1	34.5	11.4	NS	16.5	45.6	29.3	0.00
Cannabis	18.6	17.6	14.3	NS	14.9	13.8	13.6	NS	11.1	24.6	17.1	0.01
Tranquilizers, hypnotics	25.3	33.3		NS	20.7	26.9	31.0	NS	18.8	26.4	25.0	NS
Analgesics	72.8	52.9	85.7	NS	73.3	64.3	65.9	NS	68.7	75.4	73.2	NS

ental discord will express itself through higher consumption. The hypothesis is not confirmed for single children. There, among males the pattern is inconsistent. The hypothesis is supported, on the other hand, for youngest and other children; for the latter even among females. Subjects whose parents are separated or divorced are more frequently consumers than orphans or subjects from unbroken homes. Again consumption of alcohol among males is the exception. Why single children do not demonstrate an influence of the type of broken home cannot be explained by our data. There is no information on the age of the subject as the time his parent died. As the mean number of children increases with the duration of marriage, it is possible that single children have been orphaned at a younger age than children with sibs.

Still, youngest male children, whether from homes broken by divorce or separation or not, have the highest consumption of all subgroups. Among females this is true for "other children" from divorced marriages. As an analysis of variance showed that only an extremely small part of the variance in consumption is explained by birth order with control of marital status of parents, these results are not reported here.

10.5.4.3 Birth Order and Reported Educational Style of and Relations with Parents

The Battegay et al. (1977) findings (see pp. 206, 209) that, in their representative sample of Swiss conscripts, youngest and single children were overrepresented among those reporting high consumption of alcohol and drugs (in comparison with oldest and middle children) are explained by the authors with differential socialization, i.e., spoiling and subsequent frustration of the single and youngest child. On the other hand, some evidence for more acceptance of parental authority and more orientation toward parents among oldest children has been presented (see p. 93ff). In order to test the hypotheses of a differential attitude toward parents in single, youngest, and oldest children, reported educational style of and relations to parents (see Appendix) were related to birth order and sibship size in our sample (tables are not presented).

There is no consistent evidence that relations to or perceived treatment by parents deteriorate with increasing sibship size. There is also no consistent evidence that educational style is differentially evaluated by *birth order*. One finding, however, is consistent among males and females: A higher percentage of oldest sons and daughters discuss their problems with their parents than younger children. In males this is true only for subjects with one sib. The differences are small, although highly significant in the male sample. Single children do not consistently deviate in their evaluations of educational style or relations from children with sibs. Thus there is no evidence of a special position of the only and the youngest child, but *slight evidence of higher parent-relatedness in oldest children*.

The first two analyses demonstrated that only and youngest children have a different background from middle and oldest sibs and that conclusions drawn on the basis of birth order alone are not sufficiently founded. The third analysis demonstrates a very slight difference in attitudes toward parents, differentiating firstborns from subjects in other birth ranks.

10.5.4.4 Other Social Factors

On Table 81, 11 social variables that may influence consumption are presented as contingency coefficients. No consistent correlation with consumption was found for number of inhabitants in place of residence, occupation of father, habitation during childhood, and sibship size. The influence of school achievement, marital status of parents, and habitation during adolescence appears weak. The relative impact of social variables will be discussed separately for the various substances.

10.5.5 Social Factors, Personality, Birth Order, and Consumption: Multiple Classification Analysis

Because of the small number and a skewed distribution of female users, alcohol and cannabis consumption have been analyzed for males only. For similar reasons analgesic consumption could be analyzed only for the female sample. Besides the social variables mentioned in Table 63 two personality factors (extraversion and neuroticism) and either various aspects of birth order or sibship size were introduced as independent variables.

Cigarette Consumption

In Table 82, 12 predictors explain only 9% of the variance for males ($p \leqq 0.01$). Among the individual variables extraversion is the most prominent by far. It correlates positively with smoking. So does neuroticism, but to a much lower degree. An estranged relationship with parents, not having lived with parents during childhood and adolescence, and an educational style described as either overprotective or rejecting are similarly related to higher cigarette consumption, but explain only small amounts of the variance.

Among structural variables school achievement is most important. High achievers smoke less, but, unexpectedly, subjects with higher status homes smokes more. So do subjects whose home is broken by divorce, those without religious denomination, and those living in a relatively large town. The contribution of all these predictors is small.

Among females (Table 83) 12 predictors explain 12% of the variance ($P \leqq 0.01$). Only five contributions are significant. The replicate the findings for males with the difference that father's occupational status is curvilinearly related to smoking: Girls from high- and low-status homes smoke more than those from intermediate-status homes.

Birth order is significantly related to smokers' rates among both sexes, even when all the individual and structural factors mentioned above are controlled. It's impact on female smoking is relatively large. Youngest children of both sexes have

Table 81. Social factors and consumption: bivariate analysis (Contingency Coefficients, cc)

	Tobacco		Alcohol		Cannabis		Analgesics		Tranquilizers, hypnotics	
	Males cc	Females cc	Males cc	Females cc	Males cc	Females cc	Males cc	Females cc	Males cc	Females cc
Number of inhabitants in place of residence	0.05[a]	0.05	0.09[a]	0.14	0.15[a]	0.12	0.06[a]	0.09	0.07[a]	0.11
Denomination	0.07[b]	0.09[b]	0.10[a]	0.11[a]	0.25[b]	0.30[b]	0.12[a]	0.06	0.05[a]	0.10
School achievement	0.10[b]	0.12[b]	0.11[a]	0.10	0.14[a]	0.11	0.07[a]	0.09	0.08[a]	0.09
Marital status of parents	0.10[b]	0.07[b]	0.05[b]	0.12[b]	0.09[a]	0.08	0.04[b]	0.10[b]	0.06[b]	0.09[b]
Profession of father	0.01[a]	0.07	0.09[a]	0.12	0.12[a]	0.13	0.05[a]	0.07	0.08[a]	0.11
Habitation during childhood	0.09[a]	0.06	0.04[a]	0.09	0.10[a]	0.05	0.04[a]	0.04	0.04[a]	0.07
Habitation during adolescence	0.10[b]	0.06[b]	0.06[b]	0.10[b]	0.11[a]	0.06	0.04[a]	0.06	0.06[a]	0.03
Educational style of father	0.09[b]	0.11[b]	0.13[b]	0.18[b]	0.14[b]	0.21[b]	0.07[a]	0.12	0.07[a]	0.10
Educational style of mother	0.09[b]	0.09[b]	0.09[b]	0.14[b]	0.14[b]	0.17[b]	0.07[b]	0.14[b]	0.06[a]	0.10
Relationship with parents	0.12[b]	0.09[b]	0.14[b]	0.14[b]	0.21[b]	0.15[b]	0.08[a]	0.06	0.08[a]	0.09
Sibship size	0.02[a]	0.06[a]	–	0.06	0.08[a]	0.09	–	0.07	–	0.13[a]

[a] $P \leqq 0.05$
[b] In agreement for both sexes

Table 82. Social factors, personality, and cigarette consumption in males: multivariate classification analysis

Social factors	beta	P
Extraversion	0.19	0.01
School achievement	0.12	0.01
Relations with parents	0.09	0.01
Neuroticism	0.08	0.01
Marital status of parents	0.05	0.01
Denomination	0.05	0.01
Birth order	0.05	0.05
Occupational status of father	0.05	0.01
Habitation during childhood and adolescence	0.04	0.01
Educational style of mother	0.04	0.05
Number of inhabitants in place of residence	0.04	0.05
Educational style of father	0.04	NS

Multiple R^2 0.09, $P \leqq 0.01$

Table 83. Social factors, personality, and cigarette consumption in females: multivariate classification analysis

Social factors	beta	P
Extraversion	0.20	0.01
School achievement	0.12	0.01
Birth order	0.11	0.05
Occupational status of father	0.09	0.05
Neuroticism	0.08	0.05
Relations with parents	0.08	NS
Educational style of mother	0.08	NS
Denomination	0.08	NS
Educational style of father	0.07	NS
Marital status of parents	0.06	NS
Number of inhabitants in place of residence	0.05	NS
Habitation during childhood and adolescence	0.04	NS

Multiple R^2 0.12, $P \leqq 0.01$

the highest percentage of smokers. The following list gives the amount of differences by birth order:

		Sibship size two		Sibship size three or more		
	Only child	Oldest	Youngest	Oldest	Middle	Youngest
Males	50%	48%	56%	50%	51%	55%
Females	33%	35%	41%	38%	44%	50%
	$P < 0.05$					

Single children do not smoke more than subjects with sibs.
Sibship size one to six is not correlated to smoking.

Table 84. Social factors, personality, and alcohol consumption in males: multivariate classification analysis

Social factors	beta	*P*
Extraversion	0.14	0.01
Neuroticism	0.12	0.01
Relations with parents	0.07	0.01
Denomination	0.07	0.01
Number of inhabitants in place of residence	0.07	0.01
Occupational status of father	0.06	0.01
Birth order	0.06	0.01
Educational style of father	0.05	0.05
School achievement	0.05	0.01
Habitation during childhood and adolescence	0.05	0.01
Educational style of mother	0.03	NS
Marital status of parents	0.02	NS

Multiple R^2 0.06, $P \leq 0.01$

Alcohol Consumption among Males

In Table 84, the 12 predictors explain only 6% of the variance. The individual variables of extraversion and neuroticism are both positively correlated to the experience of drunkenness, as are reporting a rejecting educational style of the father and not having lived with parents during childhood and adolescence. Subjects who report discussing their problems with the father, on the other hand, unexpectedly report drunkenness at a higher rate.

Among the structural variables, men who state a religious denomination drink more, as do those with intermediate, but not high or low, school achievement, those living in smaller towns and villages, and those from low-status homes. Surprisingly, a home broken by divorce is not related to more consumption.

These are hints that among men, two patterns of drinking might be distinguished: social drinking, related to extraversion, social inconspicuousness, and good relations with the father; and neurotic drinking, related to neuroticism and reported rejection by the father.

Birth order is related to alcohol consumption. Youngest children in sibships of three or more, but not in sibships of two, have the highest rate with regard to ever having experienced drunkenness.

	Sibship size two		Sibship size three or more		
Only child	Oldest	Youngest	Oldest	Middle	Youngest
38%	40%	40%	40%	39%	47%
$P<0.01$					

Single children do not drink more than subjects with sibs.
Sibship size one to six is not correlated to drinking habits.

Table 85. Social factors, personality, and cannabis consumption in males: multivariate classification analysis

Social factors	beta	*P*
Denomination	0.15	0.01
Relations with parents	0.14	0.01
Neuroticism	0.13	0.01
Extraversion	0.10	0.01
Number of inhabitants in place of residence	0.09	0.01
Educational style of father	0.07	0.01
Occupational status of father	0.07	0.01
School achievement	0.06	0.01
Habitation during childhood and adolescence	0.06	0.01
Birth order	0.05	0.05
Educational style of mother	0.04	NS
Marital status of parents	0.01	NS

Multiple R^2 0.13, $P \leqq 0.01$

Cannabis Consumption Among Males

In Table 85, 12 predictors explain 13% of the variance. The individual variables with a high impact on cannabis use are not discussing problems with parents, neuroticism, and extraversion. A rejecting educational style of the father and not having lived with parents follow. Among the structural variables, cannabis use is most strongly correlated to not stating a denomination, to living in a relatively large town, to low school achievement, and to a low-status home.

Birth order is significantly correlated to cannabis use when all the variables mentioned above are controlled, since middle and single children are underrepresented among users. Differences are, however, small.

	Sibship size two		Sibship size three or more		
Only child	Oldest	Youngest	Oldest	Middle	Youngest
20%	25%	25%	22%	21%	24%
$P < 0.05$					

Single children do not consume cannabis at a higher rate than subjects with sibs.

Sibship size one to six is not correlated to cannabis use.

Analgesic Consumption Among Females

In Table 86, 3% of the variance is explained by 12 predictors. Neuroticism and not discussing problems with parents are associated with higher consumption. Birth order and sibship size have no demonstrable influence.

Table 86. Social factors, personality, and consumption of analgesics in females: multivariate classification analysis

Social factors	beta [a]	P [b]
Neuroticism	0.19	0.01
Relations with parents	0.11	0.01
Educational style of mother	0.09	NS
Educational style of father	0.07	NS
School achievement	0.07	NS
Birth order	0.05	NS
Extraversion	0.05	NS
Occupational status of father	0.05	NS
Marital status of parents	0.04	NS
Habitation during childhood and adolescence	0.02	NS
Number of inhabitants in place of residence	0.02	NS
Denomination	0.02	NS

[a] Multiple R^2 0.03, [b] 0.01

10.5.6 Discussion

The finding of higher rates of cigarette consumers in the male and female youngest child of small and large families and of higher alcohol consumption in the youngest male child of a large sibship correspond to results already reported (see p. 208 and 209): There, the objection was made that age, social class, sibship size, and presence of a broken home were not controlled, though all these variables may influence consumption. Our results show that even when a large number of "structural" and "individual" variables are controlled, being a youngest child still has an independent relation to consumption of cigarettes and alcohol. Among males the influence of birth order is very small (beta 0.05–0.06). Among females it is somewhat larger (beta 0.11) for cigarette consumption but nil for analgesics. It has, however, to be remembered that all variables explain merely 5%–12% of the variance in alcohol and cigarette consumption. If, for consumption of various substances, the individual variables having the strongest impact are listed, the following sequence is found:

Cigarettes	Alcohol	Cannabis	Analgesics
(Males, females)	(Males)	(Males)	(Females)
Extraversion	Extraversion	Extraversion	
	Neuroticism	Neuroticism	Neuroticism
		Relations with parents	Relations with parents

The main finding for consumption is the consistent and positive association with *extraversion and neuroticism*, which has since been confirmed by Sieber (1979) in a longitudinal study of the present sample. Only in cigarette consumption is neuroticism of secondary importance.

Social inacceptability of a substance is connected with an increasing impact of personal lability and increasing distance from parents. (Analgesic consumption is the exception, since it is associated with both without being inacceptable: As it takes place in another context, i.e., mainly to allay pain, and is not influenced by birth order, it will not be further discussed.) This relationship makes sense and is an argument for the validity of the measuring instruments used in assessing personality and consumption.

The impact of being the youngest child decreases with increasing social acceptability of the substance and increasing influence of problems of personality and familial relations. This makes the assumption that higher consumption in the youngest child could be the consequence of personality traits due to differential socialization rather improbable – the more so as no evidence for a "youngest child personality" or for youngest children reporting a special relationship with or a special educational style of parents was found.

The slight overrepresentation of youngest children among cigarette and alcohol consumers *cannot presently be explained.* A tentative hypothesis may be that youngest children have a slightly higher percentage of smokers and drinkers, because (there being less social distance between sibs than between children and parents) they *start imitating their older sibs, who smoke and drink already, at an earlier age than the latter start imitating their parents.* It is, however, inexplicable why, in the case of alcohol, this should be true only among youngest sibs in large but not in small sibships.

Single children are again in a favorable position: They have a lower rate of cannabis consumers than oldest and youngest subjects and do not deviate in consumption of other substances from subjects with sibs. This fits well with the evidence for their slightly higher school achievement and the missing evidence for a less favorable personality (see pp. 256, 266).

10.6 Summary and Conclusions

10.6.1 Survey of Results

The influence of birth order and sibship size was examined with a representative sample of 6,315 19-year-old Swiss males and a slightly less representative sample of 1,381 20-year-old Swiss females, using bivariate and multiple classification analyses.

The findings of *the bivariate analyses* are generally in agreement with the bulk of the less sophisticated literature summarized in Part I:

1. School achievement of eldest sibs from large sibships was higher than that of subjects in other birth positions, and sibship size had a slight negative influence on achievement.

2. A personality inventory did not elicit large and consistent differences for birth order or sibship size, though youngest children from large sibships of either sex were slightly lower on masculinity and subjects from large sibships were more inhibited.

3. Single and youngest children had the highest rates of consumers of the substances studied.

The multivariate classification analyses, on the other hand, introduced several structural and individual variables, such as income and occupational status of father, denomination, number of inhabitants in place of residence, present marital status of parents, habitation during childhood and adolescence, and relations with and educational style of parents. The following results were obtained:

1. While a strong correlation of school achievement with occupational status of father was found, achievement differences by birth order became insignificant with the exception of a slightly higher achievement of the male single child. Sibship size, however, retained a slight negative influence on achievement (beta 0.05).

2. Very small amounts of the variance in extraversion and neuroticism were explained. Birth order and sibship size did not contribute to the variance with the exception of single children being slightly more extraverted.

3. Consumption appeared mainly correlated to extraversion and neuroticism. Youngest children of either sex and in large and small sibships have a slightly higher rate of smokers (beta 0.05 for males, 0.11 for females). Youngest male sibs in large sibships drink very slightly more (beta 0.06). Middle male children in large sibships use cannabis slightly less often (beta 0.05). Single children are not consumers at higher rates than subjects with sibs.

Chapter 11 Relationship of the Results to the Survey of World Literature

The hypothesis was presented (see p. 53f.) that sibship size might be an indicator of background factors inhibiting school achievement rather than an inhibitor in its own right. The present investigation refutes this hypothesis. *Sibship size has a very slight independent negative influence on school achievement.*

The hypothesis was accepted (see p. 69) that firstborns achieve slightly more at school. In this large and representative sample, birth order differences in achievement did not reach significance when background variables were controlled.

It was upheld (see p. 82f.) that large sibships may be correlated to a very slightly more unfavorable socialization. On the basis of the present investigation this cannot be confirmed. *But sibs do not have a positive influence on personality.* The hypothesis of a negative impact of social class on personality was not upheld (see p. 75): Extraversion alone was very tenuously related to higher social class.

The evidence was accepted (see p. 95f.) that *firstborns have closer relations to parents.* This is confirmed by the present survey, but differences are small.

It was contended (see p. 184ff.) that birth order differences in personality, if present at all in sufficiently controlled investigations, would be small. They are nonexistent in our sample. In particular there is no evidence for a "firstborn personality."

In the preceding survey findings of a higher rate of youngest children among consumers of tobacco and alcohol were dismissed, together with results concerning the birth order – mental illness correlation (see p. 237f.), because of methodological insufficiencies. In opposition to this, with sufficient control of background variables *a very slight overrepresentation of youngest male and female sibs in large and small sibships was found among smokers, and of youngest male sibs in large sibships among those having experienced drunkeness.* It is argued that the difference is probably not due to differential socialization and personality, but to imitation of the older sibs, who are the pacemakers, at a relatively early age.

The previously expressed opinion (see p. 25f.) that the poor reputation of single children's personality is due to the frequency of broken homes among them is fully confirmed. When background variables are controlled *single children are slightly more extraverted and slightly higher achievers than children with sibs.*

Several other hypotheses put forward in the course of the survey were confirmed: *Demonination* is related to school achievement, as are *number of inhabitants* of place of residence and a *broken home.* The influence of these background variables is small in this socially rather homogeneous part of Switzerland, without cities, slums, or backward rural regions. It may be much more noticeable in a less homogeneous context.

Our representative sample demonstrates, furthermore, that there are highly significant *social class differences by birth order* and that *broken homes* and their causes are differentially distributed by birth order.

The survey of the literature produced the result that birth order differences in personality *tend to disappear with increasing control of social background variables*. This is clearly demmonstrated when the results of the bivariate and the multivariate analysis are compared (see p. 282).

The fact that our subjects are on the *threshold of adulthood* confirms our previously expressed opinion (see p. 184ff.) that birth order differences in personality, if at all present among children, are not usually durable character traits and will not be found among adults.

There are, on the other hand, *internal consistencies* in our findings that point to the reliability and validity of the measuring instruments:

- School achievement depends more on structural variables among females, more on individual variables among males.
- Extraversion depends more on structural variables, neuroticism more on individual variables.
- With increasing social inacceptability of consumption, the variance explained by neuroticism and relations with parents increases as well.

Our final conclusion is substantially the same as that of the survey of literature: *Birth order and sibship size do not have a strong impact on personality*. The present investigation points instead *to a broken home, an unfriendly educational style, and a premature disruption of relations with parents* as concomitants of neuroticism, and to *higher income and social class* (with all assets implied) and an *undisturbed home* as concomitants of higher achievement. Beside these influences, details of socialization seem to shrink to insignificance.

An environmental variable that is considered highly relevant is thus disaffirmed as a predictor for personality and behavior. This may signify that most of our opinions in the field of dynamic psychology will have to be revised.

Appendix

Definition of social variables

Structural variables

Number of inhabitants in place of residence

< 1,000 inhabitants
1,000–10,000 inhabitants
10,000–50,000 inhabitants
50,000–100,000 inhabitants
> 100,000 inhabitants

Religious denomination

Protestant
Roman-Catholic
Other
None

Present marital status of parents

Married
Separated or divorced
One or both parents dead

Father's income (monthly)

< 2,000 SFr.
2,000–3,000 SFr.
> 3,000 SFr.

Father's occupational status

High
Middle
Lower
Low

Individual variables

Habitation during childhood and adolescence (1–6 years; 7–15 years)

With parents
Elsewhere

Educational style of father and mother (during the last 3 years)

Authoritarian
Overprotective
Friendly
Rejecting
Other

Present relations with parents:

Discussing present problems with:

Father
Mother
Neither
Both

References

Asterisks indicate surveys, bibliographies, or studies that are important for methodological reasons.

Abraham A, Subramaniam K, Verghese A (1973) Birth order and psychiatric disturbance. Indian J Psychiat 15:11–19

Abramowitz SI, Abramowitz CV (1971) Birth order, sensitivity to socialization, and student activism. J Counseling Psychol 18:184–185

Abramson PR (1973) Familial variables related to the expression of violent aggression in preschool-age children. J Genet Psychol 122:345–346

Achté KA, Ginman L (1966) Suicidal attempts with narcotics and poisons. Acta psychiatr Scand 42:214–232

Adams BN (1969) Birth order and college attendance, a re-evaluation of a re-evaluation. Sociometry 32:503–504

*Adams BN (1972) Birth order: A critical review. Sociometry 35:411–439

Adams BN, Meidam MT (1968) Economics, family structure and college attendance. Am J Sociol 74:230–239

Adams RL (1967) Personality and behavioral differences among children of various birth positions. Diss Abstr Int 28-A: 1697

Adams RL, Philips BN (1972) Motivational and achievement differences among children of various ordinal birth positions. Child Dev 43:155–164

Adler A (1927) Understanding human nature. Greenberg, New York

Adler A (1928) Characteristics of the first, second, and third child. Children 3:14–52

Adler A (1958) What life should mean to you. GP Putnam's Sons, New York

Albaum G (1977) Birth order and creativity. Psychol Rep 40:792–794

Alberts CL, Landers DM (1977) Birth order, motor performance and maternal influence. Res Q Am Ass Health Phys Educ 48:661–670

Alexander CN jr (1966) Ordinal position and sociometric status. Sociometry 29:41–51

Alexander CN jr (1968) Ordinal position and social mobility. Sociometry 31:285–293

Allen CE (1967) Birth order and reaction to threat: A comparison of self-evaluation and anxiety reduction motives. Diss Abstr Int 27-A:3510

Allman TS, White WF (1968) Birth order categories and predictors of select personality characteristics. Psychol Rep 22:857–860

Allmon DE (1974) An inquiry into the interrelationship of birth order, personality, and innovativeness. Diss Abstr Int 35-A:643

Almodowar JP (1973) Existe-t-il un syndrome de l'enfant unique? Enfance 3/4:233–249

Altus WD (1959 a) Adjustment, IQ, family size, and illiteracy. Psychol Rep 5:494

Altus WD (1959 b) Birth order, intelligence, and adjustment. Psychol Rep 5:502

Altus WD (1963 a) The first-born as a conservative. Adler revisited. Am Psychol 18:356

Altus WD (1963) Some birth-order parameters related to verbal and quantitative aptitude for 1,120 college students with one sibling. Am Psychol 18:361

Altus WD (1965 a) Birth order and mean score on a ten-item aptitude test. Psychol Rep 16:956

Altus WD (1965 b) Birth order and academic primogeniture. J Pers Soc Psychol 2:872–876

Altus WD (1965 c) Birth order and scholastic aptitude. J Consult Clin Psychol 29:202–205

Altus WD (1966 a) Birth order and its sequelae. Science 151:44–49

Altus WD (1966 b) Birth order and achievement. Science 152:1181–1184

Altus WD (1967) Birth order and choice of college major. Am Psychol 22:484–485

Altus WD (1970 a) Marriage and order of birth. Proc 78th Annu Conv APA 5:361–362

Altus WD (1970 b) Sex-role dissatisfaction, birth order, and parental favoritism. Proc 78th Annu Conv APA, vol 5. American Psychological Association, Washington, DC, pp 161–162

Amir Y, Sharan S, Kovarsky Y (1968) Birth order, family structure, and avoidance behaviour. J Pers Soc Psychol 10:271–278
Anastasi A (1954) Tested intelligence and family size. Methodological and interpretative problems. Eugen Q 1:155–160
Anastasi A (1958) Heredity, environment and the question: how. Psychol Rev 65:197–204
Ando H, Tsuda K (1975) Intrafamilial incidence of autism, cerebral palsy, and mongolism. J Autism Child Schizophr 5:267–274
Andrews FM, Morgan JN, Sonquist JS, Klem L (1975) Multiple classification analysis. A report on a computer program for multiple regression using categorical predictors. 2nd edn. Ann Arbor, Michigan
Andrews R, Brown E (1974) Firstborns, only children, sex, and three dependency measures. Percept Mot Skills 39:773–774
Angelini D (1973) Birth order: Immediate elder siblings as a factor in task performance. J Individ Psychol 29:167–172
Angers WP (1974) Position in the family in relation to teaching as a career choice. J Individ Psychol 11:15–21
Angst J, Baumann U, Müller U, Ruppen R (1973) Epidemiologie des Drogenkonsums im Kanton Zürich. Eine repräsentative Umfrage bei 6315 Zürchern und 1381 Zürcherinnen (Alter 19 Jahre). Arch Psychiat Nervenkr 217:11–24
Angst J, Müller-Oswald U, Ruppen R, Baumann U (1973) Persönlichkeitsaspekte jugendlicher Drogenkonsumenten. Eine repräsentative Umfrage an 6315 neunzehnjährigen Zürchern. Arch Psychiat Nervenkr 217:207–222
Annesley PT (1961) Psychiatric illness in adolescence. Presentation and Prognosis. J Ment Sci 107:268–278
Annett M, Ockwell A (1980) Birth order, birth stress and handedness. Cortex, Milano, 16:181–187
Ansbacher HL, Ansbacher RR (1956) The individual psychology of Alfred Adler. Harper and Row, New York
Antrobus JS, Bloom BL (1965) Sibling rank among Japanese-American male schizophrenics. Transcult Psychiatr Res Rev 2:54–56
Apperly FL (1939) A study of American Rhodes Scholars. J Hered 30:493–495
Arasteh JD (1968) Creativity and related processes in the young child: A review of the literature. J Genet Psychol 112:77–108
Arnold W, Eysenck HJ, Meili R (1972) Lexikon der Psychologie. Herder, Freiburg Basel Wien, pp 398–399
Arrowood AJ, Amoroso DM (1965) Social comparison and ordinal position. J Pers Soc Psychol 2:101–104
Arthur G (1926) The relation of IQ to position in family. J Educ Psychol 17:541–550
Asbury CA (1973) Sociological factors related to discrepant achievement of white and black first graders. J Exp Educat 42:6–10
Baar PM (1977) The effect of certain variables upon affiliation in psychotherapy. Diss Abstr Int 38:(4-B) (1868)
Babladelis G (1972) Birth order and responsiveness to social influence. Psychol Rep 30:99–104
Babson SG, Kangas J, Young N, Bramhall JL (1964) Growth and development of twins of dissimilar size at birth. Pediatrics 33:327–333
Bahr HM (1971) Birth order and failure, the evidence from the skid row. Q J Stud Alcohol 32:669–686
Bahr SJ, Chadwick BA, Strauss JH (1975) The effect of relative economic status on fertility. J Marriage Family 37:335–343
Bajema CJ (1968) Relation of fertility to occupational status, IQ, educational attainment, and size of family of origin. A follow-up study of a male Kalamazoo public school population. Eugen Q 15:198–203
Bakan D (1949) The relationship between alcoholism and birth rank. Q J Stud Alcohol 10:434–440
Bakan P (1971) Birth order and handedness. Nature 229:195
Bakan P (1977) Left handedness and birth order revisited. Neuropsychologia 15:837–839
Bakan P (1978) Handedness and birth order: A critical note on a critical note. Percept Mot Skills 46:556
Bakan P, Dibb G, Reed P (1973) Handedness and birth stress. Neuropsychologia 11:363–366
Baker F, O'Brien GMSL (1969) Birth order and fraternity affiliation. J Soc Psychol 78:41–43
Baker H, Wills U (1978) School phobia, classification and treatment. Br J Psychiatry 132:492–499

Baker S (1963) Relationship of selection of nursing as a vocation to birth order. Nurs Res 12:248–249

Ballante HW (1971) Empathic ability among lower- and middle class adolescents in relation to several social psychological variables. Diss Abstr Int 31-A:4884

Barger B, Hall E (1966) The interrelationships of family size and socioeconomic status for parents of college students. J Marriage Family 28:186–187

Barker DJP, Edwards JH (1967) Obstetric complications and school performance. Brit Med J iii:695–699

* Barker DJP, Record RG (1967 a) Birth Order and the presence of disease: A comment on the Greenwood-Yule method. J Roy Statist Soc (Ser C) 16:13–16

* Barker DJP, Record RG (1967 b) The relationship of the presence of disease to birth order and maternal age. Am J Hum Genet 19:433–449

Barnes J, Fisher J, Palmer M (1979) Family characteristics and intellectual growth: an examination by race. J Educ Psychol Measurment 39:625–636

Barra JA (1973) Selected cultural variables and the reading achievement of black inner-city school children of Washington, D.C., Diss Abstr Int 34-A:1057

Barrett B (1975) Sex, birth order, and family composition as related to the sex role perceptions of male and female college students. Diss Abstr Int 36-B:4125

Barron F (1970) Heritability of factors in creative thinking and esthetic judgment. Acta Genet Med Gemellol, Roma, 19:294–298

Barry H (1945) Incidence of advanced maternal age in mothers of one thousand State Hospital patients. Arch Neurol Psychiatry 54:186–191

Barry H (1967) Birth order: Achievement, schizophrenia and culture. Int J Psychiatry 3:439–444

Barry H, Barry H (1967) Birth order, family size, and schizophrenia. Arch Gen Psychiatry 17:435–440

Barry H, Barry H (1969) Influence of family size on schizophrenic birth order. Nature, London, 223:752

Barry H, Barry H (1970) Birth order of schizophrenics. Brit J Psychiatry 116:123–124

Barry H, Barry H (1971) Birth order of psychiatric patients. Nature, London, 231:57

Barry H, Barry H, Blane HT (1969) Birth order of delinquent boys with alcoholic involvement. Q J Stud Alcohol 30:408–413

Barry H, Blane HT (1972) Birth order as a method of studying environmental influences in alcoholism. Ann NY Acad Sci 197:172–178

Barry H, Blane HT (1977) Birth positions of alcoholics. J Individ Psychol 33:62–69

Bartelt PW (1972) Birth order of siblings and differences in orientation toward parents. Ph. D. dissertation, Ohio State University. Diss Abstr Int-A 33:4556 (1973)

Barthell CN (1971) Affiliation, birth order and extraversion-introversion. Diss Abstr Int 31-B, 4324–4325

Bartlett EW, Smith CP (1966) Childrearing practices, birth order and the development of achievement-related motives. Psychol Rep 19:1207–1216

Bartow JA (1961) Family size as related to child rearing practices. Ph. D. dissertation, Pennsylvanian State University

Bassett JE, Gayton W, Blanchard EB, Ozmon KL (1977) Birth order and perceptual motor performance. Percept Mot Skills 45:1076–1078

Bathaae H, Djalili A, Azardagan F (1977) Birth order and family size in schizophrenia. Acta Med Iran 19:155–166

Battegay R, Mühlemann R, Hell D, Zehnder R, Hoch P, Dillinger A (1977) Alkohol, Tabak und Drogen im Leben des jungen Mannes. Sozialmed Pädagog Jugendkd 14, Karger, Basel

Baughman EE, Dahlstrom WG (1968) Negro and white children. A psychological study in the rural south. Academic Press, New York London

Baxter J (1965) Parental complementarity and parental conflict. J Individ Psychol 21:149–153

* Bayer AE (1966) Birth order and college attendance. J Marriage Family 28:480–484

* Bayer AE (1967 a) Birth order and attainment of the doctorate. A test of economic hypotheses. Am J Social 72:540–550

* Bayer AE (1967 b) Reply to Mr Hermalin. J Marriage Family 29:421–423

* Bayer AE, Folger JE (1967) The current state of birth order research. Int J Psychiat 3:37–39

Bayley N (1965) Comparison of mental and motor test scores for ages 1–15 months by sex, birth order, race, geographical location, and education of parents. Child Dev 36:379–411

Beck S, Lempp R (1965) Die Bedeutung der Stellung in der Geschwisterreihe für Entstehung und Art psychoreaktiver Störungen. Z Psychother Med Psychol 15:145–154

Becker G (1965) Visual acuity, birth order, achievement versus affiliation, and other Edward's Personality Preference Schedule scores. J Psychosom Res 9:277–283

Becker G (1967) Affiliate perception and the arousal of the participations-affiliation motive. Percept Mot Skills 24:991–997

Becker G (1968) Ability to differentiate message from source and birth-order and subject-sex interaction. Psychol Rep 23:658

Becker G (1970) Situational discrimination in repressor-type and sensitizer-type approval seekers and the birth order by subject and sex interaction. J Soc Psychol 82:81–97

Becker SW, Carroll J (1962) Ordinal position and conformity. J Abnorm Soc Psychol 65:129–131

Becker SW, Lerner MJ, Carroll J (1964) Conformity as a function of birth order, payoff, and type of group pressure. J Abnorm Soc Psychol 69:318–323

Becker SW, Lerner MJ, Carroll J (1966) Conformity as a function of birth order and types of group pressure. A verification. J Pers Soc Psychol 3:242–244

Becker WC (1964) Consequences of different types of parental discipline. In: Hoffman ML, Hoffman LW (eds) Review of child development, vol 1. Russell-Sage Foundation, New York, pp 169–208

Bellante HW (1971) Empathic ability among lower- and middle-class adolescents in relation to several social-psychological variables. Diss Abstr Int 31-A:4884

Beller EK (1948) Dependence and independence in young children. Ph.D. dissertation, State University of Iowa

Belmont L (1977) Birth order, intellectual competence and psychiatric status. J Individ Psychol 33:97–104

Belmont L, Marolla FA (1973) Birth order, family size, and intelligence. Science 182:1096–1101

Belmont L, Stein ZA, Susser MW (1975) Comparison of associations of birth order with intelligence test score and height. Nature 255:54–56

Belmont L, Stein ZA, Wittes JT (1976) Birth order, family size and school failure, Dev Med Child Neurol 18:421–430

Belmont L, Stein Z, Zybert P (1978) Child spacing and birth order. Science 202:995–996

Belmont L, Wittes JT, Stein Z (1977) Relation of birth order, family size and social class to psychological functions. Perc Mot Skills 45:1107–1116

Benech A, Mathieu B, Scheider E (1960) Family sizes and biological characteristics of the children. Biotypologie 21:4–36

Benjamin B (1966) Social and economic differences in fertility. In: Meade JE, Parkes AS (eds) Genetic and environmental factors in human ability. Plenum, Edinburgh London

* Bennett BM (1963) On a test for birth-order effect when several abnormalities are present. Ann Hum Genet 27:11–15

Bennett I (1960) Delinquent and neurotic children. A comparative study. Basic Books, New York (Tavistock Publications)

Berbaum ML, Moreland RL (1980) Intellectual development within the family. Dev Psychol 16:506–515

* Berelson B, Steiner GA (1964) Human behavior, an inventory of scientific findings. Harcourt Brace and World, New York, p 225

Berg I, Butler A, Mc Guire R (1972) Birth order and family size of school-phobic adolescents. Br J Psychiatry 121:509–514

Berg I, Fearnley W, Paterson M, Pollock G, Vallance R (1967) Birth order and family size of approved school boys. Br J Psychiatry 113:793–800

Berger PK, Ivancevich JM (1973) Birth order and managerial achievement. Acad Management J 16:515–519

Bernstein BE, Grambs J (1976) Sex and academic field in relation to birth order and achievement. Psychol Rep 39:659–663

Bettray R (1970) Untersuchung über die Beziehung zwischen der Stellung in der Geschwisterreihe und der Häufigkeit und Art der psychoreaktiven Störung. Med Dissertation, Tübingen

Bharathi VV, Venkatramaiah SR (1976) Birth order, family size and anxiety. Child Psychiat Quart 9:11–17

Bhushan R, Verma NK (1972) A study of social determinants of leadership preference. J Indian Acad Appl Psychol 9:81–84

Biber DC (1974) Parental attitudes and expectations towards first and second children. Diss Abstr Int 35-B:3006

Biegelsen CE (1976) The relationship of being first or laterborn and vocational academic and personality variables. Ph.D. thesis, Washington. Diss Abstr Int 37-B:1871–1872

Bies JD (1973) Environmental influences on problem solving ability in three demographic groups. Diss Abstr Int 33:4927–4928

Bigner JJ (1972) Sibling position and definition of self. J Soc Psychol 84:307–308

Bigner JJ (1972) Sibling influence on sex-role preference of young children. J Genet Psychol 121:271–282

Bigner JJ (1974a) Second borns' discrimination of sibling role concepts. Dev Psychol 10:564–573

Bigner JJ (1974b) A Wernerian developmental analysis of children's descriptions of siblings. Child Dev 45:317–323

Biles D (1971) Birth order and delinquency. Aust Psychol 6:189–193

* Birtchnell J (1970) Sibship and mental illness. Br J Psychiatry 117:303–308

* Birtchnell J (1971) Early parent death, in relation to size and constitution of sibship, in psychiatric patients and general population controls. Acta Psychiatr Scand 47:250–270

* Birtchnell J (1971a) Birth rank and mental illness. Nature, London 234:485–487

* Birtchnell J (1971b) Mental illness in sibships of two and three. Br J Psychiatry 119:481–487

* Birtchnell J (1972) Birth order and mental illness – A control study. Soc Psychiat 7:167–179

* Birtchnell J, Mayhew J (1977) Toman's theory: tested for mate selection and friendship formation. J Individ Psychol 33:18–36

Biswas M (1975) Birth order and mental retardation. Ind J Clin Psychol 2:173–174

Blake J (1965) Ideal family size among white Americans. A quarter of a century's evidence. Population Index 31:262–263

Blake J (1967) Income and reproductive motivation. Population Study 21:185–206

Blane HT, Barry H (1973) Birth order and alcoholism: a review. Q J Stud Alcohol 34:837–852

Blane HT, Barry H (1975) Sex of siblings of male alcoholics. Arch Gen Psychiatry 32:1403–1405

Blane HT, Barry H, Barry H (1971) Sex differences in birth order of alcoholics. Br J Psychiatry 119:657–661

Blau PM, Duncan OD, Tyree A (1967) The American occupational structure. John Wiley & Sons, New York London Sydney

Bleuler E (1919) Das autistisch-undisziplinierte Denken in der Medizin und seine Ueberwindung. Springer, Berlin

Bleuler M (1972) Die schizophrenen Geistesstörungen. Thieme, Stuttgart, pp 381

Blinder MG (1966) The hysterical personality. Psychiatry 29:227–235

Bliss WD (1970) Birth order of creative writers. J Individ Psychol 26:200–202

Block JH (1976) Debatable conclusions about sex difference. Contemp Psychol 21:517–522

Blustein ES (1967) The relationship of sib position in the family constellation to school behavior variables in elementary school children from 2-child-families. Ph.D. thesis, University of Maryland, Diss Abstr Int 28-B:3046–3047 (1968)

Bolte R, Gleiss J (1969) Fettsucht im Kindesalter. Kinderärztl Prax 3:123

Böök JA (1950) A clinical and genetical study of anencephaly. Am J Hum Genet 2:61–84

Böök JA, Rayner S (1953) A genetic and neuropsychiatric investigation of a North-Swedish population. Acta Genet, Basel 4:1–100

Boone SL (1979) Effects of fathers' absence and birth order on aggressive behavior of young male children. Psychol Rep 44:1223–1229

Boor M (1972) Family structure variables and need approval: Some additional data. Psychol Rep 30:204–206

Boshien R, Walkey FH (1971) Birth order and conservatism: An Adlerian myth? Psychol Rep 29:392–394

Bossard JHS (1945) Family modes of expression. Am Soc Rev 10:226–237

Bossard JHS, Boll ES (1954) Security in the large family. Ment Hyg, New York 38:531–542

Bossard JHS, Boll ES (1955) Personality roles in the large family. Child Develop 26:71–78

Bossard JHS, Boll ES (1960) Families by size. In: The sociology of child development, 3rd edn. Harper & Brothers, New York, pp 47–67

Bowerman WG (1947) Studies in genius. Philosophical Library, New York

Bradley RW (1968) Birth order and school-related behavior: a heuristic review. Psychol Bull 70:45–51

Bradley RW, Sanborn MP (1969) Ordinal position of high school students identified by their teachers as superior. J Educ Psychol 60:41–45

Bragg BWE (1969) A role theory interpretation of the effects of birth order on conformity. Diss Abstr Int 29-A:4553
Bragg BWE (1970) Academic primogeniture and sex role contrast of the second born. J Individ Psychol 26:196–199
Bragg BWE, Allen VL (1970) Ordinal position and conformity: A role theory analysis. Sociometry 33:371–381
Bragg BWE, Ostrowski MV, Finley GE (1973) The effects of birth order and age of target on use of persuasive techniques. Child Dev 44:351–354
Breland HM (1972) Birth order and intelligence. Ph.D. dissertation, State University of New York, Buffalo
* Breland HM (1973) Birth order effects: A reply to Schooler. Psychol Bull 80:210–212
* Breland HM (1974) Birth order, family configuration and verbal achievement. Child Dev 45:1011–1019
Breland HM (1977) Family configuration and intellectual development. J Individ Psychol 33:86–96
Breland NS (1972) Hereditary and environmental sources of trait variation and covariation. Diss Abstr Int 33-A:1506
Breslin PP (1968) Maternal age and birth order in mental illness. Diss Abstr Int 28–B:4182–4183
Brim OG jr (1958) Family structure and sex role learning by children. A further analysis of Helen Koch's data. Sociometry 21:1–16
Brittain CV (1966) Age and sex of siblings and conformity toward parents versus peers in adolescence. Child Develop 37:709–714
Brock TC, Becker G (1965) Birth order and subject recruitment. J Soc Psychol 65:63–66
Broman SH, Nichols PL, Kennedy WA (1975) Preschool IQ, prenatal and early development correlates. John Wiley and Sons, New York
Bronfenbrenner V (1958) Socialization and social class through time and space. In: Maccoby EE, Newcomb TM, Hartley EL (eds) Readings in social psychology. Holt, Rinehart and Wisnton, New York, pp 400–425
Bronzaft AL, Epstein GF (1972) Text anxiety, sex and ordinal position. J Soc Psychol 87:155–156
Brown C (1971) Recent trends in socio-economic fertility differentials in Japan and the United States. Proceedings International Population Conference, London, vol III. IUSSP, Liège, pp 2026–2042
Brown DG (1956) Sex role preference in young children. Psychol Monogr 70:whole No 421
Bruce WE, Sims JH (1974) Birth order among psychotherapists: A see-saw phenomenon. Psychol Rep 215–220
Bruff WK (1977) Sex, ethnicity and birth order; their effects on small group interactoin. Diss Abstr Int 38-B:958–959
Brugger C (1931) Die Stellung der Schwachsinnigen in der Geburtenreihenfolge. Z Ges Neurol Psychiatrie 135:536–554
Bryant GM, Davies KJ (1974) The effect of sex, social class, and parity on achievement of Denver Developmental Screening Test items in the first year of life. Dev Med Child Neurol 16:485–493
Bucher RE, Terzis A (1980) Birth order and sibling relations of schizophrenics. Arq Neuropsiquiatr 38:53–64
Bullough VL, Bullough B, Voight M, Kluckhohn L (1971) Birth order and achievement in 18th century Scotland. J Individ Psychol 27:80
Bumpass LL (1969) Age at marriage as a variable in socio-economic differences in fertility. Demography 6:45–54
Bumpass LL, Mburugu EK (1977) Age at marriage and completed family size. Soc Biol 24:31–33
Bumpass LL, Westoff CF (1970) The perfect "contraceptive" population. Science 169:1177–1182
Burke MO (1956) A search for systematic personality differentiae of the only child in young adulthood. J Genet Psychol 89:71–84
Buros OK (1972) The 7th mental measurement yearbook. Gryphon, New Jersey
Burton A, Bird IW (1963) Family constellation and schizophrenia. J Psychol 55:329–336
Burton D (1968) Birth order and intelligence. J Soc Psychol 76:199–206
Butler NR, Alberman ED (1966) Perinatal problems. The second report of the 1958 British Perinatal Mortality Survey. Livingstone, Edinburgh London
Button A (1953) An inquiry into the psychological effects of adrenocorticotrophic hormone administration. Diss Abstr Int 13:873
Byrdy HL, Uhlenhut WEH (1962) Ordinal sibling position and motivation toward psychiatric treatment. J Nerv Ment Dis 135:265–267

* Bytheway B (1974) A statistical trap associated with family size. J Biosoc Sci 6:67–72
* Bytheway WR (1973) Families with just two children born within a fixed sampling period. Some sampling biases. SRUS Occasional Paper No 3, Keele
Cahn P (1952) Expérimentations sociométriques apliquées au groupe fraternel. Sociometry 15:306–310
Caldwell BM (1964) The effects of infant care. In: Hoffman ML, Hoffman LW (eds) Review of child development, vol 1. Russell-Sage Foundation, New York, pp 9–87
Calnan M, Richardson K (1976) Speech problems in a national survey. Child Care Health Dev 2:181–202
Campbell DP (1971) Admissions policies: Side effects and their implications. Am Psychol 26:636–647
Campbell DT, Fiske DW (1959) Convergent and discriminant validation. Psychol Bull 56:81–105
Campbell ES, Redfering DL (1979) Relationship among environmental and demographic variables and teacher-rated hyperactivity. J Abnorm Child Psychol 7:77–81
Campbell FL (1970) Family growth and variation in family role structure. J Marriage Family 32:45–53
Cantor P (1972) The adolescent attempter: Sex, sibling position and family constellation. Life-threatening Behav 2:252–261
Capra PC, Dittes JE (1962) Birth order as a selective factor among volunteer subjects. J Abnorm Soc Psychol 64:302–306
Carlson NL (1970) Occupational choice and achievement of women graduate students in psychology as a function of early parentchild interactions and achievement as related to birth order and family size. Diss Abstr Int 31-A:2679
Carrigan WC, Julian JW (1966) Sex and birth-order differences in conformity as a function of need affiliation arousal. J Pers Soc Psychol 3:479–483
Carr-Saunders AM, Mannheim H, Rhodes EE (1942) Young offenders. An enquiry into juvenile delinquency. Cambridge University Press, Cambridge
Cartwright LK (1972) The personality and family background of a sample of women medical students at the university of California. J Am Med Womens' Ass 27:260–266
Casadebaig F, Chevalier A (1976) Etude comparative entre les caractéristiques familiales et sociales des enfants pris en charge. Psychiatrie Enf 19:302–42
Casher BB (1977) Relationship between birth order and participation in dangerous sports. Res Q 48:33–40
Catlin N (1972) Children's fears by race, sex, sibling position, grade level, and socioeconomic level. Diss Abstr Int 33-B:2788
Cattell JMcK (1917) Families of American men of science. III. Vital statistics and the composition of families. Sci Mon 5:368–377
Cattell JMcK, Brimhall DR (1921) American men of science. A biographical directory, 3rd edn. Science, Garrison, New York, p 803
Caudill W, Schooler C (1969) Symptom patterns and background characteristics of Japanese psychiatric-patients. In: Caudill W, Tsung Yi Lin (eds) Mental health research in Asia and the Pacific. East-West-Center, Honolulu
Chakraborty A (1969/70) Birth order and mental illness. Br J Soc Psychiatry 3:231–236
Chambers JA (1964) Relating personality and biographical factors to scientific creativity. Psychol Monogr 78:584
Chandrasekaran C, Talwar PP (1968) Forms of age specific birth rate by order of birth in an Indian community. Eugen Q 15:264–271
Chemers MM (1970) The relationship between birth order and leadership style. J Soc Psychol 80:243–244
* Chen E, Cobb S (1960) Family structure in relation to health and disease. A review of the literature. J Chron Dis 12:544–567
Chittenden EA, Foan WM, Zweil DM (1968) School achievement of first and second born siblings. Child Dev 39:1223–1228
Cho LJ (1968) Income and differentials in current fertility. Demography 5:198–211
Chombart de Lauwe MJ (1959) Psychopathologie sociale de l'enfant inadapté. Paris, Centre National de la Recherche Scientifique
Chopra SL (1966) Family size and sibling positoin as related to measured intelligence and academic achievement. J Soc Psychol 70:133–137
Choynowski M, Idmen P (1973) Adolescent aggressivness and its dependence on age, sex and position among siblings. Educat Psychol Interact 38.129

Christensen HT (1968) Children in the family: Relationship of number and spacing to marital success. J Marriage Family 30:283–289
Churchill JA (1965) The relationship between intelligence and birth weight in twins. J Neurol 15:341–347
Cicirelli VG (1967) Sibling constellation creativity IQ and academic achievement. Child Dev 38:481–490
Cicirelli VG (1976a) Sibling structure and intellectual ability. Dev Psychol 12:369–370
Cicirelli VG (1976b) Mother-child and sibling-sibling interactions on a problem-solving task. Child Dev 47:588–596
Cicirelli VG (1976c) Sibling influence in the development of the individual. In: Riegel FK, Mecham JA (eds) The developing individual in a changing world, vol 3. Mouton, The Hague
Cicirelli VG (1977) Childrens' school grades and sibling structure. Psychol Rep 41:1055–1058
Clark AH, Wyon SM, Richards MPM (1969) Free-play in nursery school children. J Chil Psychol Psychiatry 10:205–216
Clarke EL (1916) American men of letters, their nature and nurture. Columbia University Press, New York
Clausen JA (1965) Research note on family size, sib order and socialization influence (Unpublished paper)
*Clausen JA (1966) Family structure, socialisation and personality. In: Hoffman LW, Hoffman ML (eds) Review of child development research, vol II. Russel Sage Foundation, New York
*Clausen JA, Clausen SR (1973) The effects of family size on parents and children. In: Fawcett JT (ed) Psychological perspectives on population. Basic Books, New York
*Clausen JA, Hancock F, Williams J, Jako K (1965) Family size and birth order as influences upon socialization and personality: Bibliography and abstracts. Social Science Research Council, University of California, Berkeley
Clausen JA, Wiliams J (1963) Sociological correlates of child behavior. In: Stevenson HW, Kagan J, Spiker C (eds) Child psychology. Yearb Nat Soc Stud Educ 62:62–107
Cleland CC, Seitz S, Patton WE (1967) Birth order and ruralism as potential determinants of attendant tenure. Am J Ment Defic 72:428–434
Cleland CC, Uno T, Rago W, Case JC, McGavern M (1975) Ecology and ordinality in invention: an exploratory study. Psychol Rep 37:815–818
Clowers LE (1977) A sociological study of birth order and attitudes concerning female sex role equality. Diss Abstr Int 37-A:7348–7349
Clum GA, Clum MJ (1970) Sibling position as a factor in psychiatric illness and prognosis in a military population. J Clin Psychol 26:271–274
*Cobb JA (1913/14) The alleged inferiority of the first-born. Eugen Rev 5:357–359
Cobb S, French JRP (1966) Birth order among medical students. J Am Med Ass 195:312–313
Cohen S, Beckwith L (1976) Maternal language in infancy. Dev Ment Psychol 12:371–372
Cohen SE, Beckwith L (1977) Caregiving behaviors and early cognitive development as related to ordinal position in preterm infants. Child Dev 48:152–157
Coker RE, Back KW, Donnelly ThG, Miller N, Phillips BS (1959) Public Health as viewed by the medical student. Am J Pub Health 49:601–609
Collard RR (1968) Social and play responses of first-born and later-born infants in an unfamiliar situation. Child Dev. 39:325–334
Conley JJ (1980) Family configuration as an etiological factor in alcoholism. J Abnorm Psychol 89:670–673
Conners CK (1963) Birth order and need for affiliation. J Pers 31:408–416
Cook RC (1951) Human fertility. William Sloan, New York
Coopersmith S (1967) The antecedents of self-esteem. WH Freeman, San Francisco
Coren St, Porac C (1980) Birth Factors and Laterality. Behav Genet 10:123–138
Corneau H (1980) An examination of the relationship between sex, birth order and creativity. Creative Child Adult Q 5:251–258
Cornoldi C, Fattori LC (1976) Age spacing in firstborns and symbiotic dependence. J Pers Soc Psychol 33:431–434
Corsello P (1973) Birth order and children's perceptions of love, authority and personality adjustment. Diss Abstr Int 34-A:3132
Cowie J, Cowie V, Slater E (1968) Delinquency in girls. Heinemann, London

Crandall VC, Katovsky W, Crandall VJ (1965) Children's belief in their own control of reinforcements in intellectual-academic achievement situations. Child Dev 36:91–109
Crandall VJ, Preston A, Rabson A (1960) Maternal reactions and the development of independence and achievement behavior in young children. Child Dev 31:243–251
Critelli JW, Baldwin AC (1979) Birth order: Complementarity vs homogamy as determinants of attraction in dating relationships. Percept Mot Skills 49:467–471
Croake JW, Olson TD (1977) Family constellation and personality. J Individ Psychol 33:9–17
Cropley AJ (1964) Differentiation of abilities, socioeconomic status and the WISC. J Consult Clin Psychol 28:512–522
Cropley AJ, Ahlers KH (1975) Development of verbal skills in first-born and only boys. J Biosoc Sci 7:297–306
Crowne DP, Marlowe D (1964) The approval motive, John Wiley & Sons, New York
Crump EP, Horton CP, Masuoka J, Ryan D (1957) Growth and development. J Pediatr 51:678–697
Cullen KJ, Boundy CAP (1966) Factors relating to behavior disorders in children. Aust Paediatr J 2:70–80
Culver CM, Dunham F (1969) Birth order and spatial-perceptual ability: negative note. Percept Mot Skills 28:301–302
Cushna B (1970) Birth order and verbal mastery. In: Sutton-Smith B, Rosenberg G (eds) The Sibling, New York
Cushna B, Greene M, Snider BCF (1964) First born and lastborn children in a child development clinic. J Individ Psychol 20:179–182
Cutts NE, Moseley N (1954) The only child. A guide for parents and only children of all ages. GP Putnam's Sons, New York
Dagenais F (1979) Birth order and leadership style. J Soc Psychol 109:151–152
Dale JH (1973) The significance of sibling position and the frequency of participation by adults in group counseling activities. Diss Abstr Int 33-A:4041–4042
Damrin DE (1949) Family size and sibling age, sex and position as related to certain aspects of adjustment. J Soc Psychol 29:93–102
Dandes HM, Dow D (1969) Relation of intelligence to family size and density. Child Dev 40:641–645
Dann TC, Roberts DF (1969) Physique and family environment in girls attending a Welsh college. Br J Prev Soc Med 23:65–71
Darley JM (1966) Fear and social comparison as determinants of conformity behavior. J Pers Soc Psychol 4:73–78
Darley JM, Aronson E (1966) Self-evaluation vs direct anxiety reduction as determinants of the fear-affilation relationship. J Exp Soc Psychol Suppl 1:66–79,
Datta LE (1966) Birth order and achievement. Science 152:1181
Datta LE (1967) Birth order and early scientific attainment. Percept Mot Skills 24:157–158
Datta LE (1968) Birth order and potential scientific creativity. Sociometry 31:76–88
Dauphinais S, Leitner DW (1978) Effect of birth order, sex and family size on affiliation with encounter groups. Psychol Rep 42:673–674
David P (1973) Correlates of cheating behavior in a ghetto elementary school. Grad Res Educ Rel Disc 7:35–63
Davie R, Butler N, Goldstein H (1972) From birth to seven. Longman, London
Davies CHG (1963) The families of severely mentally retarded children: Family composition and health. Calif J Educ Res 14:121–130
* Davis A (1953) American status systems and the socialization of the child. In: Kluckhohn C, Murray HA (eds) Personality in nature, society, and culture, 2nd edn. A. A. Knopf, New York, pp 567–576
Davis DJ, Cahan S, Bashi J (1977) Birth order and intellectual development: The confluence model in the light of cross-cultural evidence. Science 196:1470–1472
Dawson B, Horobin G, Illsley R, Mitchell R (1969) A survey of childhood asthma in Aberdeen. Lancet ii: 827–830
Day RL (1967) Factors influencing offspring. Am J Dis Child 113:179–185
Dean DA (1947) The relation of ordinal position to personality in young children. Master's thesis, State University of Iowa, Iowa
De Avila-Havassy BE (1969) Birth order differences: an attempt to isolate conditions under which they occur. Dissertation, University of Colorado, Diss Abstr Int 30-A:4547 (1970)

* De Avila-Havassy BE (1971) A critical review of the approach to birth order research. Can Psychol 12:282–305

Dechêne HC (1967) Geschwisterkonstellation und psychische Fehlentwicklung. Barth, München

De Fee JF, Himelstein P (1969) Children's fear in a dental situation as a function of birth order. J Genet Psychol 115:253–255

Delaney RJ (1973) Children's role-taking ability as a function of birth order, age, sex, and mothers' parenting style. Diss Abstr Int 34-B:389–390

De Lint JEE (1964) Alcoholism, birth order and socializing agents. J Abnorm Soc Psychol 69:457–458

Dember WN (1963) Birth order and need affiliation. Am Psychol 18:356

Dember WN (1964) Birth order and need affiliation. J Abnorm Soc Psychol 68:555–557

Dentler RA, Monroe LA (1961) Social correlates of early adolescent theft. Am Sociol Rev 26:733–743

Descombey J, Roquebrune G (1953) L'enfant caractériel parmi ses frères et soeurs. Enfance 6:329–368

De Wolff P, Meerdink S (1957) La fécondité des mariages à Amsterdam. Population 12:289–318

Deutsche Forschungsgemeinschaft (1977) Schwangerschaftsverlauf und Kindesentwicklung. Bolt, Boppard

Diab L, Prothro ET (1968) Cross-cultural study of some correlates of birth order. Psychol Rep 22:1137–1142

Dickson RM (1969) A descriptive study of the relationship between specific personality factors and ordinal position in the family. Ph.D. dissertation, Stanford University, Diss Abstr Int 29-A:4278–4279

Dickson WP (1974) The development of interpersonal referential communication skills in young children using an interactional game device. Diss Abstr Int 35-A:3511

Dielman TE, Barton E, Cattell RB (1974) Adolescent personality and intelligence scores as related to family demography. J Genet Psychol 124:151–154

Dimond RE, Munz C (1968) Ordinal position of birth and self disclosure in high school students. Psychol Rep 21:829–833

Dimond RE, Hellkamp DT (1969) Race, sex, ordinal position of birth, and self-disclosure in high school students. Psychol Rep 25:235–238

Dittes JE (1961) Birth order and vulnerability to differences in acceptance. Am J Psychol 16:358

Dittes JE, Capra PC (1962) Affiliation: Comparability or compatibility? Am Psychol 17:329

Dixon RD (1980) The absence of birth order correlations among unwed and married black first conceptors. J Sex Res 16:238–244

Dohrenwend BS, Dohrenwend BP (1966) Stress situations, birth order and psychological symptoms. J Abnorm Psychol 71:215–223

Dohrenwend BS, Feldstein S, Plosky J, Schmeidler GR (1967) Factors interacting with birth order in self-selection among volunteer subjects. J Soc Psychol 72:125–128

Dolph EJA (1966) A comparative study of the ordinal position of the child and his school achievement. Diss Abstr Int 26-A:6509

* Doren MP (1972) Evaluation of studies on birth order and sibling position. Ph.D. thesis, University of Minnesota. Diss Abstr Int 33-A:5548–5549

Douglas JWB (1964) The home and the school. A study of ability and attainment in the primary school, 7th edn. McGibbon and Kee, London, pp 84–100

Douglas JWB (1966) The age of reaching puberty: some associated factors and some educational implications. In: British Postgraduate Medical Federation: The scientific basis of medicine, annual reviews. University of London, Athlone, pp 91–105

Douglas JWB (1950) Some factors associated with prematurity. The results of a national survey. J Obstet Gynaec Br Comm 57:143

Douglas JWB, Blomfield JM (1958) Children under five. Allen and Unwin, London

Douglas JWB, Ross JM, Simpson HR (1968) All our future. A longitudinal study of secondary education. Peter Davies, London

Douglas JWB, Simpson HR (1964) Height in relation to puberty family size and social class. A longitudinal study. Milbank Mem Fund Q 42:20–35

Douvan E, Adelson J (1966) The adolescent experience. J Wiley & Sons, New York Sidney London, pp 272

Dreikurs R (1950) Fundamentals of Adlerian Psychology. A Adler Institute, Chicago, pp 37–42

Dubno P, Bedrosian H, Freedman R (1969) Birth order, conformity, and managerial achievement. Pers Psychol 22:269–279

Dubno P, Freedman RD (1971/72) Birth order, educational achievement, and managerial attainment. Pers Psychol 24:63–70

Dunn J, Kendrick C (1980) The arrival of a sibling: Changes in patterns of interaction between mother and first-born child. J Child Psychol Psychiatry 21:119–132

Dunn J, Kendrick C, MacNamee R (1981) The reaction of first-born children to the birth of a sibling: Mother's reports. J Child Psychol Psychiatry 22:1–18

Dyer DT (1945) Are only children different? J Educ Psychol 36:297–302

Easterlin (1965) The decline of fertility in the United States since 1957. Population Index 31:246

Easterlin RA (1970) Towards a socioeconomic theory of fertility. In: Behrman SJ, Corsa L, Freedman R (eds) Fertility and family planning. A world view, 2nd edn. University of Michigan Press, Ann Arbor, pp 127–156

Ebert RK (1973) The reliability and validity of a mailed questionnaire for a sample of entering college freshmen. Ph.D. dissertation, Temple University

Eckstein D, Tobacyk J (1979) Ordinal position and death concerns. Psychol Rep 44:967–971

Edington G, Wilson B (1974) Children of different ordinal positions. In: Call JD et al. (eds) Basic handbook of child psychiatry, vol I. Basic Books, New York, pp 397–406

Edwards JN, Klemmack DL (1973) Birth order and the conservator of tradition hypothesis. J Marriage Family 35:619–627

Edwards RP, Thacker K (1979) The relationship of birth order, gender and sib gender in the two child family to grade point average in college. Adolescence 14:111–114

Eells K, Davis WA, Havighurst RJ, Herrick VE, Tyler RW (1951) Intelligence and cultural differences. Chicago University Press, Chicago

Ehrlich D (1958) Determinants of verbal commonality and influencibility. Ph.D. dissertation, University of Minnesota, Minnesota

Eiduson BT (1962) Scientists: Their psychological world. Basic Books, New York

Eisenman R (1965) Birth order, aesthetic preference, and volunteering for an electric shock experiment. Psychonom Sci 3:151–152

Eisenman R (1966) Birth order, anxiety and verbalizations in group psychotherapy. J Consult Clin Psychol 30:521–526

Eisenman R (1967a) Birth order and sex differences in aesthetic preference for complexity-simplicity. J Genet Psychol 77:121–126

Eisenman R (1967b) Complexity-simplicity: II. Birth order and sex differences. Psychonom Sci 8:171–172

Eisenman R (1968a) Personality and demography in complexity-simplicity. J Consult Clin Psychol 32:140–143

Eisenman R (1968b) Birth order, insolence, socialization, intelligence and complexity-simplicity differences. J Genet Psychol 78:61–64

Eisenman R (1970) Birth order, sex, self-esteem, and prejudice against the physically disabled. J Psychol 75:147–155

Eisenman R, Cherry HO (1970) Creativity, authoritarianism and birth order. J Soc Psychol 80:233–235

Eisenman R, Platt JJ (1968) Birth order and sex differences in academic achievement and internal-external control. J Genet Psychol 78:279–285

Eisenman R, Schussel NR (1970) Creativity, birth order, and preference for symmetry. J Consult Clin Psychol 34:275–280

Eisenman R, Taylor RE (1966) Birth order and MMPI patterns. J Individ Psychol 22:208–211

Elder GH jr (1962a) Adolescent achievement and mobility aspirations. Institute for Research in Social Science, University of North Carolina, Chapel Hill, NC

Elder GH jr (1962b) Structural variations in the child rearing relationship. Sociometry 25:241–262

Elder GH jr, Bowerman CE (1963) Family structure and child-rearing patterns: The effect of family size and sex composition. Am Soc Rev 28:891–905

El Islam MP (1971) Birth order and the social psychopathology of depression. J Egyp Med Ass 54:150–154

Elliott JL, Elliott DH (1970) Effects of birth order and age gap on aspiration level. Proc 78th Annu Conv APA, vol 5. American Psychological Association, Washington, DC, pp 369–370

Ellis H (1926) A study of British genius. Houghton Mifflin, Boston

Ellis A, Beechley EM (1951) A comparison of child guidance clinic patients coming from large, medium, and small families. J Genet Psychol 79:131–144

Enquête Nationale (1973) Sur le niveau intellectuel des enfants d'âge scolaire. Institut national d'études démographiques, Paris
Epstein GP, Bronzaft AL (1972) Academic primogeniture revisited. Psychol Rep 30:135–138
Erlenmeyer-Kimling L (1968) The sibships of schizophrenics. In: Vandenberg SG (ed) Progress in human behavior genetics. Johns Hopkins, Baltimore, pp 105–125
Erlenmeyer-Kimling L (1969) The problem of birth order and schizophrenia: a negative conclusion. Br J Psychiatry 115:659–677
Erlenmeyer-Kimling L (1970) Birth order of schizophrenics. Br J Psychiatry 116:124–126
Eysenck HJ, Eysenck SBG (1969a) Personality structure and measurement. Routledge & Kegan Paul, London
Eysenck HJ, Cookson D (1969b) Personality in primary school children 3. Family background. Br J Educat Psychol 40:117–131
Exner JE, Sutton-Smith B (1970) Birth order and hierarchical versus innovative role requirements. J Personality 38:581–587
Fahrenberg J, Selg H, Hampel R (1973) Das Freiburger Persönlichkeitsinventar FPI. 2. Aufl. Verlag für Psychologie Dr. C. J. Hogrefe, Göttingen
Fakouri ME (1974) Relationships of birth order, dogmatism and achievement motivation. J Individ Psychol 30:216–220
Falbo T (1977) The only child: a review. J Individ Psychol 33:47–61
Falbo T (1978) Reasons for having an only child. J Popul 1:181–184
Falbo T, Richman ChL (1979) Relationships between father's age, birth order, family size, and need achievement. Bull Psychonomic Soc 13:179–182
Falek A (1971) Differential fertility and intelligence: Current status of the problem. Soc Biol Suppl 18:50–59
Fandrich E (1976) Birth-order effects at two Canadian colleges: Residence and classroom samples. Psychol Rep 38:1183–1184
Farina A, Barry H, Garmezy N (1963) Birth order of recovered and non recovered schizophrenics. Arch Gen Psychiatry 9:224–228
Farley FH (1967) Birth order, achievement motivation and academic attainment. Br J Educ Psychol 37:256
Farley FH (1975a) Birth order and a two-dimensional assessment of personality. J Pers Assess 39:151–153
Farley FH (1975b) Family structure and approval dependency in college females. J Marriage Family 37:760–762
Farley FH (1978a) Note on creativity and scholastic achievement of women as a function of birth order and family size. Percept Motor Skills 47:13–14
Farley FH (1978b) Scholastic ability and birth order, family size, sibling age spacing and parental absence in eighth and ninth graders. An empirical study of the confluence model. Diss Abstr Int 38-A:6008
Farley FH, Farley SV (1974) Birth order and political orientation in college women. Psychol Rep 34:1045–1046
Farley FH, Hatch R, Murphy P, Miller K (1971) Sibling structure and masculinity-feminity in male adolescents. Adolescence 6:441–450
Farley FH, Smart KL, Brittain CV (1974a) Birth order, rank, and branch of service in the military. J Individ Psychol 30:227–231
Farley FH, Smart KL, Brittain CV (1974b) Implications of birth order for motivational and achievement-related characteristics of adults enrolled in non-traditional instruction. J Exp Education 42:21–24
Faust V (1976) Im Vorfeld des Alkoholismus. ZFA, Stuttgart, 52:491–499
Feeney FE, Mindlin DF, Minear VH, Short EE (1955) The challenge of the Skid Row alcoholic. Q J Stud Alcohol 16:645–667
Fehlow P (1973) Über die Ursachen und forensische Begutachtung von Sexualdelikten. Psychiatr Neurol Med Psychol 25:535–544
Feldman GC (1977) The only child as a separate entity: An attempt to differentiate only females from firstborn females. Diss Abstr Int 37-A:2633–2634
Fenton N (1928) The only child. J Genet Psychol 35:546–555
Ferguson T (1952) The young delinquent in his social setting. Oxford University Press, London

Ferguson T, Cunnison J (1951) The young wage-earner. A study of Glasgow boys. Oxford University Press, London
Fernando CPS (1952) Truancy and stealing. DPM thesis, University of London
Feshbach S (1970) Aggression. In: Mussen PH (ed) Carmichael's manual of child psychology, 3rd edn. Wiley, New York, pp 159–259
Finch FH (1933) A study of the relation of age interval to degree of ressemblance of siblings in intelligence. J Genet Psychol 43:389–404
Finley GE, Cheyne JA (1976) Birth order and susceptibility to peer modeling influences in young boys. J Genet psychol 129:273–277
Finley GE, Sølla J (1975) Birth order and field dependence-independence: A failure to replicate. J Genet Psychol 126:305–306
Finneran JAW (1969) Birth order in relation to affiliation. Diss Abstr Int 29-B:3910
Fischer A (1962) The importance of sibling position in the choice of a career in pediatric nursing. J Health Hum Behav 3:283–288
Fischer EH, Wells CF, Cohen SL (1968) Birth order and expressed interest in becoming a college professor. J Counseling Psychol 15:111–116
Fischer EH, Winer D (1969) Participation in psychological research: Relation to birth order and demographic factors. J Consult Clin Psychol 33:610–613
Floud JE, Halsey AH, Martin FM (1956) Social class and educational opportunity. Heinemann, London, pp 90–91
Fogelman KR (1975) Developmental correlates of family size: A report from the national child development study. Br J Soc Work 5:43–57
* Folger JK, Bayer AE (1966) Letter to the editor. Science 152:1177
Forbes G (1970 a) Fraternity or sorority membership and birth order: Sex differences and problems of reliability. J Soc Psychol 82:277–278
Forbes GB (1970 b) Smoking behavior and birth order. Psychol Rep 26:766
Forbes GB (1972) Birth order and political success: A study of the 1970 Illinois general elections. Psychol Rep 29:1239–1242
Forbes GB (1974) Birth order and academic behavior among seriously disadvantaged adults. J Soc Psychol 93:301–302
Forer LK (1969) Birth order and life roles. Charles C Thomas, Springfield, Illinis
Fortes M (1974) The first born. J Child Psychol Psychiatry 15:81–104
Foster JW, Archer SJ (1979) Birth order and intelligence: An immunological interpretation. Percept Mot Skills 48:79–93
Fox NA (1976) Developmental and birth order determinants of separation protest: A cross-cultural study of infants on the Israeli kibbutz. Dis Abstr Int 37-A:3515–3516
Frankel JJ (1968) The relation of a specific family constellation and some personality characteristics of children. Diss Abstr Int 28-B:2620–2621
Franklin BJ (1973) Birth order and tenedency to "adopt the sick role". Psychol Rep 33:437–438
Fraser C, Roberts N (1975) Mothers' speech to children of four different ages. J Psycholinguist Res 4:9–16
Frederking U (1975) Häufigkeiten, somatische und soziale Bedingungen von Verhaltensstörungen zehnjähriger Schulkinder. Prax Kinderpsychol Kinderpsychiatrie 24:204–213
Freedman DS, Freedman R, Whelpton PK (1960) Size of family and preference for children of each sex. AJS 66:141–146
Freud S (1938) A general introduction to psycho-analysis. Garden City, New York, p 182
Freyn W (1976) The dependence of pupil performance and grades on the siblin g-constellations of pupil and teacher. Psychologie in Erziehung und Unterricht 23:215–223
Friedman JH, Jackson BJ, Nogas C (1978) Birth order and age at marriage in females. Psychol Rep 42:1193–1194
Gallagher R, Cowen E (1977) Birth order and school adjustment problems. J Individ Psychol 33:70–77
Galton F (1874) English men of science. Macmillan, London
Galton F (1887) Hereditary genius. Appleton, New York
Gandy GL (1972) The relationship between birth order and vocational interest. Diss Abstr Int 32-A:6807
* Gandy GL (1973) Birth order and vocational interest. Dev Psychol 9:406–410
* Gandy GL (1974) Ordinal position research related to vocational interest. J Counseling Psychol 21:281–287

Gelfand S (1962) The relationship of birth order to pain tolerance. J Clin Psychol 18:406–409

Gentry WD, Shows WD, Thomas M (1974) Chronic back pain: A psychological profile. Psychosomatics 15:174–177

George EI, Devadas R (1971) Manifest anxiety as a function of birth order. J Indian Acad Appl Psychol 8:39–40

Georges A (1971/72) Influence de la séquence sur les aptitudes intellectuelles. Bull Institut National d'Etude du Travail et d'Orientation Professionelle 27:39–49

Gerard HB, Rabbie JM (1961) Fear and social comparison. J Abnorm Psychol 62:586–592

Getzels JW, Walsh JJ (1958) The method of paired direct and projective questionnaires in the study of attitude structure and socialization. Psychol Monogr 27: whole No 454

Gewirtz JL (1948) Dependent and aggressive interaction in young children. Ph.D. thesis, State University of Iowa

Gewirtz JL, Gewirtz HB (1969) Stimulus condition, infant behaviors and social learning. In: Foss BM (ed) Determinants of infant behavior III. Methuen, London, pp 161–184

Ghodsian M, Fogelman K, Lambert L (1980) Changes in behaviour ratings in a national sample of children. Br J Soc Clin Psychol 19:247–256

Gildea MCL, Glidewell JC, Kantor MB (1961) Maternal attitudes and general adjustment in school children. In: Glidewell JC (ed) Parental attitudes and child behavior. CC Thomas, Springfield, Ill, pp 42–89

Gill PE (1976) The relationship between mental ability and eight background variables. Scand J Educ Res 20:135–145

Gille H (1971) Summary review of fertility differentials in developped countries. Proceedings International Population Conference, vol III, London. IUSSP, Liège, pp 2011–2025

Gilmore JB, Zigler E (1964) Birth order and social reinforcer effectiveness in children. Child Dev 35:193–200

Glass DC, Horowitz M, Firestone I, Grinker J (1963) Birth order and reactions to frustration. J Abnorm Soc Psychol 66:192–194

Glass DC, Neulinger J, Brim jr OG (1974) Birth order, verbal intelligence, and educational aspiration. Child Dev 45:807–811

Glass DV (1970) Fertility trends in Europe since world war II. In: Behrman SJ, Corsa L, Freedman R (eds) Fertility and family planning, a world view. University of Michigan Press, pp 25–74

Glick PC (1975) A demographer looks at American families. J Marriage Family 37:15–26

Glueck S, Glueck ET (1950) Unraveling juvenile delinquency. Commonwealth Fund, New York

Gonda TA (1962) The relation between complaints of persistent pain and family size. J Neurol Neurosurg Psychiatry 25:277–281

* Goodman LA (1963) Some possible effects of birth control on the incidence of disorders and on the influence of birth order. Ann Hum Genet 27:41–52

Goodman N (1957) Relation between maternal age at parturition and incidence of mental disorder in the offspring. Br J Prev Soc Med 11:203–213

Gordon BF (1966) Influence and social comparison as motives for affiliation. J Exp Soc Psychol Suppl 1:55–65

Gorman I (1974) The relationship of mothers' achievement orientation to the academic achievement of her first and second born sons. Diss Abstr Int 34-B:5190–5191

Gormly R (1968) Birth order, family size and psychological masculinity-femininity. Proc 76th Annu Conv APA, vol 3. American Psychological Association, Washington, DC, pp 165–166

Grabill WH, Davidson M (1968) Recent trends in child spacing among American women. Demography 5:212–225

Grabill WH, Kiser CV, Whelpton PK (1958) The fertility of American women. Census Monograph Series, John Wiley & Sons, New York; Chapman & Hall, London

Grant MW (1964) Rate of growth in relation to birth rank and family size. Br J Prev Soc Med 18:35–42

Granville-Grossman KL (1966a) Parental age and schizophrenia. Br J Psychiatry 112:899–905

Granville-Grossman KL (1966b) Birth order and schizophrenia. Br J Psychiatry 112:1119–1126

Granville-Grossman KL (1968) The early environment in affective disorder. Br J Psychiatry, Special publication No 2, 65–79

Gray E, Morgan DK (1976) Desired family size and sex of children. J Hered 67:319–321

Greenberg H, Guerino R, Lashen M, Mayer D, Piskowski D (1963) Order of birth as determinant of personality and attitudinal characteristics. J Soc Psychol 60:221–230

Greenberg RA, White C (1967) The sexes of consecutive sibs in human sibships. Hum Biol 39:374–404
Greene RL, Clark JR (1968) Birth order and college attendence in a cross-cultural setting. J Soc Psychol 75:289–290
Greene RL, Clark JR (1970) Adler's theory of birth order. Psychol Rep 26:387–390
Greenwood M, Yule GU (1914) On the determination of size of family and of the distribution of characteristics in order of birth from samples taken through members of the sibships. J Roy Statist Soc 77:179–199
Greer BG, Whithley C (1971) The relationship between birth order and learning disabilities. Except Child 37:608–613
Gregory I (1958) Family size and birth order. An analysis of familial data on psychiatric patients. Br J Prev Soc Med 12:42–59
Gregory I (1959) An analysis of family data on 1,000 patients admitted to a Canadian mental hospital. Acta Genet, Basel, 9:54–96
Gregory I (1960) Family data concerning the hypothesis of hereditary predisposition toward alcoholism. J Ment Sci 106:1068–1072
Gregory I (1962) Selected personal and family data on 400 psychiatric in-patients. Am J Psychiatry 119:397–403
Gregory I (1965) Alcoholism, family size and ordinal position. Can Psychiat Ass J 10:134–140
Griffith J (1973) Social pressure on family size intentions. Fam Plann Perspect 5:237–242
Grignard B (1974) Dimension des familles et intelligence des enfants. Ann Faculté de Droit, Liège, 19:57–137
Grossman JC (1974) Birth order, sex, authorotarianism, selfreported hostility and the projection of aggression into TAT cards rated at three levels of hostile relevance. Diss Abstr Int 34-B:3497
Grossman JC, Eisenman R (1972) Birth order, authorianism, and the projection of sex and aggression. J Psychol 80:3–8
Grosz HJ (1964) Birth order, anxiety and affiliative tendency: Observations and comments regarding Schachter's hypothesis. J Nerv Ment Dis 139:588–590
Grosz HJ (1968) The depression-prone and the depression-resistant sibling. Br J Psychiatry 114:1555–1558
Grosz HJ, Miller I (1958) Sibling patterns in schizophrenia. Science 128:30
Grotevant HD (1978) Sibling constellations and sex typing of interests in adolescence. Child Dev 49:540–542
Grotevant HD, Scarr S, Weinberg RA (1977) Intellectual development in family constellations with natural and adopted children. Child Dev 48:1699–1703
Guilford RB, Worcester DA (1930) A comparative study of the only and non-only child. J Genet Psychol 38:411–426
Gunderson EKE, Arthur RJ (1968) Prognostic indicators in psychosis and neurosis. J Abnorm Psychol 73:468–473
Gunderson MM (1969) Relationships between expressed personality needs and social background and military status variables. J Psychol 71:217–224
Gundlach RH (1972) Data on the relation of birth order and sex of siblings of lesbians oppose the hypothesis that homosexuality is genetic. Ann NY Acad Sci 197:179–181
Gundlach RH (1977) Birth order among lesbians: New light on an only child. Psychol Rep 40:250
Gundlach RH, Riess BF (1967) Birth order and sex of siblings in a sample of lesbians and non-lesbians. Psychol Rep 20:61–62
Gustin MS (1972) An educational consideration of siblings ordinal position with personality and achievement dimensions. Diss Abstr Int 32-A:3786–3787
Haeberle A (1958) Interactions of sex, birth order and dependency with behavior problems and symptoms in emotionally disturbed preschool children. Unpublished paper, read at East Psychol Ass, Philadelphia. In: Clausen et al. (1965); see above.
Haldane JH, Haider I (1967) Attempted suicide in children and adolescents. Br J Clin Pract 21:587–591
* Haldane JBS, Smith CAB (1948) A simple exact test for birth-order effect. Ann. Eugen 14:117–124
Hall E (1963 a) Psychological correlates of ordinal position in the two-child Family. Ph.D. dissertation, University of Florida. Diss Abstr Int 24:2116–2117 (1964)
Hall E (1965) Ordinal position and success in engagement and marriage. J Individ Psychol 21:154–158
Hall E, Barger B (1964) Attitudinal structures of older and younger siblings. J Individ Psychol 20:59–68

Hall JR, Beil-Warner D (1977) Ordinal position, family size, and assertiveness. Psychol Rep 40:1083–1088

Hall RL (1963 b) The educational influence of dormitory roommates. Sociometry 26:294–318

Hallgren B, Sjögren T (1959) A clinical and genetico-statistical study of schizophrenia and lower grade mental deficiency in a large Swedish rural population. Acta Psych Neurol Scand Suppl 35:140

* Halperin M (1953) The use of X^2 in testing effects of birth order. Ann Eugen, Londen, 18:99

Hamid PN (1970) Birth order and family schemata. Percept Mot Skills 31:807–810

Hamilton M (1950) The personality of dyspeptics. Br J Med Psychol 23:182–198

Hancock FT (1967) An empirical investigation of the relationship of ordinal position, sex, and sex of sibling to socialization, personality, and choice behavior among adolescents in one- and two-child families. Diss Abstr Int 28-A:781–782

Hansen HA, Teilmann KA (1954) A treatment of criminal alcoholics in Denmark. Q J Stud Alcohol 15:246–287

Hansson RO (1974) The effects of test anxiety, birth order, and a confident or anxious role enactment on intellective task performance. Diss Abstr Int 34-B:4019–4020

Hansson RO, Chernovetz ME, Jones WH, Stortz S (1978) Birth order and responsibility in natural settings. J Soc Psych 105:307–308

Hansson RO, Jones WH, Chernovetz ME (1977) Birth order and political awareness. J Soc Psychol 102:151–152

Hardy RC (1972) A developmental study of relationship between birth order and leadership style for two distinctly different American groups. J Soc Psychol 87:147–148

Hardy RC, Hunt J, Lehr E (1978) Relationship between birth order and leadership style for nursery school children. Percept Mot Skills 46:184–186

* Hare EH (1967) Associations: Important or trivial. Int J Psychiatry 3:537–538

* Hare EH (1974) A note on the distribution of family sizes in the adult population of Great Britain 1972. J Biosoc Sci 6:343–346

* Hare EH, Lyster RW (1980) Sex ratio of siblings of psychiatric patients. Biol Psychiatry 15:495–498

* Hare EH, Moran PA (1979 a) Raised parental age in psychiatric patients: Evidence for the constitutional hypothesis. Br J Psychiatry 134:169–177

* Hare EH, Moran PA (1979 b) Parental age and birth order in homosexual patients: A replication of Slater's study. Br J Psychiatry 134:178–182

* Hare EH, Price JS (1969) Birth order and family size: Bias caused by changes in birth rate. Br J Psychiatry 115:647–657

* Hare EH, Price JS (1970 a) Birth rank in schizophrenia: With a consideration of the bias due to changes in birth rate. Br J Psychiatry 116:409–420

* Hare EH, Price JS (1970 b) Birth rank and schizophrenia. Nature, London, 228:1223–1224

* Hare EH, Price JS (1974) Birth order and birth rate bias: findings in a representative sample of the adult population of Great Britain. J Biosoc Sci 6:139–150

Hare EH, Shaw GK (1965) A study in family health: Health in relation to family size. Br J Psychiatry 111:461–466

Hare RT, Hare AP (1968) Social correlates of autonomy for Nigerian University students. J Soc Psychol 76:163–168

Harlap S, Davies AM, Grover NB, Prywes R (1977) The Jerusalem perinatal study: The first decade. Isr J Med Sci 13:1073–1091

Harris ID (1961) Emotional blocks to learning. Free Press of Glencoe, New York, pp 178–181

Harris ID (1964) The promised seed. A comparative study of eminent first and later sons. Free Press of Glencoe, New York

Harris ID, Howard KI (1968) Birth order and responsibility. J Marriage Family 30:427–432

Hartnett JJ (1971) Some neglected aspects of group risk taking. Diss Abstr Int 32-A:535–536

Harwood BT (1973) Expressed preferences for information seeking behaviors and their relationship to birth order. J Genet Psychol 123/1st half:123–132

Hau TF (1962) Zur Psychodynamik neurotischer Rententendenzen. Psychol Rundsch 13:208–213

Hau TF, Rüpell A (1966) Zur Familienkonstellation bei psychosomatisch Erkrankten. Z Psychother Med Psychol 16:211–219

Hawkes GR, Burchinal L, Gardner B (1958) Size of family and adjustment of children. J Marriage Family 20:65–68

Hawthorn G, Paddon M (1971) Work, family and fertility. Hum Relat, London, 24:611–628

Hayden DJ (1973) Trait oppositeness in siblings. Diss Abstr Int 33-B:3285

Hayes RF, Bronzaft AL (1979) Birth order and related variables in an academic elite sample. J Individ Psychol 35:214–244

Haywood CH jr (1969) Individual differences in reaction to psychological stress. Diss Abstr Int 29-B:3912

Heilbrun AB jr, Fromme DK (1965) Parental identification of late adolescence and level of adjustment. J Genet Psychol 107:49–59

Helmreich RL (1968) Birth order effects. Nav Res Rev 1–6, Off. Nav. Res.

Helmreich RL, Collings BE (1967) Situational determinants of affiliative preference under stress. J Pers Soc Psychol 6:79–85

Helmreich R, Kuiken D, Collinns B (1968) Effects of stress and birth order on attitude change. J Personality 36:466–473

Helson R, Crutchfield RS (1970) Mathematicians: The creative researcher and the average PhD. J Consult Clin Psychol 34:250–257

Hendershot GE (1969) Familial satisfaction, birth order, and fertility values. J Marriage Family 31:27–33

Hendrick C, Borden R (1970) Effects of extraneous fear arousal and birth order on attitude change. Psychonom Sci 18:225–226

Henry AF (1957) Sibling structure and perception of the disciplinary role of parents. Sociometry 20:67–85

* Hermalin AJ (1967) Birth order and college attendance; a comment. J Marriage Family 29:417–421

Herrell JM (1969) Birth order as a patient variable in combat zone psychiatry. USARV Med Bull Nov/Dec: 29–34

Herrell JM (1970) Birth order as a patient variable in military psychiatry. Milit Med 135:1001–1006

Herrell JM (1972) Birth order and the military: A review from an Adlerian perspective. J Individ Psychol 28:38–44

* Herrmann T (1969) Lehrbuch der empirischen Persönlichkeitsforschung, vol III. Hogrefe, Göttingen, p 363

Hess KE (1971) Ordinal position and acceptance of conventional morality. Diss Abstr Int 32-A:1073

Hetherington EM, Feldman SE (1964) College cheating as a function of subject and situational variables. J Educ Psychol 55:212–218

Hicks RA, Elliott D, Garbesi L, Martin S (1979) Multiple birth risk factors and the distribution of handedness. Cortex, Varese, 15:135–137

Hicks RA, Evans EA, Pellegrini RJ (1978) Correlation between handedness and birth order. Percept Mot Skills 46:53–54

Hilgard ER, Lauer A (1959) Birth order and presence of live siblings as affecting susceptibility to hypnosis. Unpublished paper. In: Moore et al. (1964)

Hillinger F (1958) Introversion und Stellung in der Geschwisterreihe. Z Exp Angew Psychol 5:268–276

Hilton I (1967) Differences in the behavior of mothers toward first- and later-born children. J Pers Soc Psychol 7:282–290

Himmelweit HT (1948) Intelligence and size of family. Their relationship in an adult group of high educational standard. Eugen Rev 40:77–84

Hines GH (1973) Birth order and relative effectiveness of social and nonsocial reinforces. Percept Mot Skills 36:35–38

Hinshelwood RD (1968) Schizophrenic birth order: The last but one positon. Nature 220:490

Hinshelwood RD (1970) The evidence for a birth order factor in schizophrenia. Br J Psychiatry 117.293–301

Hinshelwood RD (1972a) Schizophrenia and family function: I. Aspects of birth order. Br J Soc Psychiat Community Health 6:90–94

Hinshelwood RD (1972b) Schizophrenia and family function: II. Birth order and sources of tension. Br J Soc Psychiat Community Health 6:95–102

Ho DY (1979) Sibship variables as determinants of intellectual-academic ability in Hong Kong pupils. Genet Psychol Monogr 100:21–39

Hodapp AP, Lavoie JC (1976) Imitation by second borns in adultsibling dyads. Genet Psychol Monogr 93:113–128

Hodges A, Balow B (1961) Learning disability in relation to family constellation. J Educ Res 55:41–42

Hoffmann JA, Teyber EC (1979) Some relationships between sibling age spacing and personality. Merrill-Palmer Q 25:77–80
Hollender JW, Duke MP, Nowicki S (1973) Interpersonal distance: Sibling structure and parental affection to antecedents. J Genet Psychol 123:35–45
Hollinger CL (1976) The effects of student dependency, sex, birth order and teacher control ideology on teacher-student interaction. Diss Abstr Int 37-A:883
Hollingshead AB, Redlich FC (1958) Social class and mental illness: A community study. John Wiley & Sons, New York
Hooke R (1966) Birth order and achievement. Science 152:1177–1178
Hooker HF (1931) A study of the only child at school. J Genet Psychol 39:122–126
Horn JM, Turner RG (1975) Birthorder effects among unwed mothers. J Individ Psychol 31:71–78
Hornbostel LK, McCall JN (1980) Sibling differences in need achievement. J Individ Psychol 36:36–43
Horton AM (1977) Prediction of recidivism of adult male offenders by birth order and family size. Diss Abstr Int 37-B:3612
Horton AM, Medley DM (1978) Prediction of recidivism in a criminal population by birth order and family size. Psychol Rep 42:27–30
Horton AM, Whitesell LJ (1979) Prediction of recidivism by sex and number of siblings. Psychol Rep 45:98
Howe MG, Madgett ME (1975) Mental health problems associated with the only child. Can J Psychiatry 20:189–194
Howell FM, Malone LC (1979) Comment on Kunz and Peterson "Family size, birth order, and academic achievement". Soc Biol 26:80–84
Howells WW (1948) Birth order and body size. Am J Phys Anthropol 6:449–460 (new series)
Hoyt MF, Raven BH (1973) Birth order and the 1971 Los Angeles earthquake. J Pers Soc Psychol 28:123–128
Hreshko JL (1977) Antecedents of locus of control among young urban males. Diss Abstr Int 37-B:5354–5355
Hsaio-Hung H (1931) The status of the first-born with special reference to intelligence. Genet Psychol Monogr 9:1–118
Huback J (1957) Wives who went to college. Heinemann, London
Hubbard JI (1971) Handedness not a function of birth order. Nature 232:276–277
Hunt JM (1966) Intelligence and experience. Ronald, New York
Husaini BA, Neff JA (1981) The role of life change events and locus of control. J Nerv Ment Dis 169:638–647
Husén T (1960) Abilities of twins. Scand J Psychol 1:125–135
Iammarino NK (1975) Relationship between death anxiety and demographic variables. Psychol Rep 37:262
Ikemi Y, Ago Y, Nakagawa S, Mori S, Takahashi N, Suematsu H, Sugita M, Matsubara H (1974) Psychosomatic mechanism under social changes in Japan. J Psychosom Res 18:15–24
Illsley R (1967) Family growth and its effect on the relationship between obstetric factors and child functioning. In: Platt L, Parkes AS (eds) Social and genetic influences on life and death. Oliver Boyd, Edinburgh London, pp 29–42
Inbar M, Adler C (1976) The vulnerable age: A serendipitous finding. Sociol of Educ 49:193–200
Ingham HV (1949/50) A statistical study of family relationship in psychoneurosis. Am J Psychiatry 106:91–98
Innes JM, Sambrooks JE (1969) Paired-associate learning as influenced by birth order and the presence of others. Psychonom Sci 16:109–110
Institut national des études démographiques (1954) Le niveau intellectuel des enfants d'âge scolaire, vol 23, Presses Universitaires de France
* Irish DP (1964) Sibling interaction: A neglected aspect in family life research. Soc Forces 42:279–288
Irvin MG (1974) Self, mother and teacher perceptions of the child as related to academic readiness, sex, and sibling position in the family. Diss Abstr Int 34-A:7045–7046
Jackson TT, McGlynn RP (1977) Effect of birth order and perceived stress on social schemata. Percept Mot Skills 44:747–752
Jacobs BS, Moss HA (1976) Birth order and sex of siblings as determinants of mother-infant interaction. Child Dev 47:315–322

Jacoby J (1967) Situational anxiety and birth order as determinants of dogmatism and authoritarianism. Diss Abstr Int 27-A:4338–4339

Jacoby J (1968) Birth rank and preexperimental anxiety. J Soc Psychol 76:9–11

James WH (1969) Central nervous system malformation, still births, maternal age and birth order. Ann Hum Genet, London, 32:223–236

Jamieson BD (1969) The influences of birth order, family size and sex differences on risk-taking behavior. Br J Soc Clin Psychol 8:1–8

Janisch, RW (1973) The prediction of educational goals from selected variables. Diss Abstr Int 34-A:2301–2302

Jan-Tausch J (1963) Suicide of children, 1960–1963. Dept of Education, Trenton, NY

Jawa S (1973) Birth order and age related changes in anxiety among adolescents. Indian J Appl Psychol 10:6–11

Jayasekara R, Street J (1978) Parental age and parity in dyslexic boys. J Biosoc Sci 10:255–261

Jencks C (1972) Inequality. Basic Books, New York London

Jencks C (1979) Who gets ahead? The determinants of economic success in America. Basic Books, New York

Jensen AR (1974) Cumulative deficit: A testable hypothesis? Dev Psychol 10:996–1019

Joesting J, Joesting R (1973) Birth order and desired family size. J Individ Psychol 29:34–41

Joesting J, Joesting R (1975) Birth order and desired family size, a replication. J Individ Psychol 31:211–212

Johanson E (1958) A study of schizophrenia in the male. Acta Psych Neurol Scand Suppl 33:125

Johanson E (1968) Inmates of youth prisons compared with controls for family structure. Acta Psychiatr Scan 44:289–297

Johnson PB (1973 a) Birth order and Crowne-Marlowe social desirability scores. Psychol Rep 32:536

Johnson PB (1973 b) Birth order and college attendance Diss Abstr Int 33-A:3386

Jones AD, Seaborne AE (1974) Birth order and social class in a London college. Psychol Rep 35:467–468

Jones HE (1954) The environment and mental development. In: Carmichael L (ed) Manual of child Psychology. Wiley & Sons, New York

* Jones HE (1967) Order of birth. In: Handbook of child psychology, 2nd edn, vol 2. Russel & Russel, New York, pp 551–589

Jonsson G (1967) Delinquent boys, their parents and grandparents. Acta Psychiatr Scand Suppl 195:227–256, Appendix I

Jürgens HW (1967) Familiengröße und Bildungsweg der Kinder. Ein Beitrag zum ersten Familienbericht der Bundesregierung. Bundesministerium für Familie und Jugend, Bad Godesberg

Kaelber CT, Pugh TF (1969) Influence of intrauterine relations on the intelligence of twins. N Engl J Med 280:1030–1034

Kahn MH, Mahrer AR, Bornstein R (1972) Male psychosexual development: Role of sibling sex and ordinal position. J Genet Psychol 121:187–196

Kallmann FJ (1949) Zur Häufigkeit und psychopathologischen Motivierung des Selbstmordes bei Zwillingen und alleinigen Kindern Monatsschr Psychiatr Neurol 117:280–288

Kaltsounis B (1978) Creative performance among siblings of various ordinal birth position. Psychol Rep 42:915–918

Kamin L (1974) IQ and age confound. In: Kamin L (ed) Science and politics of IQ. John Wiley & Sons, London, pp 62–65

Kammeyer K (1966) Birth order and the feminine sex role among college women. Am Sociol Rev 31:508–515

Kammeyer K (1967 a) Sibling position and the feminine role. J Marriage Family 29:494–499

* Kammeyer K (1967 b) Birth order as a research variable. Soc Forces 46:71–80

Kanter HL (1971) Birth order, background factors, and teacher referral for emotional disturbance. Diss Abstr Int 31-A:3341–3342

Kanter VF (1970) A study of the relationship between birth order and achievement by overachieving early school starters and underachieving late school starters at the 6th grade level. Diss Abstr Int 31-A:70–71

Kaplan HB (1970) Self-derogation and childhood family structure. J Nerv Ment Dis 151:13–23

Karabenick SA (1971) On the relation between personality and birth order. Psychol Rep 28:258

Kardener SH, Fuller M (1972) The firstborn phenomenon among psychiatric residents. Am J Psychiatry 129:350–352

Kastrup M (1976) The prevalence of mental disturbances in preschool children. II. Social background and treatment (in Danish). Ugeskr Laeger 138:2391–2395

Katz CL (1973) Birth order and the effects of adult encouragement and discouragement to conformity to peers. Diss Abstr Int 33-B:5519

Katzenstein B (1957) Einfluß von Geschlecht, Lebensepoche und Stellung in der Geschwisterreihe auf das Aufsuchen einer psychologischen Beratungsstelle in Brasilien. Z Kinderpsychiatrie 24:42–48

Kayton L, Borge GF (1967) Birth order and the obsessive-compulsive character. Arch Gen Psychiatry 17:751–754

Keddie JAG (1958) The heights and weights of Scottish children of different socio-economic groups. I. Cross-sectional studies. Med Off 99:87–101

* Keeping ES (1952) The problem of birth ranks. Biometrics 6:112–119

Keetz M (1979) Social position and family correlates of study habits. J Psychol Res 23:150–153

Kellaghan T, MacNamara J (1972) Family correlates of verbal reasoning ability. Dev Psychol 7:49–53

Kellaghan T, Neumann E (1971) Background characteristics of children of high verbal ability. Irish J Educ 5:5–14

Kellock TD (1951) Childhood factors in duodenal ulcer. Br Med J ii:1117–1120

Kelsall RK, Poole A, Kuhn A (1972) Graduates; the sociology of an elite. Methuen, London

Kemper TD (1966) Mate selection and marital satisfaction according to sibling type of husband and wife. J Marriage Family 28:346–349

Kendrick C, Dunn J (1980) Caring for a second baby: Effects on interaction between mother and firstborn. Dev Psychol 16:303–311

Kennett KF (1973) Measured intelligence, family size and socio-economic status. Alberta J Educ Res 19:314–320

Kennett KF, Cropley AJ (1970) Intelligence, family size and socio-economic status. J Biosoc Sci 2:227–236

Kenyon FE (1968) Studies in female homosexuality. IV. Social and psychiatric aspects. Br J Psychiatry 114:1337–1343

Kilpatrick DG, Cauthen NR (1969) The relationship of ordinal position, dogmatism and personal sexual attitudes. J Psychol 73:115–120

Kimura S, Kagono Y, Harima Y et al. (1978) A contribution to the age-distribution and the birth order in schizophrenia and schizo-affective psychosis. J Kansai Med Univ 30 Suppl: 1–11

Kinard JE (1975) The effect of parental involvement on achievement of first and second siblings who have attended Head Start and follow through programs. Diss Abstr Int 35-A:5914

Kincaid D (1969) A study of highly gifted elementary pupils. Gifted Child Q 13:264–267

Kinsolving DL, Bone RN (1971) Firstborns, only children, sex and field independence. Psychol Rep 29:126

Kiølstad T (1964) Alcoholism among sailors. Norske Laegeforen 84:1243–1248

Kiser CV (1971) Educational differentials in fertility in relation to the demographic transition. Proceedings International Population Conference, vol III, London, IUSSP Liège, p 1926

Klebanoff HE (1976) Leadership: An investigation of its distribution in task-oriented small groups. Diss Abstr Int 36-B:3614

Kline P (1976) Psychological Testing. Malaby, London

Klockars AJ (1968) Relationships between personality dimensions and the familial variables of birth order, sex of siblings and family size. Diss Abstr Int 28-A:327

Ko Y, Sun K (1965) Ordinal position and the behavior of visiting the child guidance clinic. Acta Psychol Taiwanica 7:1016–1062

Koch HL (1954) The relation of "primary mental abilities" in five- and six-year olds to sex of child and characteristics of his sibling. Child Dev 25:209–223

Koch HL (1955a) Some Personality Correlates of sex, sibling position, and sex of sibling among five- and six-year-old children. Genet Psychol Monogr 52:3–50

Koch HL (1955b) The relation of certain family constellation characteristics and the attitudes of children toward adults. Child Dev 26:13–40

Koch HL (1956a) Sissiness and tomboyishness in relation to sibling characteristics. J Genet Psychol 88:231–244

Koch HL (1956b) Attitudes of young children toward their peers as related to certain characteristics of their siblings. Psychol Monogr 70:426

Koch HL (1956c) Children's work attitudes and sibling characteristics. Child Dev 27:289–310

Koch HL (1956d) Some emotional attitudes of the young child in relation to characteristics of his siblings. Child Dev 27:393–426

Koch HL (1956e) Sibling influence on children's speech. J Speech Dis 21:322–328

Koch HL (1957a) Der Einfluß der Geschwister auf die Persönlichkeitsentwicklung junger Knaben. Jb Psychol Psychother 5:211–225

Koch HL (1957b) The relation in young children between characteristics of their playmates and certain attributes of their siblings. Child Dev 28:175–202

Koch HL (1960a) Einige Ursachen von Eifersucht, Bewunderung, Ablehnung und von Überlegenheitsgefühlen, wie sie bei jüngeren Geschwistern auftreten. Psychol Beitr 4:38–53

Koch HL (1960b) The relation of certain formal attributes of siblings to attitudes held toward each other and toward their parents. Monogr Soc Res Child Dev 25(4):78

Koch HL (1966) Twins and twin relations. University of Chicago Press, Chicago London

Koenig F (1969) Definition of self and ordinal position of birth. J Soc Psychol 78:287–288

Kohn ML (1969) Class and conformity. A study in values. Dorsey, Homewood, Ill

Kohn ML, Schooler C (1969) Class, ocupation and orientation. Am Sociol Rev 34:659–678

Koller KM (1971) Parental deprivation, family background and female delinquency. Br J Psychiatry 118:319–327

Koller KM, Castanos JN (1969a) Family background and life situation in alcoholics. Arch Gen Psychiatry 21:602–610

Koller KM, Castanos JN (1969b) Parental deprivation and attempted suicide in prison populations. Med J Aust 1:858–861

Konig K (1963) Brothers and sisters. A study in child psychology. St George Books, Blanvelt, New York

Korté SD (1975) Student teacher performance as measured by a scale of observed teacher behaviors. Diss Abstr Int 35-A:4302

Kosugi Y, Tanaka M (1975) Parental deprivation, birth order and alcoholism. Jpn J Studies in Alcohol 10:70–77

Krauthamer CM (1974) The personality of alcoholic mothers and their children. Diss Abstr Int 34-B:5198

Kreutz H (1975a) Lernumwelt, intellektuelle Leistungsfähigkeit und Lernmotivation. In: Walter H (ed) Sozialisationsforschung, vol II. Fromann-Holzboog, Stuttgart, pp 131–146

Kreutz H (1975b) Die zeitliche Dimension von Sozialisationsumwelten. Schulbildung, Zukunftsbezug, Selbsteinschätzung und soziale Anpassung von Jugendlichen aus verschiedenen sozialen Schichten. In: Walter H (ed) Sozialisationsforschung, Problemata, vol III, Fromann-Holzboog, Stuttgart, pp 107–150

Krinsky SG (1963) The relationship amongst birth order, dimensions of independence – dependence and choice of a scientific career. In: Cooley WW (ed) Career development of scientists, an overlapping longitudinal study. Harvard University Grade School Educ, Cambridge, MA, pp 157–170

Krumboltz UB, Krumboltz JD (1958) Birth rank and family size: relationship to certain qualities of prospective teachers. J Teach Educ 9:171–178

Kunz PR (1965) The relation of income and fertility. J Marriage Family 27:509–513

Kunz PR, Peterson ET (1972) Family size and academic achievement. In: Bahr HM, Chadwick BA, Thomas DL (eds) Population, resources, and the future: Non-Malthusian perspectives. Brigham Young University Press, Provo, Utah, pp 159–173

Kunz PR, Peterson ET (1973) Family size and academic achievement of persons enrolled in high school and the university. Soc Biol 20: 454–459

Kunz PR, Peterson ET (1977) Family size, birth order, and academic achievement. Soc Biol 24:144–148

* Kushnir T (1978) A review of the evidence for birth order differences in anxiety and affiliation in stressful situations. Soc Behav Pers 6:179–186

Lahey BB, Hammer D, Crumrine PL, Forehand RL (1980) Birth order sex interactions in child behavior problems. Dev Psychol 16:608–615

Laitman RJ (1975) Family relations as an intervening variable in the relationship of birth order and self-esteem. Diss Abstr Int 36-B:3051

Lamke LK, Bell NJ, Murphy C (1980) Sibling constellation and androgynous sex role development. J Psychol 105:139–144

Landers DM (1970) Sibling-sex-status and ordinal position effects on females' sport participation and interests. J Soc Psychol 80:247–248

Landers DM, Martens R (1971) The influence of birth order and situational stress on motor performance. Psychonom Sci 24:165–167

Langenmayr A (1975a) Familiäre Umweltfaktoren und neurotische Struktur. Suppl 15 to Praxis der Kinderpsychologie und -psychiatrie. Vandenhock & Ruprecht, Göttingen, p 32

Langenmayr A (1975b) Geschwisterkonstellation und Neurosestruktur. Prax Kinderpsychol 24:41–46

Langenmayr A (1976) Family constellation and behavioral judgements in group dynamics. Gruppendynamik 7:46–60

Laniel Y, Chagnon G (1975) Rang de naissance et intelligence: Un effort méthodologique. Can Counsellor 10:20–24

Laosa LM, Brophy JE (1970) Sex birth order interaction in measures of sex typing and affiliation in kindergarten children. Proc 78th Annu Conv APA, vol 5. American Psychological Association, Washington DC, pp 363–364

Laosa LM, Brophy JE (1972) Effects of sex and birth order on sexrole development and intelligence among kindergarten children. Dev Psychol 6:409–415

Lapouse R, Monk MA (1964) Behavior deviations in a representative sample of children: Variation by sex, age, race, social class and family size. Am J Orthopsychiatry 34:436–446

Lasko JK (1954) Parent behavior toward first and second children. Genet Psychol Monogr 49:97–137

Latané B, Eckman J, Joy V (1966) Shared stress and interpersonal attraction. J Exp Soc Psychol Suppl 1:80–94

Lavoie JC (1973) Individual differences in resistance-to-temptation behavior in adolescents: An Eysenck analysis. J Clin Psychol 29:20–22

Lawler RH, Nakielny W, Wright NA (1963) Suicidal attempts in children. Can Med Ass J 89:751–754

Lawson A, Ingleby JD (1974) Daily routines of pre-school children: Effects of age, birth order, sex and social class, and developmental correlates. Psychol Med 4:399–415

Layman WA, Saueracker A (1978) Birth order and sibship size of medical school applicants. Soc Psychiatry 13:117–123

Lees JP (1952) The social mobility of a group of eldest born and intermediate adult males. Br J Psychol 43:210–221

Lees JP, Newson LJ (1954) Family or sibship position of some aspects of juvenile delinquency. Br J Delinq 5:46–55

Lees JP, Stewart AH (1957) Family or sibship position and scholastic ability: An interpretation. Soc Rev 5:173–189

Legg C, Sherick I, Wadland W (1974) Reaction of preschool children to the birth of a sibling. Child Psychiatry Hum Dev 5:3–39

Lehr U (1970) Die Familie im Sozialisationsprozeß. Gutachten erstattet dem Bundesministerium für Jugend, Familie und Gesundheit, Bonn

Lemay ML (1968) Birth order and college misconduct. J Individ Psychol 24:167–169

Lemay ML (1970) Birth order and scholastic aptitude and achievement. J Consult Clin Psychol 34:287

Lempp R (1967) Die Bedeutung der Situation in der Familie für Entstehung und Art psychischer Störungen im Kindesalter. Jb Jugendpsychiatrie 6:71–77

* Lenz W (1959) Der Einfluß des Alters der Eltern und der Geburtennummer auf angeborene pathologische Zustände beim Kind. Acta Genet, Basel, 9:169–201

Leonhard K (1976) Bedeutung von Geschwisterkonstellationen für die Entstehung systematischer Schizophrenien. Arch Psychiatr Nervenkr 222:27–45

Lerner SE, Linder RL (1975) Birth order and polydrug abuse among heroin addicts. J Drug Educ 5:285–291

Lessing EE, Oberlander M (1967a) Developmental study of ordinal position and personality adjustment of the child as evaluated by the California test of personality. J Pers 35:487–497

Lessing EE, Oberlander M (1967b) Ordinal position and childhood psychopathology as evaluated from four perspectives. Proc 75th Annu Conv APA, vol 2. American Psychological Association, Washington, DC, pp 179–180

Lessing EE, Oberlander M (1972) Birth order and personality adjustment as evaluated by the California test of personality and the IPAT children's personality questionnaire. Psychol Rep 31:23–27

Lester D (1966) Sibling position and suicidal behavior. J Individ Psychol 22:204–207

Lester D (1970) Suicide and sibling position. J Individ Psychol 26:203–204

Leventhal GS (1970) Influence of brothers and sisters on sex-role behavior. J Pers Soc Psychol 16:452–465

Levinger G (1965) Complementarity in marital adjustment: Rejoinder. J Individ Psychol 21:147–148

Levinger G, Sonnheim M (1965) Complementarity in marital adjustment: Reconsidering Toman's family constellation hypothesis. J Individ Psychol 21:137–145

Levinson P (1963) The relationship between birth order and reading ability. Diss Abstr Int 24:2614

Leviton A, Kilty T (1976) Birth order and left-handedness. Arch Neurol 33:664

Lewis BD (1975) Birth order and religiosity. Psychol Rep 37:809–810

Lewis BD (1976) Borth order, religiosity, college major, and attitudes toward women in the work force. Psychol Rep 39:993–994

Lewis M, Kreitzberg VS (1979) Effects of birth order and spacing on mother-infant interactions. Dev Psychol 15:617–625

Lichtenwalner JS, Maxwell JW (1969) The relationship of birth order and socioeconomic status to the creativity of preschool children. Child Dev 40:1241–1247

Lidberg L (1976) Family constellation and psychosexual disturbance. Acta Psychiatr Scand 54:125–130

Lilienfeld AM, Pasamanick BP (1956) The association of maternal and fetal factors with the development of mental deficiency. Am J Ment Defic 60:557–569

Lilliston L (1970) Birth order and schizophrenia. Schizophr Bull 3:40–42

Linarducci RP (1972) Birth order incidence among institutionalized drug addicts compared to national norms. J Drug Educ 2:297–302

Linder RL, Lerner SE (1972a) Self-medication: An only child syndrome? J Psychedelic Drug 5:62–66

Linder RL, Lerner SE (1972b) Self-medication and the only child. J Drug Educ 2:361–370

Linder RL, Lerner SE (1975/76) Birth order and psychoactive drug use among students. Drug Forum 5:1–3

Lindsay JSB (1971) Sex distribution in sibships. Aust NZ J Psychiatr 5:286–288

Lipset SM, Bendix R (1959) Social mobility in industrial society. University of California Press, Berkeley Los Angeles, pp 238–243

Lisansky ES (1957) Alcoholism in women; social, and psychological concomitants. I. Social history data. Q J Stud Alcohol 18:588–623

Ljungberg L (1957) Hysteria. A clinical, prognostic and genetic study. Acta Psychiatr Scand Suppl 32:112

Lloyd B, Archer J (1976) Exploring sex differences. Academic Press, London New York San Francisco

Lobl M, Welcher DW, Mellits ED (1971) Maternal age and intellectual functioning of offspring. Bull Johns Hopkins Hosp 128:347–361

Longstreth LE (1970) Birth order and avoidance of dangerous activities. Dev Psychol 2:154

Looft WR (1971) Conservatives, liberals, radicals, and sensation-seekers. Percept Mot Skills 32:98

Looft WR, Baranowski MD (1971) Birth order and complexity-simplicity. Percept Mot Skills 32:303–306

Lord CG, Veliger WF (1975) Effects of sex, birth order, target's relationship and target's sex on self-disclosure by college students. Psychol Rep 37:1167–1170

Lowe LH (1966) Families of children with early childhood schizophrenia. Arch Gen Psychiatry 14:26–30

* Loxton GE (1962) Birth rank and maternal age. Lancet i:271

Lubin B, Brady JP, Levitt EE (1962) Volunteers and non-volunteers for a hypnosis experiment. Dis Nerv Syst 23:642–643

Lukesch H (1976) Elterliche Erziehungsstile. Psychologische und soziologische Bedingungen. Kohlhammer, Stuttgart

Lunneborg PW (1968) Birth order, aptitude and achievement. J Consult Clin Psychol 32:101

Lunneborg PW (1971) Birth order and sex of sibling effects on intellectual abilities. J Consult Clin Psychol 37:445

Lunsford JE (1977) Factors related to the seriousness of offenses of juvenile law violators. Diss Abstr Int 37-A:5611

Luria AR, Yudovich FJ (1959) Speech and development of mental processes in the child. An experimental investigation. Staples, London

Macbeth BL (1975) Birth order, personality and scholastic aptitude. Thesis Dept Psychology, University of Oregon. Diss Abstr Int 36-B:4757 (1976)

Maccoby EE, Jacklin NE (1975) The psychology of sex differences. Stanford University Press, Stanford, pp 104–105

MacDonald AP jr (1967) Birth order effects in marriage and parenthood; affiliation and socialization. J Marriage Family 29:656–661

MacDonald AP jr (1969 a) Birth order and religious affiliation. Dev Psychol 1:628

MacDonald AP jr (1969 b) Manifestations of different levels of socialization by birth order. Dev psychol 1:485–492

MacDonald AP jr (1970) Anxiety, affiliation and social isolation. Dev Psychol 3:242–254

MacDonald AP jr (1971 a) Relation of birth order to morality types and attitudes toward the poor. Psychol Rep 29:732

MacDonald AP jr (1971 b) Birth order and personality. J Consult Clin Psychol 36:171–176

MacDonald AP jr (1972 a) Characteristics of volunteer subjects under three recruiting methods: Pay, extra credit and love of science. J Consult Clin Psychol 39:222–234

MacDonald AP jr (1972 b) Does required participation eliminate volunteer differences? Psychol Rep 31:153–154

MacFarlane JW, Allen L, Honzik MP (1954) A developmental study of the behavior problems of normal children between 21 months and 14 years. Child Dev 2

* MacMahon B, Pugh TF, Ipsen J (1960) Epidemiologic methods. Little, Brown, Boston Toronto; J & A Churchill, London p 187

* Magaud J, Henry L (1968) Le rang de naissance dans les phénomènes démographiques. Population, Paris, 23:879–920

Malzberg B (1950 a) Statistical aspects of mental deficiency, due to birth traumas. Am J Ment Defic 54:427–433

Malzberg B (1950 b) Statistical aspects of mental deficiency with congenital cerebral spastic infantile paralysis. Am J Ment Defic 55:99–104

Malzberg B (1973) Order of birth and size of family among epileptics. Acta Psychiatr Scand 49:341–352

Manaster G (1977) Birth order, an overview. J Individ Psychol 33:3–8

* Mantel N, Halperin M (1963) Analyses of birth-rank data. Biometrics 19:324–340

Marjoribanks K (1972) Environment, social class, and mental abilities. J Educ Psychol 63:103–109

Marjoribanks K (1976) Birth order, family environment, and mental abilities: A regression surface analysis. Psychol Rep 39:759–765

Marjoribanks K (1978) Birth order, age spacing between siblings and cognitive performance. Psychol Rep 42:115–123

Marjoribanks K (1979) Social attitudes: Social status and sibling constellation correlates. Psychol Rep 45:995–1000

Marjoribanks K, Walberg HJ (1975 a) Ordinal position, family environment, and mental abilities. J Soc Pschol 95:77–84

Marjoribanks K, Walberg HJ (1975 b) Birth order, family size, social class, and intelligence. Soc Biol 22:261–268

Marjoribanks K, Walberg HJ, Bargen M (1975 c) Mental abilities: Sibling constellations and social class correlates. Br J Soc Clin Psychol 14:109–116

Marks E (1972) Sex, birth order, and beliefs about personal power. Dev Psychol 6:184

Markus GB, Zajonc RB (1977) Family configuration and intellectual development: A simulation. Behav Sci 22:137–142

Marquette CH (1972) The birth order socialization hypothesis: A validation study. Diss Abstr Int 32-B:7317

Martensen-Larsen O (1956) Family constellation analysis and male alcoholism. Acta Psychiat Scand Suppl 106:241–247

Martensen-Larsen O (1957) The family constellation analysis and alcoholism. Acta Genet Statist Med 7:441–444

Martensen-Larsen O (1963) Kann der Unterschied in der Familienkonstellation der Alkoholiker, Epileptiker und Schizophrenen psychodynamische Ursachen enthüllen? Acta Psychiatr Scand 39 Suppl 169:193–196

Mascie-Taylor CG (1980) Family size, birth order and IQ components: A survey of a Cambridge suburb. J Biosoc Sci 12:309–312

Masling J (1965) Birth order and the need for affiliation. Psychol Rep 16:631–632
Masling J, Weiss L, Rothschild B (1968) Relationships of oral imagery to yielding behavior and birth order. J Consult Clin Psychol 32:89–91
Maslow AH, Sakoda JM (1952) Volunteer error in the Kinsky study. J Abnorm Soc Psychol 47:259–63
Masterson ML (1971) Family structure variables and need approval. J Consult Clin Psychol 36:12–13
Matejcek Z, Dytrych Z, Schüller V (1978) The Prague study of children from unwanted pregnancies. Int J Ment Health 7:63–77
Mathews KE jr (1973) Helping behavior in crisis intervention as a function of the severity of the crises and the helper's empathy and birth order. Diss Abstr Int 33-A:4530
Matheny AP jr, Brown AM (1971) The behavior of twins: Effects of birth weight and birth sequence. Child Dev 42:251–257
Mauco G, Rambaud P (1951) Le rang de l'enfant dans la famille. Rev Franc Psychanal 15:253–260
Maxwell J (1961) The level and trend of national intelligence. Publications of the Scottish Council for Research in Education 46. University of London Press, London
Maxwell J (1969 a) Sixteen years on: A follow-up of the 1947 Scottish survey. University of London Press, London
Maxwell J (1969 b) Intelligence, education and fertility: A comparison between the 1932 and 1947 Scottish surveys. J Biosoc Sci 1:247–271
Maxwell J, Pilliner AEG (1960) The intellectual resemblance between sibs. Ann Hum Genet, London, 24:23–32
May JC (1978) The relationship between locus of control, achievement, and demographic variables among Blacks in a personalized instructional program. Diss Abstr Int 39:1398–1399
McAllister P, Shannon-Stockes C, Knapp M (1974) Size of family of orientation, birth order, and fertility values. J Marriage Family 36:337–342
McArthur C (1956) Personalities of first and second children. Psychiatry 19:47–54
* McCall JN (1973) Birth order differences in special ability: Fact or artifact? Psychol Rep 33:947–952
* McCall JN (1980) Limitations of the single age sample for research on birth order. Percept Mot Skills 51:831–837
* McCall JN, Johnson OG (1972) The independence of intelligence from family size and birth order. J Genet Psychol 121:207–213
McCall RB (1970) Intelligence quotient pattern over age: Comparisons among siblings and parent-child pairs. Science 170:644–648
McClure RF (1969) Birth order and school related attitudes. Psychol Rep 25:657–658
McClure RF (1971) Birth order, income, sex, and school related attitudes. J Exp Educ 39:73–74
McCormick K, Baer DJ (1975) Birth order, sex of subject and sex of siblings as factors in extraversion and neuroticism in two-child families. Psychol Rep 37:259–261
McCutcheon LE (1974) Birth order and selected student characteristics. Catalogue of selected documents. Psychol Rep 4:44–45
McCutcheon LE (1977) Dumber by the dozen? Not necessarily! Psychol Rep 40:109–110
McCutcheon LE, Sweet M (1976) Birth order of volunteers under varying conditions of recruitment incentive. Psychol Rep 38:431–436
McDonagh JM (1971) The relationship between familial characteristics and two measures of dependency. Diss Abstr Int 32-B:542
McDonald A (1964) Intelligence of children of very low birth weight. Br J Prev Soc Med 18:59–74
McGervey JD (1966) Birth order and achievement. Science 152:1178–1181
McGlynn FD (1969) Academic performance among first-born students. J Individ Psychol 25:181–182
McGurk H, Lewis M (1972) Birth order: A phenomenon in search of an explanation. Dev Psychol 7:366
McKeithen JE (1965) Patterns of motivation as related to ordinal position in the family. Diss Abstr Int 25:4845–4846
McKeown T (1970) Prenatal and early postnatal influences on measured intelligence. Br Med J iii:63–67
* McKeown T, Record RG (1956) Maternal age and birth order as indices of environmental influences. Am J Hum Genet 8:8–23
McKeown T, Record RG (1971) Early environmental influences on the development of intelligence. Br Med Bull 27:48–52
McKissack IJ (1974) A less delinquent cohort. Br J Criminol 14:158–164
McPherson BD (1978) Success in sport: The influence of sociological parameters. Can J Appl Sport Sci 3:51–59

Mealiea WL, Farley FH (1973) The relationship between ordinal position in females and the expression of extreme fear. J Soc Psychol 90:333–334
Mechanic D (1966) Response factors in illness: The study of illness behavior. Soc Psychiatry 1:11–20
Medawar PB (1959) The future of man: Intelligence and fertility. Listener 62:1067–1069
Mehta PH, Juneja S (1969) Birth order, vocational preference and vocational expectation. Indian J Psychol 44:57–70
Meiners GA (1975) Geschwisterkonstellation and psychosomatische Krankheit im Erwachsenenalter. Med Dissertation, Freiburg i. Breisgau
Melican GJ (1978) The effects of age spacing to next-younger and age-spacing to next-older on academic achievement. Diss Abstr Int 39.3535
Mendelsohn MB (1973) Successful heterosexual pairing, sibling configuration and social expectancy. Diss Abstr Int 33:4521
Mendelsohn MB, Linden J, Gruen G, Curran J (1974) Heterosexual pairing and sibling configuraton. J Individ Psychol 30:202–210
Mentzos, Knödler, Pittrich (1972) Die Stellung in der Geschwisterreihe als Umweltfaktor in der Pathogenese endogener Psychosen. Zbl Ges Neurol Psychiatrie 204:119–120
Meredith HV (1950) Birth order and body size. Am J Phys Anthropol 8:195–224 (new series)
* Miley CH (1969) Birth order research 1963–1967: Bibliography and index. J Individ Psychol 25:64–70
Miller N, Maruyama G (1976) Ordinal position and peer popularity. J Pers Soc Psychol 33:123–131
Miller N, Zimbardo PG (1966) Motives for fear-induced affiliation. Emotional comparison as interpersonal similarity? J Personality 34:481–503
Millis J, Seng YP (1954) The effect of age and parity of the mother on birth weight of the offspring. Ann Hum Genet 19:58–73
Misovich S (1973) Birth order, affiliation, and membership in weight watchers. Psychol Rep 32:94
Misra SL (1969) Effect of birth order, education and rank status on insecurity. Psychol Ann 3:17–19
Mitchell S (1965) A study of the mental health of school children in an English country. Ph. D. thesis, London University, London
Monson RG, Gorman B (1976) Sibling set composition and female occupational achievement. Sociol Symp 15:65–79
Montagu MFA (1948) Sex, order of birth and personality. Am J Orthopsychiatry 18:351–353
Montgomery RL, Puetz L, Montgomery SM (1975) Birth order, graduate school, and marriage. Psychol Rep 37:746
Moore NV, Evertson CM, Brophy JE (1974) Solitary play: Some functional reconsiderations. Dev Psychol 10:830–834
Moore RK (1964) Susceptibility to hypnosis and susceptibility to social influence. J Abnorm Soc Psychol 68:282–294
Moran G (1967) Ordinal position and approval motivation. J Consult Clin Psychol 31:319–320
Motlagh H (1968) Selected non-academic factors related to creativity. Diss Abstr Int 29-A:1453
Mueller-Oswald U, Ruppen R, Baumann U, Angst J (1973) Persönlichkeitaspekte jugendlicher Drogenkonsumenten. Arch Psychiat Nervenkr 217:207–222
Mukherjee K, Kundu S (1961) A study of birth order and family positions of the criminals. Indian J Psychol 36:127–132
Munro A (1966) Some familial and social factors in depressive illness. Br J Psychiatry 112:429
Munroe RL, Munroe RH (1971) Overrepresentation of firstborns in East African secondary schools. J Soc Psychol 84:151–152
Munz DC, Smouse AD, Letchworth G (1968) Achievement motivation and ordinal position of birth. Psychol Rep 23:175–180
Murdoch PHJ (1966) Birth order and age at marriage. Br J Soc Clin Psychol 5:24–29
Murdoch PHJ, Smith GF (1969) Birth order and affiliation. Br J Soc Clin Psychol 8:235–245
Murray C (1971) The effects of ordinal position on measured intelligence and peer acceptance in adolescence. Br J Soc Clin Psychol 10:221–227
Murrell SA (1974) Relationships of ordinal position and family size to psychosocial measures of delinquents. J Abnorm Child Psychol 2:39–46
Muzekari LH (1972) Birth order and social behavior among chronic schizophrenics. J Clin Psychol 28:483–484
Myers RC (1952) Biographical factors and academic achievement: An experimental investigation. Educ Psychol Measurements 12:415–426

Myrianthopoulos NC, Nichols PL, Broman SH (1976) Intellectual development of twins compared with singletons. Acta Genet Med Gemellol, Roma, 25:376–380

Nasanow ES (1976) Communicator adaptability as related to selfconcept, personal adjustment, social adjustment, and birth order in children. Diss Abstr Int 37-B:979–980

Nash JC (1970) The relationship of ordinal status to sex-role identity, father-identification and self-esteem amoung university males. Diss Abstr Int 31-A:1916

Natsis M (1977) The impact of family structure on self-esteem, alienation and hostility among college students. Diss Abstr Int 35-A:7422–7423

Navar I, Helmreich R (1971) Prior social setting, type of arousal, and birth order as determinants of affiliative preference for a working situation. Represent Res Soc Psychol 2:32–42

Navratil L (1956) Alkoholismus und Geburtennummer. Klin Wochenschr, Wien, 68:158–160

Navratil L (1959) On the etiology of alcoholism. Q J Stud Alcohol 20:236–244

Neetz VM (1974) Birth order and leadership in the elementary school: A cross-cultural study. J Soc Psychol 92:143–144

Neisser EG (1957) The eldest child. Harper, New York

Neligan GA, Prudham D (1976) Family factors affecting child development. Arch Dis Child 51:853–858

Newbert N (1969) A study of certain personality correlates of the middle child in a three-child family. Diss Abstr Int 29-A:4333–4334

Newcombe HB (1964) Screening for effects of maternal age and birth order in a register of handicapped children. Ann Hum Genet, London, 27:367–382

Newcombe HB (1965) Environmental versus genetic interpretations of birth-order effects. Eugen Q 12:90–101

Newcombe HB, Tavendale OG (1964) Maternal age and birth order correlations. Problems of distinguishing mutational from environmental components. Mutation Res 1:446–467

Newhouse RC (1974) Locus of control and birth order in school children. J Clin Psychol 30:364–365

Newhouse RC (1974) Reinforcement-responsibility differences in birth order, grade level, and sex of children in grades 4,5 and 6. Psychol Rep 34:699–705

Nichols RC (1964) Birth order and intelligence. Unpublished research, National Merit Scholarship Corporation, Evanston, Ill

Nichols RC (1968) Heredity, environment and school achievement. Meas Eval Guid 1:122–129

Nichols RC, Davis JA (1964) Characteristics of students of high academic aptitude. Pers Guid J 42:794–800

Nie NH (1975) SPSS: Statistical package for the social sciences. McGraw-Hill Book Company, New York

Nisbet JD (1953) Family environment and intelligence. Eugen Rev 45:31–40

Nisbet JD (1958) Intelligence and family size 1949–1956. Eugen Rev 49:201–202

Nisbet JD, Entwistle NJ (1967) Intelligence and family size 1949–1965. Br J Educ Psychol 37:188–193

Nisbet JD, Illesley R (1963) The influence of early puberty on test performance at age eleven. Br J Educ Psychol 33:169–176

Nisbet RD (1968) Birth order and participation in dangerous sports. J Pers Soc Psychol 8:351–353

Nisbett RE, Schachter S (1966) Cognitive manipulation of pain. J Exp Soc Psychol 2:227–236

Nishiura N, Takeuchi K (1967) A study of birth-rank-effect in schizophrenia and neurosis. In: Mitsuda H (ed) Clinical genetics in psychiatry. Igaku Shoin, Tokyo, pp 242–245

Nissen G (1971) Depressive Syndrome im Kindes- und Jugendalter, vol 4. Monogr Gesamtgeb Psychiatrie, Springer Verlag, Berlin

Norton A (1952) Incidence of neurosis related to maternal age and birth order. Br J Soc Med 6:253–258

Nowicki S (1967) Birth order and personality, some unexpected findings. Psychol Rep 21:265–267

Nowicki S jr (1971) Ordinal position, approval motivation, and interpersonal attraction. J Consult Clin Psychol 36:265–267

Nuttall EV, Nuttall RL (1971) Effect of size of family on parent-child relationships. Proc 79th Annu Conv APA, vol 6. American Psychological Association, Washington, DC, pp 267–268

Nuttall EV, Nuttall RL (1979) Child-spacing effects on intelligence, personality, and social competence. J Psychol 102:3–12

Nuttall EV, Nuttall RL, Polit D, Hunter JB (1976) The effects of family size, birth order, sibling separation and crowding on the academic achievement of boys and girls. Am Educ Res J 13:217–223

Nuttall RL, Smith DH, Nuttall EV (1970) Family background, parentchild relationships, and academic achievement among Puerto Rican junior and senior high school students. Proc 78th Annu Conv APA, vol 5, American Psychological Association, Washington, DC, pp 307–308

Nye FI, Carlson J, Garrett G (1970) Family size, interaction, affect and stress. J Marriage Family 32:216–226

Nystul MS (1974) The effects of birth order and sex on selfconcept. J Individ Psychol 30:211–215

Oberlander MI, Frauenfelder KJ, Heath H (1970) Ordinal position, sex of sibling, sex, and personal preferences in a group of eighteen-year-olds. J Consult Clin Psychol 35:122–125

Oberlander MI, Frauenfelder KJ, Heath H (1971) The relationship of ordinal position and sex to interest patterns. J Genet Psychol 119:29–36

Oberlander M, Jenkin N (1967) Birth order and academic achievement. J Individ Psychol 23:103[1]10

Oberlander M, Jenkin N, Houlihan K, Jackson J (1970) Family size and birth order as determinants of scholastic aptitude and achievement in a sample of 8th graders. J Consult Clin Psychol 34:19–21

Ohlson LE (1974) The effects of the female-based family and birth order on the ability to self-disclose. J Psychol 87:59–69

Oldman D, Bytheway B, Horobin G (1971) Family structure and educational achievement. J Biosoc Sci Suppl 3:81–91

Oliver LW (1975) The relationship of familial variables to career and homemaking orientation in college women. Diss Abstr Int 36-B:893

Olneck MR, Bills DB (1979) Family configuration and achievement: Effects of birth order and family size in a sample of brothers. Soc Psychol Q 42:135–148

Olsen GP (1969) Need for approval, expectancy set, and volunteering for psychological experiments. Diss Abstr Int 29-B:4382

Olson TD (1973) Family constellation as related to personality and achievement. Diss Abstr Int 33-B:5000–5001

Oscherwitz M, Krasnow SO, Moretti L (1968) The relationship of myocardal infarction to parental mortality and longevity. J Chron Dis 21:341–348

Osler SF, Cooke RE (1965) The biosocial basis of mental retardation. Johns Hopkins, Baltimore, Maryland

Osofsky JD, Oldfield S (1971) Children's effects on parental behavior: Mothers' and fathers' responses to dependent and independent child behaviors. Proc 79th Annu Conv APA, vol 6, American Psychological Association, Washington DC, pp 143–144

Otto W (1965) Family position and success in reading. Reading Teacher 19:119–123

Owens AG (1968) Some biographical correlates of assessed performance in small antarctic groups. Aust Mil Forces Res Rep 12-68:1–24

Owyang WN (1971) Ordinal position, frustration, and the expression of aggression. Diss Abstr Int 31-B:6243

Pacini A, Martinotti A (1975) Ordine di nascita ed alcoolismo. Lav Neuropsichiat 57:261–290

Padan-Eisenstark D (1972) Career women in Israel: Their birth order and their sibling groups' sex composition. J Marriage Family 34:552–556

Paffenbarger RS, Asnes DP (1966) Chronic disease in former college students. III. Precursors of suicide in early and middle life. Am J Publ Health 56:1026–1036

Paffenbarger RS, Thorne MC, Wing AL (1968) Chronic disease in former college students. VIII: Characteristics in youth predisposing to hypertension in later years. Am J Epidemiol 88:25–32

Page EB, Grandon GM (1979) Family configuration and mental ability: Two theories contrasted with US data. Am Educ Res J 16:257–272

Pakrasi K, Halder A (1971) Sex ratios and sex sequences of birth in India. J Biosoc Sci 3:377–387

Palmer RD (1966) Birth order and identification. J Consult Clin Psychol 30:129–135

Parker FB (1959) A comparison of the sex temperament of alcoholics and moderate drinkers. Am Sociol Rev 24:366–374

Parson ER (1978) The capacity for empathy: An investigation of the relationship between interpersonal sensitivity and patterning of psychological type as a function of race, sex, birth order, and other variables. Diss Abstr Int 39:1052

Parsons J (1977) The socialisation argument: The fallacy of the large family. In: Parsons J (ed) Population fallacies. Elek-Peberton, London, pp 74–96

Parsons KR (1978) Violence on the road. Dept Justice, Wellington, New Zealand

Payne DL (1971) Birth-order, personality and performance at the Air Force Academy. J Individ Psychol 27:185–187
Pearson K (1914) On the handicap of the first born. Eugen Lab Lect, ser No 10; Dulan, London
Pedersen DM (1973) Correlates of behavioral personal space. Psychol Rep 32:828–830
Penn JR (1973) Sibling position and the development of personal values. Psychology 10:40–43
* Pepper FC (1972) Birth Order. In: Nikelly AG (ed) Techniques for behavior change: Applications of Adlerian theory. CC Thomas, Springfield, Ill
Perkins MW (1978) On birth order among lesbians. Psychol Rep 43:814
Perris C (1966) A study of bipolar and unipolar manic-depressive psychosis. Acta Psychiatr Scand Suppl 194:15–44
Perry CJG (1965) Psychiatric selection of candidates for space missions. JAMA 194:841–844
Perry SL, Goldin GJ, Stotsky BA, Margolin RJ (1970) The rehabilitation of the alcohol dependent; an exploratory study. Heath, Lexington, MA
Peskin H, Giora Z, Kaffman M (1974) Birth order in child psychiatric referrals and kibbuz family structure. J Marriage Family 36:615–618
Peterson RA, Sharpe LK (1972) Effects of ordinal position: Tripartite analysis. Psychol Rep 30:890
Peterson M (1971) Birth order effects in juvenile patients with diabetes mellitus. Diss Abstr Int 31-B:5004
Petroni FA, Griffin C (1970) The influence of social class and family size on adult psychiatric outpatients. Bull Menninger Clin 34:148–160
* Peuckert R (1974) Zum Erkenntniswert empirischer Generalisierungen. Z Soziol 3:189–199
Pfouts JH (1980) Birth order, age-spacing, IQ differences, and family relations. J Marriage Family 42:517–531
Phatak P (1974) Mental development patterns during infancy and some related factors. Psychol Stud (Mysore University) 19:1–7
Phillips EL (1956) Cultural versus intrapsychic factors in childhood behavior problem referrals. J Clin Psychol 12:400–401
Piepmeier KB, Adkins TS (1973) The status of women and fertility. J Biosoc Sci 5:507–520
Pierce JV (1959) The educational motivation patterns of superior students who do and do not achieve in high school. US Office of Education, Dept Health, Education, Welfare, Washington, DC
Pinsky HJ (1974) The effect of sibling constellation on mateselection. Diss Abstr Int 35-B:3031–3032
Platt JJ, Eisenman R, DeGross E (1969) Birth order and sex differences in future time perspectives. Dev Psychol 1:70
Platt JJ, Moskalski DD, Eisenman R (1968) Sex and birth order, and future expectations of occupational status and salary. J Individ Psychol 24:170–173
Polirstok SR (1975) The relationship between birth order and reading ability in urban ninth grade junior high school students. Graduate Res Educ Relat Discip 8:68–97
* Poole A (1974) Bytheway's stastitical trap. J Biosoc Sci 6:73–74
Poole A, Kuhn A (1973) Family size and ordinal position: Correlates of academic success. J Biosoc Sci 5:51–59
Poor D (1967) The social psychology of questionnaires. Bachelor's thesis, Harvard College
Powers EA (1960) Children's adjustment to a sibling birth and its relations to ego functions. Diss Abstr Int 30:5B:2406
Prabhu GG, Ramachandran K (1973) Birth order and schizophrenia. Indian J Psychiatr 15:1–10
Prakash J, Srivastava PK (1963) The effect of family size, economic condition and order of birth on adolescent adjustment. Manas, Delhi, 10:83–88
Prasad Singh K (1972) Anxiety and birth order. J Psychol Res 16:64–66
* Price J (1969) Personality differences within families. Comparison of adult brothers and sisters. J Biosoc Sci 1:177–205
* Price JS, Hare EH (1969) Birth order studies: Some sources of bias. Br J Psychiatry 115:633–646
Purpura PA (1971) A study of the relations between birth-order, self-esteem and conformity. Diss Abstr Int 31-B:6266
Query WT, Query JM (1973) Birth order: Urban-rural effects on need affiliation and school activity participation among high school male students. J Soc Psychol 90:317–320
Racamato CP (1969) The relationship of birth order to seeking counseling. Diss Abstr Int 29-A:4294
Radloff R (1961) Opinion evaluation and affiliation. J Abnorm Soc Psychol 62:578–585
Rainwater L (1965) Family design. Marital sexuality, family size, and contraception. Aldine, Chicago

Ramey CT, Stedman DJ, Borders-Paterson A, Mengel W (1978) Predicting school failure from information available at birth. Am J Ment Def 82:525–534

Ranking RJ, Gaite AJH, Heiry T (1979) Cultural modification of effect of family size on intelligence. Psychol Rep 45:391–397

Rao BSS, Sundaraj N (1964) A preliminary report on the statistical and genetical survey of cases with schizophrenia and other mental disorder. Trans All-India Inst of Mental Health 4:33–36

Rao MSS (1969) Sibling position and mental disorders. Psychiatr Q Suppl 39:27–47

Rassidakis N, Kelepouris M, Sparros L, Trichopoulos D (1971) La relation de la schizophrénie avec l'ordre de la naissance des enfants selon leur sexe. Arch Un Méd Balkan 9:303

Rathod NH, Gregory E, Blows D, Thomas GH (1966) A two-year follow-up study of alcoholic patients. Br J Psychiatry 112:683–692

Ray RE, Walker CE (1973) Biographical and self-report correlates of female guilt responses to visual erotic stimuli. J Consult Clin Psychol 41:93–96

* Raychaudhuri AK (1956) Are the first born more susceptible to functional mental disease. J Nerv Ment Dis 124:478–486

Record RG, McKeown T, Edwads JH (1969) The relation of measured intelligence to birth order and maternal age. Ann Hum Genet 33:61–69

Record RG, McKeown T, Edwards JH (1969) The relation of measured intelligence to birth weight and duration of gestation. Ann Hum Genet, London, 33:71–79

Record RG, McKeown T, Edwards JH (1970) An investigation of the difference in measured intelligence between twins and single births. Ann Hum Genet, London, 34:11–20

Reddy NY (1967) A study of the relationship between ordinal position of adolescents and their adjustment. Psychol Studies 12:91–100

Reed EW (1971) Mental retardation and fertility. Soc Biol Suppl 18:42–49

Reed EW, Reed SC (1965) Mental retardation: A family study. WB Saunders, Philadelphia London

Rees AH, Palmer FH (1970) Factors related to change in mental test performance. Dev Psychol Monogr 3, No 2, part 2

Rehberg RA, Westby DL (1967) Parental encouragement, occupation, education, and family size: Artifactual or independent determinants of adolescents educational expectations. Soc Forces 45:362–374

Reighard PB, Johnson DT (1973) Effects of birth order and sex on field independence-dependence. Percept Mot Skills: 223–226

Reinhardt RF (1970) The outstanding jetpilot. Am J Psychiatry 127:732–736

Rhine WR (1968) Birth order differences in conformity and level of achievement arousal. Child Dev 39:987–996

Rhine WR (1969) Birth order differences in resistance to conformity pressure related to social class and level of achievement arousal. Proc 77th Annu Conv APA, vol 4. American Psychological Association, Washington, DC, pp 265–266

Rhine WR (1974) The relation of birth order, social class, and need achievement to independent judgment. J Soc Psychol 92:201–208

Richardson SK (1936) The correlation of intelligence quotients of siblings of the same chronological age levels. J Juv Res 20:186–198

Riess BF, Safer J (1973) Birth order and related variables in a large outpatient population. J Psychol 85:61–68

Rin H (1965) Family study of Chinese schizophrenic patients: Loss of parents, sibling rank, parental attitude and short-term prognosis. Transcul Psychiatr Res Rev 2:24–27

Ring K, Lipinski CE, Braginsky D (1965) The relationship of birth order to self-evaluation, anxiety reduction and susceptibility to emotional contagion. Psychol Monogr 79, No 603

Roach DA (1979) Effects of some social variables on field dependence. Percept Mot Skills 48:559–562

Roach DA (1980) Some social variables in conceptual style preference. Percept Mot Skills 50:452–454

Roach JL, Gurrslin O, Hunt RG (1958) Some social-psychological characteristics of a child guidance clinic caseload. J Consult Clin Psychol 22:183–186

Robbins LC (1963) The accuracy of parental recall of aspects of child development and of child rearing practices. J Abnorm Soc Psychol 66:261–270

Roberts CJ, Rowley JR (1972) A study of the association between quality of maternal care and infant development. Psychol Med 2:42–49

Roberts JAF (1947/48) Birth order, maternal age and intelligence. Br J Psychol 1:35–51

Robertson A (1971) Social class differences in the relationship between birth order and personality development. Soc Psychiatry 6:172–178

Robertson LS, Dotson LE (1969) Perceived parental expressivity, reaction to stress, and affiliation. J Pers Soc Psychol 12:229–234

Robins LN (1966) Deviant children grown up. Williams & Wilkins, Baltimore

Roe A (1953) A psychological study of eminent psychologists and anthropologists and a comparison with biological and physical scientists. Psychol Monogr, No 352

Romanoff JJS (1976) Birth order, family size, and sibling spacing as influences on intelligence and academic abilities of Jewish adolescents. Diss Abstr Int 37-A:2086–2087

Roodin PA (1971) Birth order and cooperativeness: Peer ratings. Psychol Rep 29:590

Roodin PA, Broughton A, Vaught GM (1974) Effects of birth order, sex, and family size on field dependence and locus of control. Percept Mot Skills 39:671–676

Roodin PA, Vaught GM (1972) Birth order and conservatism. Psychol Rep 31:814

Roodin PA, Broughton A, Vaught GM (1978) Birth order of volunteers for group and individual psychological experiments: A negative note. Psychol Rep 42:575–580

Roodin PA, Vaught GM (1974) Birth order, volunteering, and status of the experimenter: A negative note. J Psychol 87:119–122

Roost A (1976) A Q sort analysis of family ordinal position. Diss Abstr Int 37-B:443–444

Rosen BC (1961) Family structure and achievement motivation. Am Soc Rev 26: 574–585

Rosen BC (1964) Family structure and value transmission. Merrill-Palmer Q Behav Dev 10:59–76

Rosenberg BG, Sutton-Smith B (1964 a) The relationship of ordinal position and sibling sex status to cognitive abilities. Psychonomic Sci 1:81–82

Rosenberg BG, Sutton-Smith B (1964 b) ordinal position and sex role identification. Gen Psychol Monogr 70:297–328

Rosenberg BG, Sutton-Smith B (1968) Family interaction effects on masculinity-femininity. J Pers Soc Psychol 8:117–120

Rosenberg BG, Sutton-Smith B (1969) Sibling age spacing effects upon cognition. Dev Psychol 1:661–668

Rosenberg CM (1969) Determinants of psychiatric illness in young people. Br J Psychiatry 115:907–915

Rosenberg M (1965) Society and the adolescent self-image. Princeton University Press, Princeton, pp 107–127

Rosenberg PH, Latimer R (1966) Suicide attempts by children. Ment Hyg, New York, 50:354–359

Rosenblatt PC, Skoogberg EL (1974) Birth order in cross-cultural perspective. Dev Psychol 10:48–54

Rosenbluh ES, Haarman GB (1970) Birth order, need for achievement, college attendence and sociocultural learning. Psychology 7:8–13

Rosenfeld HM (1966) Relationships of ordinal position to affiliation and achievement motives: Direction and generality. J Personality 34:467–480

Rosenthal R, Rosnow RL (1975) The volunteer subject. John Wiley & Sons, New York, pp 25–30

Rosnow RL, Rosenthal R, McConochie RM, Arms RL (1969) Volunteer effects on experimental outcomes. Educ Psychol Measurement 29:825–846

Rossi AS (1965) Naming children in middle-class families. Am Soc Rev 30:499–513

Rothbart MK (1971) Birth order and mother-child interaction in an achievement situation. J Pers Soc Psychol 17:113–120

Rothbart MK, Maccoby EE (1966) Parents' differential reactions to sons and daughters. J Pers Soc Psychol 4:237–243

Rothbart M, Horner S, Yackley A (1970) Sibling configuration and interpersonal dominance. Proc 78th Ann Conv APA, vol 5. American Psychological Association, Washington, DC, pp 367–368

Roy A (1979) Hysteria: A case note study. Can J Psychiatry 24:157–160

Rubin KH, Hultsch DF, Peters DL (1971) Non-social speech in four-year-old children as a function of birth order and interpersonal situation. Merrill-Palmer Q 17:41–50

Ruch FL, Zimbardo PG (1975) Lehrbuch der Psychologie, Springer, Berlin Heidelberg New York, pp 342–343

Rückert GR (1976) Die Kinderzahl der Ehen in der Bundesrepublik Deutschland im Intergenerationenvergleich. Z Bevölkerungswiss 2:36–52

Ruesch J, Christiansen C, Harris RE, Dewes S, Jacobson A, Loeb M (1948) Duodenal ulcer. University of California Press, California

Ruff CF, Ayers JL, Templer DI (1975) Birth order and hysterical versus obsessive-compulsive continuum. Catal Select Docum Psychol 5:332

Ruppen R, Müller U, Baumann U, Angst J (1973) Zur Prüfung der Aussagegenauigkeit bei einer Befragung über Drogenkonsum. Z Präventivmed 18:173–181

Russell-Davis D (1962) Birth order and maternal age of homosexuals. Lancet i:540–541

Rutter M, Madge N (1976) Cycles of disadvantage. Heinemann, London

Rutter M, Tizard J, Whitmore K (eds) (1970) Education, health and behavior. Longman, London

Rutter M, Yule B, Quinton D, Rowlands O, Yule W, Berger M (1975) Attainment and adjustment in two geographical areas. Br J Psychiatry 126:520–533

* Ryder NB (1965) The cohort as a concept in the study of social change. Am Sociol Rev 30:843–861

Sagi PC (1959) A component analysis of birth intervals among two-child white couples in Metropolitan America. In: Thirty years of research in human fertility; retrospect and prospect. Papers presented at the 1958 annual conference of the Milbank Memorial Fund. Milbank Memorial Fund, New York, pp 135–148

Sampson EE (1962) Birth order, need achievement and conformity. J Abnorm Soc Psychol 64:155–159

* Sampson EE (1965) The study of ordinal position: Antecedents and outcomes. In: Maher B (ed) Progress in experimental personality research, vol 2. Academic Press, New York, pp 1–53

Sampson EE, Hancock FT (1967) An examination of the relationship between ordinal position, personality and conformity: An extension, replication, and partial verification. J Pers Soc Psychol 5:398–407

Sandler BE, Scalia FA (1975) The relationship between birth order, sex, and leadership in a religious organization. J Soc Psychol 95:279–280

Sandler PC, Sandler EH (1978) Schizophrenia and birth order. Arq Neuropsyquiatr 36:46–66

Sankar DV, Chuda R (1977) Birth order and family size in child mental health. Res Commun Psychol Psychiatr Behav 1:511–522

Sarason IG (1969) Birth order, test anxiety, and learning. J Personality 37:171–177

Sarason IG, Smith RE (1971) Personality. Ann Rev Psychol 22:393–446

Sarnoff I, Zimbardo PG (1961) Anxiety, fear, and social affiliation. J Abnorm Soc Psychol 62:356–363

Satz P (1973) Left-handedness and early brain insult: An Explanation. Neuropsychologia 11:115–117

Saunders M (1977) A review of studies of the socio-familiar background and educational facilities of the homes of moderately educational subnormal children. Child Care Health Dev 3:407–423

Scarr S, Weinberg RA (1979) Intellectual similarities in adoptive and biologically related families of adolescents. In: Willerman L, Turner RG (eds) Readings about individual and group differences. Freeman, San Francisco, pp 61–75

Scott EM, Nisbet JD (1955) Intelligence and family size in an adult sample. Eugen Rev 46:233–235

Scott JA (1962) Intelligence, physique, and family size. Br J Prev Soc Med 16:165–173

Scottish Council for Research in Education (1949) The trend of Scottish intelligence. A comparison of the 1947 and 1932 surveys of the intelligence of eleven-year-old pupils. London University Press, London

Scottish Council for Research in Education (1953) Social implications of the 1947 Scottish Mental Survey. University of London Press, London

Searleman A, Tsao YC, Balzer W (1980) A reexamination of the relationship between birth stress and handedness. Clin Neuropsychology 2:124–128

Sears PS (1951) Doll play aggression in normal young children: Influence of sex, age, sibling status, father's absence. Psychol Monogr 65:6 (whole No 323)

Sears RR (1950) Ordinal position in the family as a psychological variable. Am Sociol Rev 15:397–401

Sears RR (1961) Relation of early socialization experiences to aggression in middle childhood. J Abnorm Soc Psychol 63:466–492

Sears RR (1970) Relation of early socialization experiences to self-concepts and gender role in middle childhood. Child Dev 41:267–289

Sears RR, Maccoby EE, Levin H (1957) Patterns of child rearing. Row Peterson, Evanston, Ill

Sechrest I, Flores I (1969) Sibling position of Philippine psychiatric patients. J Soc Psychol 77:135–137

Sells SB, Roff M (1963) Peer acceptance-rejection and birth order. Am Psychologist 18:355

Sellwood RM (1975) Birth order and creativity. Diss Abstr Int 35-B:3598

Selvin S, Garfinkel J (1976) Paternal age, maternal age and birth order and the risk of a fetal loss. Hum Biol 48:223–230

* Senn MJE, Hartford C (1968) The firstborn. Harvard University Press, Cambridge, MA

Sethi BB, Gupta SC (1973) Sibling position in India. Psychiatric and nonpsychiatric patients. Am J Psychother 27:61–69

Shapiro AH (1974) Effects of family density and mothers' education on preschoolers motor skills. Percept Mot Skills 38:79–86

Shapiro S, Ross LJ (1965) Relationship of selected prenatal factors to pregnancy outcome and congenital anomalies. Am J Pub Health 55:268–282

Sharan S, Amir Y, Kowarsky J (1969) Birth order and level of task performance: A cross-cultural comparison. J Soc Psychol 78:157–163

Shaver P, French JR jr, Cobb S (1970) Birth order of medical students and the occupational ambitions of their parents. Int J Psychol 5:197–207

Sheldon PM (1954) The families of highly gifted children. J Marriage Family 16:59–60, 67

Sheldrake P, Cormack M (1976) Variation in menstrual cycle symptom reporting. J Psychosom Res 20:169–177

Sheldrake P, Cormack M, McGuire J (1976) Psychosomatic illness, birth order and intellectual preference. J Psychosom Res 20:37–49

Shepherd M, Oppenheim B, Mitchel S (1971) Childhood behavior and mental health. Grune & Stratton, New York

Sherman JA (1974) Field articulation, sex, spatial visualization, dependency, practice, laterality of the brain and birth order. Percept Mot Skills 38:1223–1235

Sherman SE (1971) Empathy, attraction, and birth order. Diss Abstr Int 32-B:2989–2990

Shrader WK, Leventhal T (1967) Birth order of children and parental report of problems. Child Dev 39:1164–1175

Shrivastava SS (1977) Creativity as related to birth order and number of siblings. Indian Psychol Rev 14:1–4

Shrivastava SS, Usha S (1977) The influence of ordinal position and school performance on the popularity of 7th, 8th and 9th grade children. Manas, Madras, India, 24:33–46

Sieber M, Angst J (1977) Zur Epidemiologie des Drogen-, Zigaretten- und Alkoholkonsums junger Männer. Schweiz Med Wochenschr 107:1912–1920

Sieber MF (1979) Social background, attitudes and personality in a three year follow-up study of alcohol consumers. Drug Alc Dep 4:407–417

Siegelman M (1973) Birth order and family size of homosexual men and women. J Consult Clin Psychol 41:164

Simon JL (1974) The effect of income on fertility. Monogr 19, Carolina Population Centre, Chapel Hill, NC

Simon JL (1975) The mixed effects on income upon successive births may explain the convergence phenomenon. Population Stud 29:109–122

Simon WE (1973) Ordinal position of birth in the family constellation and adult smoking behavior. J Soc Psychol 90:157–158

Simon WE, Primavera LH, Klein B, Cristal RM (1972) Personality and nonverbal rigidity: Some preliminary findings. J Psychol 82:127–132

Simon WE, Primavera LH, Simon MG, Orndoff RK (1974) A comparison of marijuana users and nonusers on a number of personality variables. J Consult Clin Psychol 42:917–918

Simon WE, Sands B, Forman MR (1971) Ordinal position of birth and perceived popularity for sixth graders. Percept Mot Skills 33:1097–1098

Simon WE, Wilde V (1971) Ordinal position of birth, field dependency and Forer's measure of gullibility. Percept Mot Skills 33:677–678

Sims A (1975) Factors predictive of outcome in neurosis. Br J Psychiatry 127:54–62

Singer E (1967) Birth order, educational aspirations, and educational attainment. Diss Abstr Int 27-A:2638

Singer E (1971) Adult orientation of first and later children. Sociometry 34:328–345

Singer JE (1964) The use of manipulative strategies: Machiavellianism and attractiveness. Sociometry 27:128–150

Singer JE, Lamb PF (1966) Social concern, body size, and birth order. J Soc Psychol 68:143–151

Singer JE, Shockley VL (1965) Ability and affiliation. J Pers Soc Psychol 1:95–100

Singh A (1978) A study of personality of truants. Indian J Clin Psychol 5:179–184

Sinha Jai BP (1967) Birth order and sex differences in n-achievement and n-affiliation. J Psychol Res 11:22–27

Skipper JK jr, McCaghy CH (1970) Stripteasers: The anatomy and career contingencies of a deviant occupation. Soc Probl 17:391–405
Skovholt T, Moore E, Wellman F (1973) Birth order and academic behavior in first grade. Psychol Rep 32:395–398
Slater E (1962) Birth order and maternal age of homosexuals. Lancet 13:69–71
Slavney PR, McHugh PR (1974) The hysterical personality: A controlled study. Arch Gen Psychiatry 30:325–329
Smart RG (1963 a) Alcoholism, birth order, and family size. J Abnorm Soc Psychol 66:17–23
Smart RG (1963 b) The relationship between birth order and alcoholism among women. Ontario Psychol Ass Q 16:10–16
* Smart RG (1964) A response to Sprott's "use of chi square". J Abnorm Soc Psychol 69:103–105
Smart RG (1965) Social-group membership, leadership, and birth order. J Soc Psychol 67:221–225
Smelser WT, Stewart LH (1968) Where are the siblings? A re-evaluation of the relationship between birth order and college attendance. Sociometry 31:294–303
Smith CB (1964) An investigation on the relationship between birth order and parental acceptance. Master's thesis, Brigham Young University
Smith CM (1965) Family size in alcoholism. J Abnorm Psychol 70:230
Smith CM, McIntyre S (1963) Family size, birth rank and ordinal position in psychiatric illness. Can Psychiatr Ass J 8:244–248
Smith TE, Goodchilds JD (1963) Some personality and behavioral factors related to birth order. J Appl Psychol 47:300–303
Smith TE (1971) Birth order, sibship size and social class as antecedents of adolescents' acceptance of parents' authority. Soc Forces 50:223–232
Snowdon J (1979) Family size and birth-order in obsessional neurosis. Acta Psychiatr Scand 60:121–128
Solomon D (1965) Birth order, family composition and teaching style. Psychol Rep 17:871–874
Solomon D, Hirsch JG, Scheinfeld DR, Jackson JC (1972) Family characteristics and elementary school achievement in an urban ghetto. J Consult Clin Psychol 39:462–466
Solomon F (1977) The influence of sibling position, family size and sex upon initial requests for mental health services. Diss Abstr Int 37-A:7550–7551
Solomon L, Nuttall R (1967) Sibling order, premorbid adjustment and remission in schizophrenia. J Nerv Ment Dis 144:37–46
Sonstegard M (1973) Life style identification and assessment. Individ Psychologist 10:1–4
Sontag LW, Baker CT, Nelson VL (1958) Mental growth and personality development: A longitudinal study. Monogr Soc Res Child Dev 23: No 2, serial No 68
* Spiegel JP, Bell NW (1959) The family of the psychiatric patient. In: Arieti S (ed) American handbook of psychiatry, vol 1, chap 5, Basic Books, New York, pp 114–149
* Sprott DA (1964) Use of chi square. J Abnorm Soc Psychol 69:101–303
Sprowls FS (1978) A study of the relationships among birth order, family size, and sibship constellation and high school behavioral and academic adjustment. Diss Abst Int 39:3483
Srivastava ML, Sinha AK (1975) Sex sequences of births in India. J Biosoc Sci 7:233–241
Srole L, Fischer AK (1973) Smoking behavior 1953 and 1970: The midtown Manhattan study. In: Smoking behavior: Motives and incentives. Winston, Washington, DC, pp 255–265
Suchman EA (1965) Social patterns of illness and medical care. J Health Hum Behav 6:2–16
Suedfeld P (1964) Birth order of volunteers for sensory deprivation. J Abnorm Soc Psychol 68:195–196
Suedfeld P (1968) Anticipated stress in sensory deprivation as a function of orientation and ordinal position. J Soc Psychol 76:259–263
Suedfeld P (1969) Sensory deprivation stress: Birth order and instructional set as interacting variables. J Pers Soc Psychol 11:70–74
Süllwold F (1971) Schultests. Handbuch der Psychologie, 3rd edn, vol 6. Hogrefe, Göttingen
Sundaraj N, Rao BSS (1966) Order of birth and schizophrenia. Br J Psychiatry 112:1127–1129
* Sutton-Smith B, Roberts JM, Rosenberg BG (1964) Sibling associations and role involvement. Merrill-Palmer Q 10:25–38
Sutton-Smith B, Rosenberg BG (1965) Age changes in the effects of ordinal position on sex role identification. J Genet Psychol 107:61–73
Sutton-Smith B, Rosenberg BG (1970) The sibling. Holt, Rinehart & Winston, New York
Sutton JM, McIntire WG (1977) Relationship of ordinal position and sex to neuroticism in adults. Psychol Rep 41:843–846

Svalastoga K (1959) Prestige, class and mobility. W Heinemann, London Melbourne Toronto, pp 404–406

Svanum S, Bringle RG (1980) Evaluation of confluence model variables on IQ and achievement test scores in a sample of 6- to 11-year-old children. J Educ Psychol 72:427–436

Swanson B (1971) Note on the relationship of ordinal position, dogmatism, and personal sexual attitudes. J Psychol 77:213–215

Swanson BR, Massey RH, Payne IR (1972) Ordinal position, family size, and personal adjustment. J Psychol 81:53–58

Sweeney DR, Fine BJ (1970) Note on pain reactivity and family size. Percept Mot Skills 31:25–26

Sweet PR, Nuttall RL (1971) Predicting family size from parental characteristics. Proc 79th Annu Conv APA. American Psychological Association, Washington, DC

Szaklo M, Tonascia J (1976) Psychological factors and the risk of myocardial infarction in white women. Am J Epidemiol 103:313–320

Schachter FF, Gilutz G, Shore E, Adler M (1978) Sibling deidentification judged by mothers: Cross-validation and developmental studies. Child Dev 49:543–546

Schachter FF, Shore E, Feldman-Rotman S, Marquis RE, Campbell S (1976) Sibling deidentification. Dev Psychol 12:418–427

Schachter S (1959) The psychology of affiliation. Experimental studies of the sources of gregariousness. Stanford University Press, Stanford

Schachter S (1963) Birth order, eminence, and higher education. Am Soc Rev 28:757–767

Schachter St (1964) Birth order and sociometric choice. J Abnorm Soc Psychol 68:453–456

Schaller J (1972) Ordinal position and parental control. Psychol Rep 2:17, Göteborg

Scheidt FJ, Smith ME (1974) Same-sex dyads and Toman's theory of birth-order compatibility. Psychol Rep 34:1174

Scheidt FJ, Smith ME (1976) Birth-order compatibility and same-sex dyads: A replication. J Soc Psychol 99:291–292

Schell RE, Silber JW (1968) Sex-role discriminatin among young children. Percept Mot Skills 27:379–389

Schettino AP, Borden RJ (1976) Sex differences in responses to naturalistic crowding: Affective reactions to group size and group density. Pers Soc Psychol Bull 2:67–70

Schildhaus D (1975) The role of ordinal position in the psychological development of children. Diss Abstr Int 35-B:4634

Schindler S (1974) Familienkonstellation und aggressives Verhalten. Z Klin Psychol Psychother 22:180–182

Schlichting UU (1968) Einige Persönlichkeitszüge von Gymnasiasten mit hoher Testintelligenz. Arch Ges Psychol 120:125–150

* Schmidt CW, Tölle R (1977) Familienkonstellation von psychisch Kranken. Ergebnisse und Methoden statistischer Untersuchungen der Familiengröße, Geburtenfolge und Geschwisterposition. Fortschr Neurol Psychiatr 45:20–52

Schmidt R, Schreier K (1978) Der Einfluß einer mäßigen intrauterinen Mangelernährung auf die spätere körperliche und geistige Entwicklung von Zwillingen. Mschr Kinderheilk 126:81-86

Schmuck R (1963) Sex of sibling, birth order position, and female dispositions to conform in two-child families. Child Dev 34:1913–1918

Schneewind KA (1978) Eltern-Kind-Beziehung als Dominante des generativen Verhaltens. Unpublished Paper, München

Schooler C (1961) Birth order and schizophrenia. Arch Gen Psychiatry 4:91–97

Schooler C (1964) Birth order and hospitalization for schizophrenia. J Abnorm Soc Psychol 69:574–579

* Schooler C (1972 a) Birth order effects: Not here, not now: Psychol Bull 78:161–175

* Schooler C (1972 b) Childhood family structure and adult characteristics. Sociometry 35:255–269

* Schooler C (1972 c) Social antecedents of adult psychological functioning. Am J Sociol 78:299–322

* Schooler C (1973) Birth order effects: A reply to Breland. Psychol Bull 80:213–214

Schooler C, Caudill W (1964) Symptomatology in Japanese and American schizophrenics. Ethnology 3:172–178

Schooler C, Long J (1963) Affiliation among chronic schizophrenics: Factors affecting acceptance of responsibility for the fate of another. J Nerv Ment Dis 137:173–179

Schooler C, Scarr S (1962) Affiliation among chronic schizophrenics: relation to intrapersonal and birth order factors. J Personality 30:178–192

Schoonover SM (1959) The relationship of intelligence and achievement to birth order, sex of sibling, and age interval. J Educ Psychol 50:143–146

Schopler E (1966) Birth order and preference between visual and tactual receptors. Percept Mot Skills 22:74

Schramm CO (1978) Maternal acceptance of toddler behavior. Child gender and ordinal position comparison. Diss Abstr Int 38(9-A) 5301

* Schubert DSP, Wagner ME, Schubert HJP (1976) One thousand references on sibling-constellation variables: Ordinal position, sibship size, sibling age-spacing, and sex of sibling. JSAS Catalogue of select Documents in Psychol 6:73

Schubert DSP, Wagner ME, Schubert HJP (1977) Family constellation and creativity: Firstborn predominance among classical music composers. J Psychology 95:147–149

Schubert DSP, Wagner MB, Schubert HJP (1977) Interest in creativity training by birth order and sex. J Creat Beh 11:144–145

Schubert HJP, Wagner ME, Riess BF (1976) Sibship size, sibsex, sibgap, and homosexuality among male outpatients. Transnat Ment Health Res Newsl 18:1, 3–8

Schuckit MA, Gunderson EK (1977) Early identification of alcoholics in Navy psychiatric out-patients. Dis Nerv Syst 38:397–400

Schuh JH, Williams OJ (1977) The effect of birth order on room-mate compatibility. Coll Students J 11:285–286

Schultz DP (1967) Birth order of volunteers for sensory restriction research. J Soc Psychol 73:71–73

Schwab MR, Lundgren DC (1978) Birth order, perceived appraisals by significant others, and self-esteem. Psychol Rep 43:443–454

Schwartz BA (1976) The relationship between birth order, sex of sibling and Kohlberg's stages of moral development in a sample of college freshman males from two-child families. Diss Abstr Int 36-B:3625

Schwartz M (1977) Left-handedness and high-risk pregnancy. Neuropsychologia 15:341–344

Schwartzman S (1962) Birth order and social conditioning. Diss Abstr Int 23:2222–2223

Schwarzbeck C (1977) Role-taking abilities as functions of family constellations. Diss Abstr Int 37-B:4227

Stäcker KH, Bartmann U (1974) Psychologie des Rauchens. Quelle Meyer, Heidelberg

Staffieri JR (1970) Birth order and creativity. J Clin Psychol 26:65–66

Staffieri JR, Basset JE (1970) Birth order and perception of facial expressions. Percept Mot Skills 30:606

Stagner R, Katzoff ET (1936) Personality as related to birth order and family size. J Appl Psychol 20:340–346

Staples FR, Walters RH (1961) Anxiety, birth order and susceptibility to social influence. J Abnorm Soc Psychol 62:716–719

Stark S (1964) Geschwisterposition und Charakterentwicklung. Psychol & Praxis 13:134–140

Start A, Start KB (1974) The relation between birth order and effort or conscientiousness among primary school children. Res Educ 12:1–8

Stecker RM (1957) Documenta rheumatologica. Western Reserve University Medical School, Cleveland, Ohio

Steelman LC, Mercy JA (1980) Unconfounding the confluence model. Am Soc Rev 45:571–582

Steen PG (1966) Alkoholmissbrukares placering: syskonskaren. Social-Medicinsk Tidskrift 43:318–23

Stein AH, Bailey MM (1973) The socialization of achievement orientation in females. Psychol Bull 80:345–366

Stein KB (1971) Psychotherapy patients as research subjects: Problems in cooperativeness, representativeness, and generalizability. J Consult Clin Psychol 37:99–105

Steiner JD; Vannoy JS (1966) Personality correlates of two types of conformity behavior. J Pers Soc Psychol 4:307–315

Stenger JE (1975) A study of the relationship of family constellation to work values, occupational choice and psychological factors among college students. Diss Abstr In 35-A:4170

Stenning WF (1968) The relationship of birth order to affiliation and achievement in children of two cultures: Mexico and USA. Diss Abstr Int 28-B:4286–4287

Stenstedt A (1959) Involutional melancholia. Acta Psychiatr Scand Suppl 127

Stephens JH, Kamp M (1962) On some aspects of hysteria: A clinical study. J Nerv Ment Dis 134:305–315

Sterner GA (1973) Birth order and self-esteem as determinants of affiliative behavior under ego-threatening conditions. Diss Abstr Int 33-B:5501

Sternlicht M, Staaby J, Sullivan I (1975) Birth order, maternal age, and mental retardation. Ment Retard, New York, 13:3–6

Steuber H (1973) Zur Häufigkeit von Verhaltensstörungen im Grundschulalter. Praxis Kinderpsychol 22:246–250

Stewart L (1970) The politics of birth order. Proc 78th Annu Conv APA, vol 5. American Psychological Association, Washington, DC, pp 365–366

Stewart M (1962) The success of the firstborn child. Workers Educational Association, London

Stewart RH (1967) Birth order and dependency. J Pers Soc Psychol 6:192–194

Stokes CS, Johnson NE (1977) Birth order, size of family of orientation and desired family size. J Individ Psychol 33:42–46

Stone LA (1963) Birth order and curricular choice. Is there a relationship? Vocational Guid Q 11:209–211

Stotland E, Cottrell NB (1962 a) Similarity of performance as influenced by interaction, self-esteem, and birth order. J Abnorm Soc Psychol 64:183–191

Stotland E, Dunn RE (1962 b) Identification, "oppositeness", authoritarism, self-esteem, and birth order. Psychol Monogr 76:9 (whole No 528)

Stotland E, Dunn RE (1963) Empathy, self-esteem, and birth order. J Abnorm Soc Psychol 66:532–540

Stotland E, Sherman SE, Shaver KG (1971) Empathy and birth order. Some experimental explorations. University of Nebraska Press, Lincoln

Stotland E, Walsh JA (1963) Birth order and an experimental study of empathy. J Abnorm Soc Psychol 66:610–614

Stout AM (1960) Parent behavior toward children of differing ordinal position and sibling status. Ph.D. Dissertation, University of California

Strickland BR, Crowne DP (1963) Need for approval and the premature termination of psychotherapy. J Consult Clin Psychol 27:95–101

Strodtbeck FL, Creelan PG (1968) Interaction linkage between family size, intelligence, and sex-role identity. J Marriage Family 30:301–307

* Stroup AL, Jamison HK (1965) Sibling position in the family and personality of offspring. J Marriage Family 27:65–68

Strudler BM (1976) The relationship to occupational achievement of birth order, education and ethnicity in middle-aged adults. Diss Abstr Int 37-A:2652

Struempfer DJ (1973) Failure to find relationships between family constellation and achievement motivation. J Psychol 85:29–36

Strunk P, Berger M (1973) Psychische Störungen im Kindesalter und Geschwisterposition. Z Kinder-u. Jugendpsychiatrie 1:18–24

Tabah L, Sutter J (1954) Le niveau intellectuel des enfants d'une même famille. Ann Hum Genet 19:120–150

Tähkä V (1966) The alcoholic personality. A clinical study. The Finnish Foundation for Alcohol Studies, vol 13, Helsinki

Taintor Z (1970) Birth order and psychiatric problems in boot camp. Am J Psychiatry 126:1604–1610

Takuma T (1971) Einige japanische Untersuchungen zur Zwillingsforschung. Z Exp Psychol 18:670–677

Tanner JM (1955) Growth at adolescence. Blackwell Scientific Publications, Oxford

Tanner JM (1966) Galtonian eugenics and the study of growth: The relation of body size, intelligence test score, and social circumstances in children and adults. Eugen Rev 58:122–135

Tanner JM (1968) Earlier maturation in man. Sci Am 218:21–27

Taylor L (1945) The social adjustment of the only child. Am J Soc 51:227–232

Taylor MK, Kogan KL (1973) Effects of birth of a sibling on mother-child interactions. Child Psychiat Hum Dev 4:53–58

Taylor RE, Eisenman R (1968) Birth order and sex differences in complexity-simplicity, color-form preference and personality. J Project Techn Pers Ass 32:383–387

Teepen NS (1963) Sibling relationship in sex role identification. Master's thesis, Ohio State University

Teitelbaum MS (1970) Factors affecting the sex ratio in large populations. J Biosoc Sci Suppl 2:61–71

Teja JS (1967) Birth order and schizophrenia. Indian J Psychiatry 9:203–207

Templeton JA (1962) Influence of family size on some aspects of teen-agers' attitudes, behavior and perception of home life. Family Life Coordinator 3:51–57

Teng EL, Lee BH, Yang KS, Chang PC (1976) Handedness in a chinese population: Biological, social, and pathological factors. Science 193:1148–1150

Tennent TG (1970) Truancy and steeling. A comparative study of education act cases and property offenders. Br J Psychiatry 116:587–592

Terhune KW (1973) Fertility values: Why people stop having children. Proc 81st Annu Conv APA, vol 8. American Psychological Association, Washington, DC, pp 351–352

Terman LM et al. (1925) Genetic studies of genius: The mental and physical traits of a thousand gifted children, vol 1. Stanford University Press, Standford

Thoman EB, Turner AM, Leiderman PH, Barnett CR (1970) Neonate-mother interaction; effects of parity on feeding behavior. Child Dev 41:1103–1111

Thoman EB, Leiderman PH, Olson JP (1972) Neonate-mother interaction during breast-feeding. Dev Psychol 6:110–118

Thomas A, Birch HG, Chess S, Robbins LC (1961) Individuality in response of children to similar environmental situations. Am J Psychiatr 117:798–803

Thomas DL (1972a) Family size and children's characteristics. In: Bahr HM, Chadwick BA, Thomas DL (eds) Population, resources and the future: Non-Malthusian perspectives. Brigham Young University Press, Provo, Utah, pp 137–157

Thomas DL (1972b) Family size and personal welfare. An analysis of conformity, religiosity and self-esteem. Washington State University, St Louis

Thomas JH jr (1976) The influence of sex and birth order on Parent-adolescent interaction. Diss Abstr Int 37-B:2532

Thompson VD (1974) Family size: Implicit policies and assumed psychological outcomes. J Soc Issues 30:93–124

Thurstone LL, Jenkins RL (1929) Birth order and intelligence. J Educ Psychol 20:641–651

Thurstone LL, Jenkins RL (1931) Order of birth, parent-age and intelligence. Behavior research fund monographs. University of Chicago Press, Chicago, Ill

Tienari P (1966) On intrapair differences between male twins, with special reference to dominance-submissiveness. Acta Psychiatr Scand Suppl 42:188

Timsit M, Urbain E, Sabatier J, Timsit-Berthier M (1975) Statistische Untersuchung der psychosomatischen Kopfschmerzen. Med Wochenschr, München, 117:1515–1520

* Tölle R (1972) Methodologische Probleme bei statistischen Untersuchungen der Beziehungen zwischen Familienkonstellation und psychischen Störungen. Zbl Ges Neurol Psychiatrie 203:248

Tolstrup K (1953) On psychogenic obesity in children IV. Acta Paediat Scand 42:289–304

Toman W (1960) Haupttypen der Familienkonstellation. Psychol Rdsch 11:273–284

Toman W (1961) Familienkonstellationen. Ihr Einfluß auf den Menschen und seine Handlungen. CH Beck, München

Toman W (1962) Family constellations of the partners in divorced and married couples. J Individ Psychol 18:48–51

Toman W (1963a) Die prägenden Wirkungen der Geschwisterkonstellation auf den Charakter. Z Psychother Med Psychol 13:113–117

Toman W (1963b) Large age differences among spouses and their family constellations. Psychol Rep 13:386

Toman W (1964) Choices of marriage partners' by men coming from monosexual sibling configurations. Br J Med Psychol 37:43–46

Toman W (1965) Complementarity in material adjustment: Comment. J Individ Psychol 21:145–147

Toman W (1966) Familienkonstellationen. Schule und Psychologie 13:33–39

Toman W (1968) Motivation, Persönlichkeit, Umwelt. Hogrefe, Göttingen

Toman W (1970) Birth order rules all. Psychol Today. Dec

Toman W (1971a) A minimal data system for comparative social psychiatric documentation. Soc Sci Med 5:169–172

Toman W (1971b) The duplication theorem of social relationships as tested in the general population. Psychol Rev 78:380–390

Toman W, Gray B (1961) Family constellation of "normal" and "disturbed" marriages: An empirical study. J Individ Psychol 17:93–95

Toman W, Preiser S (1973) Familienkonstellationen und ihre Störungen. Ferdinand Enke, Stuttgart

Toman W, Toman E (1970) Sibling positions on a sample of distinguished persons. Percept Mot Skills 31:825–826

Tomeh AK (1969) Birth order and kinship affiliation. J Marriage Family 31:19–26

Tomeh AK (1970) Birth order and friendship associations. J Marriage Family 32:360–369

Tomeh AK (1971) Birth order and familial influences in the middle east. J Comparat Family Stud 2:88–106

Tomeh AK (1972) Birth order and dependence patterns of college students in Lebanon. J Marriage Family 34:361–374

Torrance EP (1954) A psychological study of American jet aces. In: Schachter S (1959)

Touhey JC (1971 a) Birth order and mate selection. Psychol Rep 29:618

Touhey JC (1971 b) Birth order and virginity. Psychol Rep 28:894

Touliator J, Lindholm BW, Rich A (1978) Influence of family background on scholastic achievement. J Exp Educ 46:22–27

Trasler G (1973) Criminal behaviour. In: Eysenck HJ (ed) Handbook of abnormal psychology. Pitman Medical, London, pp 67–96

Trémolières J, Boulanger JJ (1950) Contribution à l'étude du phénomène de croissance et de stature en France de 1940 à 1948. Recueil Trav Inst Nat Hyg 4:117–212

Trudewind C (1972) Versuch einer Taxonomie von leistungsmotivationsgenetischen Bedingungen des nicht-schulischen Lebensraumes. Dissertation Psychologisches Institut Universität Bochum, Bochum

Trudewind C (1975) Leistungsmotivgenese und Umwelt. In: Walter H (ed) Sozialisationsforschung, vol III. Problemata, Frommann-Holzboog, Stuttgart, p 55–79

Tsuang MT (1966) Birth order and maternal age of psychiatric in-patients. Br J Psychiatry 112:1131–1141

Tsuang MT (1972) Psychiatric genetics in Taiwan. Int J Ment Health 1:221–230

Tucker GJ, Reinhardt RF (1966) Suicide attempts. US Naval Aerospace Medical Institute, NAM 1:975

Tuckman J, Regan RA (1967 a) Ordinal position and behavior problems in children. J Health Soc Behav 8:32–39

Tuckman J, Regan RA (1967 b) Size of family and behavioral problems in children. J Genet Psychol 111:151–160

Tulkin SR, Kagan J (1970) Mother-child interaction: Social class differences in the first year of life. Proc 78th Annu Conv APA, vol 5. American Psychological Association, Washington, DC, pp 261–262

Turner RH (1962) Some family determinants of ambition. Sociol & Soc Res 46:397–411

Uddenberg N (1974) Psychological aspects of sexual inadequacy in women. J Psychosom Res 18:33–47

Uddenberg N, Almgren PE, Nilsson Å (1971 a) Birth order and sex of siblings: Influence on parental identification. Acta Psychiatr Scand 47:324–333

Uddenberg N, Almgren PE, Nilsson Å (1971 b) Preference for sex of the child among pregnant women. J Biosoc Sci 3:267–280

Udjus JG (1964) Anthropometrical changes in Norwegian men in the 20th century. Universitetsforlaget, Olso

United Nations (1973) The determinants and consequences of population trends. Population Studies No 50, Dept of Economic and Social Affairs, New York, pp 96–105

Unruh S, Grosse ME, Ziegler E (1971) Birth order, number of siblings, and social reinforcer effectiveness in children. Child Dev 42:1153–1163

Van Krevelen A (1946) Het eenige kind. Utrecht

Varela JA (1964) A cross-cultural replication of an experiment involving birth order. J Abnorm Soc Psychol 69:456–457

Vaughn CS (1975) Birth order effects on personality dimensions. Diss Abstr In 36-B:3017

* Veevers JE (1971) Rural-urban differences in distribution of birth orders. Rural Sociol 38:219–227

* Veevers JE (1973) Estimating the incidence and prevalence of birth orders: A technique using census data. Demography 10:447–458

Velandia W, Grandon GM, Page EB (1978) Family size, birth order, and intelligence in a large South American sample. Am Educ Res J 15:399–416

Verger D (1968) Birth order and sibling differences in interests. J Individ Psychol 24:56–59

Vernon DTA (1974) Modeling and birth order in responses to painful stimuli. J Pers Soc Psychol 29:794–799

Vernon DTA, Foley JM, Schulman JL (1967) Effect of mother-child separation and birth order in young children's responses to two potentially stressful experiences. J Pers Soc Psychol 5:162–174

Vernon PE (1951) Recent investigation of intelligence and its measurement. Eugen Rev 43:125–137

Very PS, Goldblatt RB, Monacelli V (1973) Birth order, personality development, and vocational choice of becoming a carmelite nun. J Psychol 85:75–80

Very PS, Prull RW (1970) Birth order, personality development, and the choice of law as a profession. J Genet Psychol 116:219–221

Very PS, VanHine NP (1969) Effects of birth order upon personality development of twins. J Genet Psychol 114:93–95

Very PS; Zannini JA (1969) Relation between birth order and being a beautician. J Appl Psychol 53:149–151

Vinoda KS (1966) Personality characteristics of attempted suicide. Br J Psychiatry 112:1143–1150

Visher SS (1947) American men of science. Johns Hopkins, Baltimore, p 537

Visher SS (1948) Environmental background of leading american scientists. Am Sociol Rev 13:65–72

Vockell EL, Bennett B (1972) Birth order, sex of siblings, and incidence of learning disabilities. Exceptional Children 39:162–166

Vockell EL, Felker DW (1971) Self-classification by subjects using Toman's birth-order categories. Psychol Rep 29:1010

* Vockell EL, Felker DW, Miley CH (1973) Birth order literature 1967–1971: Bibliography and index. J Individ Psychol 29:39–53

Vogel HP (1979) Fertility and sibship size in psychiatric patients. Acta Psychiatr Scand 60:483–503

Vogel W, Lauterbach CG (1963) Sibling patterns and social adjustment among normal and psychiatrically disturbed soldiers. J Consult Clin Psychol 27:236–242

Vogel-Sprott M (1962) Birth order and personality characteristics of alcoholics. Toronto Alcoholism Research Foundation, Toronto

Volksdorf NR (1970) The relationship of ego-strength to ordinal position and sex. Diss Abstr Int 31-B:403

Vonderheide S (1978) Birth order and college grade point average. Psychol Rep 42:150

Vroegh K (1971) The relationship of birth order and sex of siblings to gender role identity. Dev Psychol 4:407–411

Vuyk R (1959) Das Kind in der Zweikinderfamilie. Suppl 38 to Schweiz Z Psychol, Huber, Bern Stuttgart

Vuyk R (1961) Eltern vergleichen ihre beiden Kinder. Schweiz Z Psychol 20:224–237

Vuyk R (1963) Eltern vergleichen ihre beiden Kinder zum zweiten Mal. Schweiz Z Psychol 22:220–231

Wagner ME, Schubert HJP (1977) Sibship variables and United States Presidents. J Individ Psychol 33:78–85

Wagner NN (1968) Birth order of volunteers. Cross-cultural data. J Soc Psychol 74:133–134

Wahl CW (1954) Some antecedent factors in the family histories of 392 schizophrenics. Am J Psychiatry 110:668–676

Wahl CW (1956a) Some antecedent factors in the family histories of 562 male schizophrenics of the US navy. Am J Psychiatry 113:201–210

Wahl CW (1956b) Some antecedent factors in the family histories of 109 alcoholics. Q J Stud Alcohol 17:643–654

Waldrop MF, Bell RQ (1964) Relation of preschool dependency behavior to family size and density. Child Dev 35:1187–1195

Waldrop MF, Bell RQ (1966) Effects of family size and density on newborn characteristics. Am J Orthopsychiatry 36:544–550

Walker CE, Tahmisian J (1967) Birth order and student characteristics: A replication. J Consult Clin Psychol 31:219

Walker LV, Johnson DL, Goolishian H (1973) Ordinal position and psychopathology in two-child families. Tex Rep Biol Med 31:777–790

Waller JH (1971) Differential reproduction: Its relation to IQ test score, education, and occupation. Soc Biol 18:122–136

Walsh BM (1973) Marital status and birth order in a sample of Dublin males. J Biosoc Sci 5:187–193

Walter DA, Ziegler CA (1980) The effects of birth order on locus of control. Bull Psychonomic Soc 15:293–294

Walters RH, Ray E (1960) Anxiety, social isolation and reinforcer effectiveness. J Personality 28:358–367
Warburton FW (1951/52) Relationship between intelligence and size of family. Eugen Rev 43:36–37
Ward CD (1964) A further examination of birth order as a selective factor among volunteer subjects. J Abnorm Soc Psychol 69:311–313
Ward CD, Castro A, Wilcox AH (1974) Birth-order effects in a survey of mate selection and parenthood. J Soc Psychol 94:57–64
Ward CD, Ward KM, Randers-Pehrson SB, Runion L (1973) Birth order and dreams. J Soc Psychol 90:155–156
Wark DM, Swanson EO, Mack J (1974) More on birth order: Intelligence and college plans. J Individ Psychol 30:221–227
* Warren JR (1966) Birth order and social behavior. Psychol Bull 65:38–49
Waters LK, Kirk WE (1967) Birth order and EPPS affiliation. J Psychol 67:241–243
Waters LK, Kirk WE (1969) Characteristics of volunteers and non volunteers for psychological experiments. J Psychol 73:133–136
Watkins D, Astilla E (1980) Birth order, family size, and self-esteem: A Filipino study. J Genet Psychol 137:297–298
Watkins TR (1976) Sibling relationships of children entering reatment in mental health centers: A descriptive study. Diss Abstr Int 37-A:3190
Wattenberg WW (1949) Delinquency and only children: Study of a "category". J Abnorm Psychol 44:356–366
Weiner H (1973) Birth order and illness behavior. J Individ Psychol 29:173–175
Weintrob Z (1976) Personality integration as related to family constellation. Diss Abstr Int 37-B:481–482
Weiss JH (1968) Birth order and asthma in children. J Psychosom Res 12:137–140
Weiss JH (1970) Birth order and physiological stress response. Child Dev 41:461–470
Weiss JH, Wolf A, Wiltsey RG (1963) Birth order, recruitment conditions, and preferences for participation in group versus non-group experiments. Am Pschologist 18:356
Weiss RL (1966) "Acquiescence" response set and birth order. J Consult Clin Psychol 30:365
Weiss RL (1966) Some determinants of emitted reinforcing behavior: Listener reinforcement and birth order. J Pers Soc Psychol 3:489–492
Welch BL (1977) A psychological study of only children. Diss Abstr Int 37-B:4174
Weller GM (1965) Arousal effects on the new born infant of being first or later born. Am J Orthopsychiat 35:341–342
Weller L (1962) The relationship of birth order to anxiety: A replication of the Schachter findings. Sociometry 25:415–417
Weller L (1964) The relationship of birth order to cohesiveness. J Soc Psychol 63:249–254
Weller L, Hazi O, Natan O (1975) Birth order and the feminine sex role of married women. J Individ psychol 31:65–70
Weller L, Eytan R, Solel M (1976a) Birth order and risk taking among kibbutz and city youth. Br J Soc Clin Psychol 15:103–104
Weller L, Shlomi A, Zimont G (1976b) Birth order, sex, and occupational interest. J Vocational Behav 8:45–50
Weller L, Miller S (1978) Birth order, country of origin and schizophrenia in Israel. Int J Soc Psychiatry 24:195–198
Weller L, Natan O, Hazi O (1974) Birth order and marital bliss in Israel. J Marriage Family 36:794–797
Weller RH (1974) Excess and deficit fertility in the US 1965. Soc Biol 21:77–87
West DJ, Farrington DP (1973) Who becomes delinquent? Second report of the Cambridge study on delinquent development. Heinemann's Educational Books, London
West SS (1960) Sibling configurations of scientists. Am J Sociol 66:268–274
Westoff CF, Potter RG jr, Sagi PC (1963) The third child. A study in the prediction of fertility. Princeton University Press, Princeton, NJ
Westoff CF, Potter RG jr, Sagi PC, Mishler EG (1961) Family growth in metropolitan America. Princeton University Press, Princeton, NJ
White LF (1969) Relationship between ordinal position and mental disorders. Diss Abstr Int 29-B:2643
Whitelaw AGL (1971) The association of social class and sibling number with skinfold thickness in London schoolboys. Hum Biol 43:414–420

Wiedl KH (1977) The relationship of interest for visual complexity to birth order, sex, and personality characteristics: A genetic analysis. Genet Psychol Monogr 96:143–162

Wiener DN, Stiper DR (1959) Psychometric prediction of length and outcome of outpatients therapy. In: Schachter S (1959). See above

Wild CM, Shapiro LN, Abelin T (1974) Sampling issues in family studies of schizophrenia. Arch Gen Psychiatry 30:211–215

Wile IS, Davis R (1948) The relation of birth order to behavior. In: Kluckhohn C, Murray HA (eds) Personality in nature, society and culture, 2nd edn. HA Knopf, New York, pp 403–420

Wilks L, Thompson P (1979) Birth order and creativity in young children. Psychol Rep 45:443–449

Willems LFM, Van Gelderen MH, Defares PB (1972) Anxiety, affiliation-need and social contact. Ned T Psychol 27:221–246

Wilsnack SC (1972) Psychological factors in female drinking. PH.D. dissertation, Harvard University

Wilson PR, Patterson J (1965) Sex differences in volunteering behavior. Psychol Rep 16:976

Wilson PR, Patterson J, Lysons AM (1966) Sex, birth order and volunteering behaviour. Aust J Psychol 18:158–159

Winett RA, Nerviano VJ (1978) Birth order effects and their implications for child care research and programs. J Commun Psychology 6:173–174

Wisdom G, Walsh RP (1975) Dogmatism and birth order. J Individ Psychol 31:32–36

Witchell BM (1966) A study of teachers' ordinal position with respect to anxiety and teacher role. Diss Abstr Int 26:7171–7172

Wohlwill JF (1970) The age variable in psychological research. Psychol Rev 77:49–64

Wolf A (1966) Recruitment pressure, birth order and sex as possible sources of bias in the recruitment of volunteer subjects. Unpubl. paper presented at the 1966 Eastern Psychology Association Convention (1967)

Wolf A, Weiss JH (1970) Birth order, recruitment conditions and volunteering preference. J Person Soc Psychol 2:269–273

* Wolf A, Wolf GE (1965) First born and last born: A critique. J Individ Psychol 21:159–165

Wolf KA (1967) A comparison of sibling position and academic achievement in elementary school. Diss Abstr Int 28-A:1222

Wolkon GH (1964) A comment on alcoholism, birth order and family size. Report from mental health rehabilitation research. Hill House, Cleveland

Wolkon GH (1968) Birth order and desire for and participation in psychiatric post-hospital services. J Consult Clin Psychol 32:42–46

Wolkon GH, Levinger G (1965) Birth order and need for achievement. Psychol Rep 16:73–74

Wood CH, Bean FD (1977) Offspring gender and family size implication from a comparison of Mexican Americans and Anglo Americans. J Marriage Family 39:129–139

Wray JD (1971) Population pressures on families: Family size and child spacing. In: Rapid population growth: Consequences and policy implications, vol 1. Johns Hopkins, Baltimore London

Wrigthsman LS jr (1960) Effects of waiting with others on changes in level of felt anxiety. J Abnorm Soc Psychol 61:216–222

Wudel P, Loo R (1979) Birth order and person variables. Psychol Rep 45:280

Wuebben PL (1967) Honesty of subjects and birth order. J Pers Soc Psychol 5:350–352

Wyshak G (1969) Intervals between births in families containing one set of twins. J Biosoc Sci 1:337–351

Yamaguchi T, Makihara H, Nagai H, Hagiwara N, Ishikawa T, Anazama U, Yano S, Kobayashi T (1964) Sibling rank in schizophrenia and neurosis. Seishinigaku 6:578–586

Yando R, Zigler E, Litzinger S (1975) A further investigation of the effects of birth order and number of siblings in determining children's responsiveness to social reinforcement. J Psychology 89:95–111

Yang KS, Liang WH (1973) Some correlates of achievement motivation among Chinese high school boys. Acta Psychol Taiwanica 15:59–67

Yarrow MR, Campbell JD, Burton RV (1964) Recollections of childhood; a study of the retrospective method. Monogr Soc Res Child Dev 35, No 5

Yaryan RB, Festinger L (1961) Preparatory action and belief in probable occurence of future events. J Abnorm Soc Psychol 63:603–606

Yasuda S (1964) A methodical inquiry into social mobility. Am Soc Rev 29:16–23

Yerushalmy J (1945) On the interval between successive births and its effect on survival of the infant. Hum Biol 17:65–106

Yiannakis A (1976) Birth order and preference for dangerous sports among males. Res Q Am Ass Health Phys Educ 47:62–67

Yoda A, Fukatsu A (1963) Ordinal positon, birth order and personality. Jpn J Educat Psychol 11:239–246

Zajonc RB (1976) Family configuration and intelligence. Science 192:227–236

Zajonc RB, Bargh J (1980) Birth order, family size, and decline of SAT scores. Am Psychol 35:662–668

Zajonc RB, Bargh J (1980) The confluence model: parameter estimation for six divergent data sets on family factors and intelligence. Intelligence 4:349–361

Zajonc RB, Markus GB (1975) Birth order and intellectual development. Psychol Rev 82:74–88

Zajonc RB, Markus H, Markus GB (1979) The birth order puzzle. J Pers Soc Psychol 37:1325–1341

Zazzo R (1960) Les jumeaux, le couple et la personne. Presses Universitaires de France, Paris

Ziegler FJ, Imboden JB, Meyer E (1960) Contemporary conversion reactions: A clinical study. Am J Psychiatry 116:901–909

Zielinski W (1966) Schulleistung, Intelligenz und Familienkonstellation. Ph.D. dissertation, Universität Erlangen-Nürnberg

Ziesat HA (1978) Are family patterns related to the development of chronic back pain? Percept Mot Skills 46:1062

Zimbardo P, Formica R (1963) Emotional comparison and self-esteem as determinants of affiliation. J Pers 31:141–162

Zucker RA, Horn H van (1972) Sibling social structure and behavior: Drinking and smoking in adolescence. Q J Stud Alcohol 33:193–197

Zucker RA, Manosevitz M, Lanyon RI (1968) Birth order, anxiety, and affiliation during a crisis. J Pers Soc Psychol 8:354–359

Zuckerman M, Barrett BH, Bragiel RM (1960) The parental attitudes of parents of child guidance cases. Child Dev 31:401–417

Zuckerman M, Link KE (1968) Expectancy and birth order as determinants of affective response to isolation. Percept Mot Skills 27:279–286

Zuckerman M, Schultz DP, Hopkins TR (1967) Sensation-seeking and volunteering for sensory deprivation and hypnosis experiments. J Consult Clin Psychol 31:358–363

Zuger B (1974) Effiminate behavior in boys: Parental age and other factors. Arch Gen Psychiatry 30:173–177

Zybert P, Stein Z, Belmont L (1978) Maternal age and children's ability. Percept Mot Skills 47:815–818

Postscript:

Touliatos J, Lindholm BW (1980) Birth order, family size and behavior problems in children. Child Psychiat Quart 13:1–8

Author Index

Subject Index